with a new introduction
and afterword by the author

Doctors & Rules

A Sociology of Professional Values

Expanded Second Edition

Joseph M. Jacob

Transaction Publishers
New Brunswick (U.S.A.) and London (U.K.)

This book is printed on acid-free paper that meets the American National Standard for Permanence of Paper for Printed Library Materials.

Library of Congress Catalog Number: 98-27095
ISBN: 0-7658-0477-8
Printed in the United States of America

Library of Congress Cataloging-in-Publication Data

Jacob, Joseph M., 1943-
    Doctors and rules : a sociology of professional values / Joseph M. Jacob. — Expanded 2nd ed.
        p. cm.
    Originally published: London ; New York : Routledge, 1988.
    "With a new introduction and afterword by the author."
    Includes bibliographical references and index.
    ISBN 0-7658-0477-8 (pbk.: alk. paper)
    1. Medical ethics. 2. Medical laws and legislation. I. Title.
R724.J28   1998
174'.2—dc21   98-27095
                                                            CIP

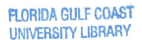

This work is for all who might read it

except

Miriam, Emily, and Nicholas
who know when enough is enough

Contents

Introduction to the Transaction Edition   ix

Foreword   xiii

Preface   xvii

1 An introduction   1

    The purpose and structure   1

    The method and the argument   13

    The use and limits of history   15

    A critique and justification   21

2 Medical practice   28

    A topography   28

    The medical clinic   32

    Scientific and Hippocratic medicine   35

    Scientific medicine   36

    Hippocratic medicine   41

3 Theories of medicine   46

    Participatory and classical medicine   46

    Rival health-based theories   56

    An explanation   67

    Some history: the scientific imperative and medical
science   81

4   The profession of medicine: Some more history   88

5   Professionalism   109

    Professionalism   109

    The ideal-typical gentleman   117

    Professional morality   123

    Professional privilege and the bargain with the State   134

    The external regulation   136

6   Administration and medicine   143

    Still more history: The growth of public health
    institutions   143

    Public regulation – bureaucracy and law   147

    The British National Health Service   153

    The untoward   156

    Litigation   165

    The patient's place: situation liability, consent, and
    self-determination   168

7   Conclusion   173

    Selves: Singulars and plurals   173

    Incommensurables and social cohesion   181

Appendix: The Hippocratic Oath   192

Afterword to the Transaction Edition   193

Notes   243

Bibliography   267

Index   289

Introduction to the
Transaction Edition

Aldous Huxley wrote a foreword to the 1946 edition of his *Brave New World*. He began:

> Chronic remorse, as all the moralists are agreed, is a most undesirable sentiment. If you have behaved badly, repent, make what amends you can and address yourself to the task of behaving better next time. On no account brood over your wrongdoing. Rolling in the muck is not the best way of getting clean.
>
> Art also has its morality, and many of the rules of this morality are the same as, or at least analogous to, the rules of ordinary ethics. . . . To pore over the literary shortcomings of twenty years ago, to attempt to patch a faulty work into the perfection it missed at its first execution, to spend one's middle age in trying to mend the artistic sins committed and bequeathed by that different person who was oneself in youth—all this is surely vain and futile. . . . And so, resisting the temptation to wallow in artistic remorse, I prefer to leave both well and ill alone and to think about something else.

Like Huxley's, my work is art portraying reality. It is not fiction but more than most works coming out of the academy it is informed by the imagination. I return to such methods later. I begin by thanking Professor Ann Greer of the University of Wisconsin, Milwaukee, and Professor Irving Horowitz of Rutgers University, New Jersey, for making this reissue possible.

It is appropriate now, as it was not ten years ago, to confess how this book came to be written. There were a number of wholly separate problems that I felt needed addressing. It was a long time in the writing. First, I began it shortly after the Conservative election victory in 1979 and did not finish until after Mrs Thatcher had won her third term in 1987. The puzzle of the 1980s was how and why the audacious social experiment of the democratic caring State should have been so decisively rejected. Second, just before this, in the late 1970s, I edited a text on hospital law. Although I thought it sufficient at a technical level, I found it uninspiring, even boring, and did not know why. Third, a number of legal academics were beginning to write of law and medicine and were beginning to tell doctors how they ought to behave. My instinct questioned whether these lawyers had the tools to do that. There were other inputs, too. For a long time, we, in Britain, had smugly watched the transatlantic explosion in medical malpractice actions and thought it could not happen to us. But nineteen years ago there was reason to doubt the foundation of that complacency. So too, it was gradually becoming clear that the pace of change in technology, in social relations, and in social ideas was beginning to diverge in ways that were fracturing the old social order. The work then had a variety of parents. It was a mongrel of a book: it never was, to mix the metaphor, a thoroughbred, single disciplinary effort. And in that, it confused at least some of my readers.

The caring State had risen Aphrodite-like at least since the Great War of 1914-18 and maybe before. In the years immediately after 1945 the Nation had been enchanted by it. Through the 1950s and 1960s, like a love affair, the magic waned but no one was really prepared for the jaded reaction against it of the 1970s and 1980s. This book hardly addressed the problem but rather left it to brood.[1] Later, I returned more directly to the issue of its rise and fall in my history of the constitution, *The Republican Crown*, which carried the subtitle *Lawyers and the Making of the State in Twentieth Century Britain*. There I discovered that 1979 was not the watershed it was thought to be. The seeds of the 1980s and 1990s had not only been planted long before but some were already sprouting before the advent of the Thatcher government. One reason why this book could afford to ignore the waning love for the caring state was that, despite all else, the NHS continued to give a stable pride in a real and lasting achievement. Because 1979 was not the great turning point, the election of 1997, important as it may turn out to be, was not as decisive as first appeared. Perhaps, in fact, before the term 'New Labour' appeared, 'Old Labour' was no longer old.

Selfishly, but inevitably, the first publication of this book sought explanations that would satisfy me. It is reprinted here in all its complexity. Here I have added one new chapter, the Afterword. In the

Preface to the first printing I adopted Darwin's aphorism that I should have liked to have held off publication for a long interval because only then 'a man can criticise his own work, almost as well as if it were that of another person'. The main reason that I am grateful to Professors Horowitz and Greer is that I can now return to seek to simplify the complexity and make my own criticism of what I was when younger. I also have taken the chance to respond to my critics and to reflect again on the issues that preoccupied me then.

Reading the book again, I am surprised that I still hold much the same opinions, although at this distance of time I can now apologize for the density of the language. At times, it is difficult to see the wood for the trees, and I might add the undergrowth as well! Now is no time to be unfaithful to the work's heterogeneous ancestry. I have not tried to survey the literature of the last ten years if only because in its original form the book itself was eclectic in the works it discussed. Amongst other things, the new chapter sorts out some of the various themes of the book. It avoids the byways that were necessary to its colour but detracted from its thesis. It reflects on what the past decade has meant for the argument. The current reader who is impatient to get to the point is advised to go straight to the Afterword and only then to return to those parts of the text that need amplification. As this edition was being prepared, I learned of the death of my friend Donald MacRae. Accordingly, I have kept his kind, but enigmatic, Foreword.

Joe Jacob
London School of Economics
July 1998

Note

1. But see my discussion of Hirschman at pp. 69ff.

Foreword

Joe Jacob has produced an *apologia pro vita sua*, but it is in a sense
disguised. Just as John Henry Newman's *Apologia* is not a mere
apology nor a defence, but a criticism of this world so also is this
book. Only a sceptic trained in the law but also deeply concerned
by our fate and circumstances could have produced it. It is also a
contribution both to the sociology of law and the sociology of
medicine. It is in law and medicine that meet and diverge many of
the unexamined paths of our lives.

Sociologists of law in the 'classical age' of sociology did not
think of themselves as practitioners of a specialized technique. At
the turn of the century Durkheim, Weber, Hobhouse, Sumner, all
insouciantly reflected on and studied 'law and justice', law as an
index of social solidarity, law as an index of (for example) bureaucratization, law as an index of rationality and efficiency in distri-
butive, retributive justice. Law to them was a third in the great
symbolic institutions of society along with language and exchange
– in particular money. These concerns have, alas, altered. By his
own route Jacob, doing much else, returns one to them. He adds
to this work, congruently, but in the same tradition, by his foray
into the once unthinkable world of the institutionalization of the
body, itself in great part a social construct.

The sociology of medicine quite legitimately means many
things. Some of these border on epidemiology, or on demography,
and are highly quantitative and positivist. Others involve – we
come closer to Jacob here – the comparative study of institutions
and the idea of the profession, the vocation, and the clinic, hospital, and lazar-house. Doctors and lawyers stand in an asymmetrical relationship to others: they are metaphorically and literally
agents more than patients. Power, influence, and fear are part of
their roles – and the roles are many, even contradictory, and never

constitute a verity. In these things, and in the concepts of rationality, individualism, and the collective Jacob is imaginative, quirky, informative, and novel. He is also as near to being right in original work as is possible. It is not the last word – even to the last sentence – but I hope the first. I also find reading him a pleasure.

Jacob does not always use the technical vocabularies of either sociology or (as I understand it) philosophy. To attack him for this would be to miss not merely the point, which is his total thrust, but also the important places passed through on his journey. Let me now comment on these not as a reviewer but as someone playing a kind of maieutic part in making a difficult and valuable birth possible. (Of course Jacob is not responsible for what I say – and the attentive reader will discover how well he can speak for himself.)

If I am anything I am a sociologist and it is both flattering and frightening to be asked to preface a book by a trained lawyer but which takes the possibility of sociology seriously.

Jacob's sociology is about how those devices by which humankind defines itself and the social world – not least in its relation to the various disciplines and manners which we call medicine – can solve some of our problems, can locate some of our quarrels and even resolve them, and make the difficult matter of being both animals and rational animals tolerable in society. Society is at once external to every individual, but it is what has been achieved by the interaction of individuals through institutions larger than any individual but essentially part of our 'social structure' of reality.

This way of looking at the world has a long history, going back at least to the Italian philosopher, Vico, in the early eighteenth century. But it is still unfamiliar; one of the important things about this book is that Jacob has rediscovered this approach for himself. He is therefore unfashionable in terms of the concepts which have been regarded as avant-garde since the 1960s.

So it is not that Joseph Jacob is not central to rising concerns, but that he has come to these concerns by an original route which gives him great strength. There is a sense in which this work is a contribution to public understanding, but, as was also true of Vico, it must be in some measure autobiography.

Or, to state these points in a different way and perhaps add to them, Jacob's style is perfectly transparent although sometimes a rapid reader will not see the density and different aspects of what he is saying – in a word, this is not a book to be read rapidly any more than it is a book to be dismissed because of what might be thought of as solecisms at the present stage of social thought. Again, I insist Jacob is not idiosyncratic nor is he self-indulgent, but that with his eye he is all at once innocent, intelligent, and informed. In the institution and world of learning lies a world increasingly bureaucratized and philistine, so he risks I think, being ignored by the learned establishments of the law, of medicine, and social science. It is for this reason that with difficulty and temerity I have agreed to his flattering imputation that I might do something to introduce his work. What I plead for, as he is too proud to do so, is that his text should be approached slowly, although it is not technical, and with reflection. Our world is full of journals and monographs. Most of their readers, certainly in the Academy, therefore, read rapidly, and look for institutional markers to help them to do so. This won't work for Jacob. I have no doubt that in other work he fits into the institutional structures. No writer is likely to write two books so original as this, and at the same time both so objective and subjective. Radical novelty in art, science, or scholarship is disturbing and can easily be dismissed. I am delighted that Routledge is publishing something so unorthodox but also so central to our humanity in what is increasingly an oversocialized world.

I am nearly at the end of my encomium. As the Latin proverb tells us 'little books have their fates', but this is not a little book and I can only guess at who will be its discriminating readers and who will therefore gain from its freshness and its acuity.

I am writing as a Scotsman who has lived most of his life in England and other countries of the common law. I realize therefore that some of Jacob's formulations will not necessarily be equally familiar to readers based on different legal traditions from France to Japan. Again, in the fields of our therapies, he naturally starts from essentially British assumptions. However, there is a sufficient convergence of the cultures of civilized societies for his messages to be relevant in all such societies and there is nothing parochial even though there is much that is personal in his text.

As will be clear I am not attempting to write a review of Jacob. I would not find this difficult: after all it is my trade. What I am trying to do is to explain something about the feel and texture of what we are given and to explain why it is valuable. A review should always try to put the work which is reviewed into a context, then to simplify and suggest all the thrust of its argument, and finally to appraise it. In a Foreword I do not think it appropriate to do this, but I hope I have been in some way helpful to the readers which this unusual volume deserves. I hope I shall live long enough to see its influence widely diffused, and its ideas so accepted that they have become the conventional wisdom of a better management of our affairs.

Donald Gunn MacRae
Professor Emeritus of Sociology in the University of London
Highgate, December 1987

Preface

Michel Foucault once wrote:[1]

Each time I have attempted to do theoretical work, it has been on the basis of elements from my experience – always in relation to processes that I saw taking place around me. It is in fact because I thought I recognized something cracked, dully jarring, or disfunctioning in things I saw, in the institutions with which I dealt, in my relation with others, that I undertook a particular piece of work.

One may think how can it be otherwise? But . . . . There is always a 'but'; there is always another way. In the case of the work in the social sciences, a great deal, but not all, can be and is achieved without the benefit of even vicarious experience. It is done out of the soulless, passionless – we might say, humanless – application of discipline. This book does not take this other way. Emphatically, it is done out of experience.

Although I am trained as a lawyer, as I began the first plan for this book I was uncomfortable with a common view of legal rules: the view that they can be respected merely because they exist and because they play a part in centralizing the organization of society. I had similar doubts regarding the equally widespread notion that a 'test case' here or a piece of law reform there could achieve very much or, more seriously, all and no more than it intends. Those who have not felt similar dissatisfactions can live in their world. I am envious of them. This work is not for them. It regards such ideas as naïve and such strategies as often more likely to do more harm than good: something is not always better than nothing. This century, if no other, has taught that change does not always improve things and that much arises out of exaggerated reaction to error.

It will become apparent that I have ranged over a number of specialties and intruded into a number of almost private debates, in each of which doubt is cast on those all too common views of law. As I have indicated the enquiry postulates a rejection of the notion that the courts always or even often offer useful mechanisms for defining and settling disputes. On the contrary, it sees in their formalism many things which hinder the common cause of humanity. It casts doubt on the regime of rational economic man. The method it uses is to assess the current importance of the Hippocratic tradition. Because of this the enquiry is focused on medical practice not only as an end in itself but as the inspiration for other occupations. So also because that tradition is not economic, it recasts the history of that practice outside bounds imposed by economic theory. It implies a particular method of looking at human relations based both in the self and the group. It examines the continuing influence of some formerly religious ideas in this secular age.

A word of warning. Before anything else, this work has to be approached in a spirit of enjoyment, even adventure. These are times of rapid change and such times are the best to rethink established values. This work, then, spends much space reasserting old values – but, as so often with reactionary efforts based in an idealized past, out of that conservatism, it presents a novel view of the present, and of the future.

It follows from the nature of my central field – biomedicine – and the eclectic and kaleidoscopic method of discussion I have adopted that scholars from several or even many other disciplines may, or will, regard the parts they recognize as facile or outdated. So be it. So also they may think I have ignored whole libraries of commonplace works. So be that also. These are vices of interdisciplinary study. A Marx or a Weber or a Dewey might have been more easily able to write in this field. It is no longer possible to write with the same intellectual breadth and the same relative depth. But, in order to give reality to interdisciplinary study rather than to genuflect at its shrine, occasional books must, unless thought is to ossify, take these risks. The approach of this book seeks one viewpoint for phenomena which commonly are not seen together. An important rationale is that some of them have not been studied in traditional academia.

In some ways I should have liked to follow the precept of Charles Darwin and hold off publication:[2] 'for a man after a long interval can criticise his own work, almost as well as if it were that of another person'. But that cannot be. I am aware that my enterprise has faults. For this reason, it is almost ingratitude to acknowledge all those with whom I have discussed parts of it or who have seen this work develop. And indeed there are very many on whom I have inflicted my thoughts during its writing, among these are many students, former students, colleagues and friends. David Smith, Alison Real of Brunel University and R.W. Rawlings of the LSE saw much earlier drafts and set me on useful lines of enquiry. Robert Dingwall of the Socio-Legal Centre at Wolfson College saw a relatively late version. I am grateful to Philip Windsor for correcting some of the more glaring errors in the references to Aristotle and Kant. W.T. Murphy, although he has seen none of this work, will recognize much of the thinking from discussions we have had and many of the references are the result of his suggestions. It is otiose, but customary and true, to acknowledge that none of these are responsible for anything that follows. In this acknowledgement I can go beyond custom. I too know that in almost every place, my work is improvable: of its nature a work such as this can never be complete, and all things must come to some sort of end.

Joe Jacob
London School of Economics
September 1987

I

An introduction

Although the art of healing is the most noble of all the arts, yet, because of the ignorance both of its professors and of their rash critics, it has fallen at this time into the least repute of them all. The chief cause for this appears to me to be that it is the only science for which states have laid down no penalties for malpractice. Ill-repute is the only punishment.... Holy things are revealed only to holy men. Such things must not be made known to the profane until they are initiated into the mysteries of the science.

(The Canon of Hippocrates)

The purpose and structure

There are several levels in this book. It is a study of politics and of the constitution; it reflects the argument of the American sociologist, Everet Hughes:[1]

> The power of an occupation to protect its licence and maintain its mandate, the circumstances in which they are attacked, lost or changed; all these are matters for investigation. Such investigation is study of politics in the very fundamental sense of studying constitutions.

It is a way of approaching the relationships between rules and those subjected to them.[2] In particular, it uses the foundations of contemporary debates concerning the relation of law and medicine. It seeks to understand how the current worries of doctors about law have come about. Indeed, in some ways the core of my intended audience is in the rather narrow field of medical sociology. That field is important in its own right but it has wider lessons, and I seek them. Rules, I shall suggest, may be power enhancing rather than power limiting. My work, then, is about power and rules and what can be done with them.

The method adopted is to seek a definition of medicine and hence of its practice and to distinguish it from health. Because the concern is with rule-makers and their aspirations, the place of patients is (unfashionably) relegated. Because the majority of general practitioners are dispersed, their place in this work is small. In an early work Freidson assumed,[3] 'that the analytical variables of social organization are more useful discriminants than those of norms, attitudes, ethics'. His concentration[4] was not on spokesmen who might be the models of the profession but on the individuals who are the profession. I, by contrast, seek to describe rules: my concerns are with norms and models. My interest is similar to but not identical with his. So also his works are centred on the United States; my description stays in England.

This book proposes various models of practice. They include: an ideal based in the reciprocal duties of patient and doctor; a clinic-based one, arising out of a duality of mind and body; a scientific medicine limited by a contrast between its quantitative style and the other purposes of medicine; and, participatory and Classical (Hippocratic) medicine. These last will be seen to differ concerning the moral agency of the patient. In the former, it is equal to, although different from that of the doctor. In the latter, it is suspended during the relationship.

These models will be distinguished from health-based theories which, it will be argued, although they have a contemporary influence, do not explain medical practice. What they have to say in this respect is largely negative. In so far as there has been a shift from power based in medicine as an art to power based in the objectivities of science, medicine has changed the doctor from encompassing the uniqueness of the disease-carrier in front of him to the generalizations of science. This shift to impersonal medicine has caused patients to look for their own objectivity in the relationship by the assertion of claims to self-determination. In turn, this is reinforced by modern ideas of the paramountcy of the consumer. However, it is the models of medicine, particularly participatory and Classical medicine, which are important in understanding the regulation of practice. Through them some of the limits of consumerism are to be seen.

A considerable part of the argument of this book is based in histories of medical practice, science, and technology. Emphasis is placed on the changes of the Renaissance. Cure became natural.

The individual began to become conscious of himself. Manners could be cultivated. New sources of information challenged the extant sources of knowledge. The foundations were laid of the institutions which still dominate medicine. The Royal College of Physicians in particular developed a tradition of advising government on public health matters. In the 1800s, the rise of the élite in London led to the rise of aspirations among others. Scientific and professional organizations were founded, including the one which became the British Medical Association. The Medical Act of 1858 ratified the trends towards increased competence, status, formality, and joinder of function.

The book rejects economic models of professionalism and particularly the 'bargain' theory. These ideas do not appreciate that a profession requires a separation of service and reward. The bargain theory is itself ahistorical; it opposes group cohesion and the concept of the guild. Further, it suggests an external capacity to review standards and competence. A bargain would cause major changes in the meaning of medicine and hence its regulation.

What is relevant in considering regulation is not what doctors and patients do but what they think they have done and are doing. In place of economic models, a theory based in the ideal-typical gentleman is proposed. An account of the application of this idea is offered from the time when its mode was seen as capable of being acquired. This theory is itself linked to the idea of efficient sanctions being based in the occupational group, with those externally imposed being corrosive. Internal rules are only vaguely understandable from the outside because they relate to activities which by definition are not common.

It is argued that the actual legal forms adopted in Britain give reality to the classical theory of medical practice and that they recognize the ideal-typical gentleman in medicine as an occupational group. The statutes regulating the professions (a detailed analysis appears in the *Encyclopedia of Health Services and Medical Law*)[5] are assessed and seen to support this view. It is noted that groups lower in social status seek to adopt the forms and prestige of higher groups and commonly they succeed to a remarkable extent, except, significantly, where they are in trade.

To this point the argument is concerned with practice as an occupation. It is also necessary to examine the way in which the bureaucratic organization of medicine copes with untoward events. The circumstances leading to the Public Health Acts of the mid-nineteenth century and the Board of Health and the development of the early voluntary hospitals and their doctors are outlined. Altruism could grow within the structure of institutions. Eventually doctors became able to influence resource allocation.

Bureaucracy and legal rules are to be distinguished. It is noted that in terms of formal instruments there is often a failure to distinguish advice from coercion. The rationality of bureaucracy is associated with, *inter alia*, objectivity, and its consequences for medicine are, once again, a reduction in the effects of medicine as an art. The typical models of medical practice have to be modified.

The *Encyclopedia* identifies twelve distinct mechanisms for coping with the untoward in British health care. Of these, only two – civil and criminal litigation – are based in the traditional concerns of lawyers. This book follows that analysis. The variety is explained by theories based on historico-anthropological, economic, administrative, and psychological considerations. As this book turns to the most formal of the mechanisms, litigation, it follows the *Encyclopedia* in proposing a situation basis of liability in place of the more usual application of contract, trespass, and negligence. This work leaves aside the strictly legal consequences of that proposal and concentrates on its theoretical justification and consequences. It supports the classical theory of medical practice in ways the others do not. The usual contract and tort dichotomy is a response to economic theory current in the nineteenth century and to academic attempts to classify the law. It misunderstands the place of the professions. In particular, science, the medical guilds, and their public responsibilities were in opposition to the economic fashions of the time.

The consequences of situation liability are: that the courts can apply the customs of the profession without becoming an arbiter of standards; that the same standards can be applied with or without contract or agreement; mistakes leading to no liability can be recognized; and, criminal liability can be restricted. In short, it recognizes the current state in England of medical liability.

In keeping with this professionally dominated view, it is only at this point that it becomes appropriate to discuss the place of the patient by way of the law of consent and J.S. Mill's dictum concerning what he calls the 'freedom' of the individual. This last will be shown to assume static relationships between men. Ideas of consent which were important in a religious age have been secularized. As subservience has declined generally so requirements of disclosure have increased. These differences underlie the corresponding differences in, for example, the American and English law, and cultures.

But there is also another difference of importance. It is based in the greater emphasis on individualism in the United States. In an English sort of way, I have regarded patients as objects and out of this adopt an argument that in any two person relationship there is another party to which each of them has a dynamic relation: the 'joint-party'. By not recognizing oscillation, the psychology of Mill and his followers misconstrues the structure of human thought. Objective scientific medicine, in part arising out of a general culture and in part out of specific organizational character-istics – themselves both more greatly emphasized in the United States – breaks the links to the 'joint-party', and so causes the claims to informed consent. It also sharpens loneliness. It is thus possible to distinguish liberty (looking to individual self-determination) and freedom (as part of society). It will be sug-gested that it is necessary, not so much to build institutions, as to refurbish them, and that the law is not well suited to that task.

In his *ABC of Relativity*, Bertrand Russell[6] postulated a bal-loonist sailing over England on the night of the fifth of November or over America on the night of the fourth of July. The balloonist was drugged so that his memory was gone but not his reasoning powers. Seeing the fireworks, Russell asked[7] what sort of picture of the world would be formed and concluded his answer by saying:

> The theory of relativity depends, to a considerable extent, upon getting rid of notions which are useful in ordinary life but not to our drugged balloonist. Circumstances on the surface of the earth, for various more or less accidental reasons, suggest con-ceptions which turn out to be inaccurate, although they have come to seem like necessities of thought.

In this book I have tried to be like Russell's drugged balloonist in rejecting ideas merely because they are 'useful in ordinary life or seem like necessities of thought': 'the most radical doubt is the father of knowledge'.[8] In seeking to understand 'regulation', the discussion goes beyond law into other normative systems, and to the relation between them and law. In seeking to bring these areas together, the learning of many disciplines is seen just as the drug-ged balloonist saw fireworks. And just as his reasoning would lead him to conclusions different from those on conventional Earth, so this book differs from the traditional, the comfortable, or the conventional. To take two examples: as I have indicated, im-plicit in the argument is a rejection of the assumptions that indi-vidual health and liberty are in the economists' sense fundamental goods. So also I have not adopted the now fashionable ideas that intellectual recognition of mysticism and intuition are necessarily insufficient explanations of social phenomena.

It is useful at this point to expand the description of the argument. At bottom it is an account of a particular set of aspirations. There are seven chapters, namely: (1) this introduction which sets out the scope and method of the work; (2) a discussion of medical practice; (3) a description of theories of medicine; (4) and (5) discussions of professionalism; (6) discussions of the effects of administration; and finally, (7) conclusions which go beyond the mere regulation of medicine.

The practice of medicine is used as the organizing tool. To do this it is necessary to set out a theoretical understanding of what it has been thought to be and a history of its formative ideas: in order to use the tool it is necessary to get to know it. I describe 'the medical act' in terms of the 'clinical encounter', and define this idea. However, if 'medicine' were to be limited in this way, important areas of the study would be omitted. Neither the doctor, nor the patient, is confined in space or time to 'the clinic'. There is a continuum from 'medicine' to 'health'. It encompasses fuller ranges of issues which include social security, education, housing, employment, and the rest. These are not my concern, except to note that often if a social or individual problem is not solved it will, in time, be redefined as medical, with particular consequences. Thus to be destroyed in nuclear war is unhealthy, a fact which has aroused the active concern of the European Office of the World Health Organisation. Generally, we may say that what can be called 'iatrocracy' (rule by doctors) – prescriptions by doctors defining the proper way of life for individuals and the correct State policy on the grounds that health will or may be promoted – is more obvious outside the clinic than in it.

The study, then, is not of the content of the controls of, and by, medicine but of the forces which mould them. Both within and externally, as they operate on the wider population, these controls have a variety of types. In many of its important areas what is sometimes called 'biomedicine' is governed by more than one of them. For convenience these types of regulation are called 'norms'.[9] They have more or less specific definition; more or less specific sanctions to support them; interact with each other; and, moreover, at times, they are also to greater or lesser degree in conflict with each other. Further, some of the other values underlying these 'medical norms' are in conflict, again to a greater or lesser extent, with other values that society recognizes and whose source is independent of medical ideology (for example, the pursuit of health is not always the pursuit of liberty, or of freedom).

The main systems of rules against which I place my considerations are: professional ethics; the law as developed in the courts; and administrative structures determined by the State. Because on occasion my terminology departs from that of other authors (for example, professional philosophers in jurisprudence, morality, and ethics), it is helpful here to say something of the way in which I use these terms. *Morality* and *ethics* are taken to be the processes of distinguishing right and wrong: they create or assume judgmental criteria. To the individual, the former is externally validated and the latter, internally. *Etiquette* describes certain conventional rules of personal and professional behaviour, particularly those which affect the interests of other members of the profession or its dignity. On this view *professional codes of ethics* are laid down by the governing bodies of the profession. They may for brevity be described as a formal, but crude, mixture of morality and etiquette, which often contain some legal comment. For reasons which will appear I reject Leake's view[10] that professional ethics (as defined in such codes) relate to etiquette and are thus *hedonistic* (self-interested) rather than *idealistic* (community interested). These normative systems must be distinguished from behaviour which is regulated solely by self-interest, or habit, or custom. I spend little space on conventional behaviour as such because to do so would be to confuse the aspirations of groups with individual action.

I have taken the *law* to be more, rather than less, well defined rules with generally clear but limited sanctions which are external to the individual and imposed by the State. It is neither the same, nor as wide, as social relations but it is connected with them; at times, it conditions them. It cannot exist, and has no meaning, without them; whether they can exist without law is a separate issue to be debated with other means (which I suspect are in part anthropological and in part linguistic). At any rate, in order to know about the law in a particular field, at least at a level other than the technical, it is necessary to become acquainted with a more general understanding of that field. Within the field of law, we may include *Rules of conduct* laid down by employers which gain their *sanction* through the general law of contract; they gain their *meaning* through an understanding of the professional or occupational practices involved.

I should at this stage make it clear that I accept much of Hyde's criticism[11] that the concept of 'legitimation' is not helpful as an analytical tool. That is to say, behaviour can be analysed without postulating 'law to belief to action'. Often 'legitimation' means no more than 'formal acceptance'. There are indeed many causes of acceptance of prescriptions for behaviour. In the field on which I focus, I shall argue one of the causes is the shared traditions and customs which arise out of the working and living arrangements of the élite group which practises medicine. Although I want to avoid discussing conventional behaviour *simpliciter*, the effects of the traditions of medical activity on existing custom are considerable. The extent of their effects varies, however, over time and between cultures. The fact that particularly in England the group was historically, and still is, relatively tightly knit indicates that it is to be expected that its traditions are also relatively more important in the regulation of medical practice.

Before turning to matters of regulation – the law and other normative systems – I must explain, as I have said, in some detail my understanding of the images of the sociology and philosophy of medical practice which are regulated. That is, regulation cannot be considered without first seeking to understand what is to be regulated, and it may not always be a reality. The principal sociologists and philosophers in the field have given a particular and limited meaning to the word 'medicine'. To authors such as Talcot Parsons,[12] Michel Foucault,[13] Edmund Pellegrino, and David Thomasma,[14] the idea of the clinical interaction is implicit in the concept. I shall rest on the ideal model of medical practice offered by Parsons (and some of his more empirical successors) and a philosophy I have derived from the work of Pellegrino and Thomasma.

Having described medicine as an ideal (an image) I am in a position to explore the different theoretical approaches to its practice which in turn influence its regulation. I shall suggest that there are three rival established theories of medicine: the scientific, the participatory, and the classical. Because my approach is infused with an explicit rejection of discussion of the world as it ought to be, it will appear to some as old-fashioned. I contend this method is justifiable except possibly in one respect: if the mechanisms for the transmission of traditions are altered and types of entrant to the profession are different, then possibly one may expect to find consequential changes in the new practices. I doubt that, at least yet in England, there has been sufficient change to alter the ethos of the here and now.

However, even leaving aside this caveat, thus far the analysis is not complete. It does not begin to cope with rival theories of care not based in a clinical interaction but rather in health. True for Pellegrino and Thomasma 'health' is a 'foundational good'; but what they have described is based upon the doctor–patient relationship. I therefore need to consider what has been called 'the radical critique of medicine' and seek an explanation for it. For authors such as Thomas McKeown, the basis and purpose of medicine is health. Indeed they judge clinical interaction by its measure. Thus to them the hospital and the tobacconist are equal parts of the discourse. My account uses two apparently contradictory ideas: on the one hand the emphasis on health with, for example, the common idea of choice of life-style, can be seen as biomedicine's consumerism; on the other, because we are so often told in order to survive we must do this and not that, medicine can be seen as coercive.

Although I speak of the 'function' of, for example, a regulation, I do not use the word in a strictly utilitarian sense. My meaning is often closer to 'cause'. In considering the causes of medicine's regulations, it is as necessary to look at the history of their imperatives as it is at their theory. Both are essential to the method of looking at law through medicine. Thus armed with a method, it is possible to begin to describe the regulation of medicine. As the discussion unfolds, other more general matters continue to intrude. Health care is not simply a matter of 'doctors' 'prescribing' 'medicines' for 'sick' people: each of those terms is problematic. More to the current point are the facts: that health care exists as part of a structured social system, which at the point of action is applied by a professional group, and which is in part bureaucratic and in part subjected to other methods of government; and because law and conflict are often so close, the relevant methods of dispute resolution and responding to unwanted events, which are as diverse and confusing in this field as anywhere else, need to be examined.

Accordingly, I describe within theoretical frameworks and, from the point of view of regulation, the nature of the profession and the bureaucracy within which it largely operates. At points I am concerned with the structure of the health care system. My emphasis in this respect is on rules made externally to the profession. I will note that health professionals, and administrators with whom they work, are only infrequently concerned with the *form* of regulation. Both within the National Health Service and outside it, their main interest is in *content*. For most practical purposes, it does not matter to them whether the instruction which they recognize as coming from a superior (for example, an employer) is laid down in a statute, statutory instrument, ministerial circular, or management directive. What they are concerned with is what it says. The questions which arise are, what is the relationship between the varying forms of instruction and the content, and how do these systems cope with the untoward? Neither here, nor elsewhere in the book, do I adopt the facile assumptions of the modern fashion of consumerism.

A mode of considering each human being as an autonomous, separate individual whose actions are not responsible for reaction in others is sufficient for many of life's purposes. However, it is not axiomatic that it is sufficient for them all. I attempt therefore to look at procedures for complaints, dealing with grievances, and coping with the untoward, not only as facilitating isolated redress for an individual (which they may do) but also as something else. Of course, these procedures are usually set within a framework fashioned by the 'rational economic man' of the later utilitarians and neo-classical economists. My endeavour is also to locate them within a whole social environment.

Consideration of externally made rules and decisions could not be sufficient. I must also consider those made internally by the profession; and indeed this will become a central part of the argument. But also of course I am concerned with the fact that for some of their content and for some of their sanction they depend upon the machinery of the State. Thus I need to consider whether the profession's rules are to be regarded as a part of a bargain with the State in return for the sanctions it offers (which I dispute) or whether they are regarded as an autonomous area of regulation.

One of the conclusions which I shall draw is that medicine is organized by a group of initiates who necessarily better understand their own forms and modes of regulation than anyone else can. In this the argument is similar to Durkheim's concept of a political society as a federation: as a 'whole network of representations, symbols, exchanges and obligations unknown to the individual in isolation':[15] it is a study of group regulation. It asserts that in respect of the understanding of a large number of social phenomena – of which medicine provides many examples – it is necessary to look at several centres of power[16] and that professional power is not exercised in some way as the delegated authority of the State.

However, the regulation of medicine is not a merely modern

phenomenon. It follows that rules (whose direct links with the modern law can be traced) were devised to regulate some phenomena different from modern practice. As we turn to 'the past' and to 'the modern unorthodox' the modern doctor becomes differentiated to a greater extent than are the rules governing medical practice: the relative coarseness of rules cannot reflect the subtlety of practice. I argue that western medicine, as it is usually practised, is centred on a classical theory which is as old as its civilization and still embosomed in mystification; that it is conducted by an élite, fundamentally secret society; that within it, patients are regarded, not so much as selves, as the carriers of objects of discourse; and, that in all this it is given support by the law which thus differs to medicine's ideology.

But there is also a further set of issues which must be considered: what are the rules concerning the relationship of this group to those with which it deals – the patients? Once again, I shall argue that the technical legal view (itself informed by 'rational economic man' rather than the whole social environment) provokes more questions than it solves. Thus I shall assert that the doctor's legal liability to the patient depends upon whether what the 'law' regards as objective standards have been fulfilled but nevertheless a range of questions present themselves:

- Is it a matter of the skills and science the doctor has learnt or ought to have learnt and, in either case, when? In other words, is there a duty on a doctor to undergo continuous training and, if so, how far does the duty extend?
- What is meant by a 'patient'? Is it someone whom the doctor perceives as ill, or someone who sees himself as ill, or must there be agreement between them as to the nature and extent of the illness?
- What is 'consent'? For example, is it legally possible to give a general consent or must it always be specific to the doctor or to the treatment regime proposed? In any event, what is the relationship between consent and diagnostic procedures? Who is to judge whether a patient's 'health' improves? Is this for the doctor's science or the patient's own perception or are these two inevitably linked? Does the doctor's legal liability arise if the patient's health does not improve or only if it is as a result of the failure to use the skills he had, or ought to have had? Is the patient liable to pay only if the doctor has cured him, or even when without cure the doctor has exercised his skills?

- Who is to make the choice if the doctor's skill or science point to choices of diagnostic or therapeutic regime? And on what basis? If the involvement of the patient will alter the nature of the choice, is it necessary in law for him to be consensual, or to be consulted? What if the patient is unconcious, mad, or a child? By what right, or what machinery, can others consent for him?

- How does a duty of confidence arise and what is its extent? What indeed is a medical record? Is the duty of confidence altered if the patient's illness presents a threat to others or if the doctor learns of it in the course of a consultation? How does the duty alter if in order to provide the requisite medical care the doctor must consult with other members of the therapeutic team or if the patient's illness is merely interesting to others? Or instructive to them? To what extent, if at all and why, does the duty of confidence extend beyond matters relevant to treatment?

- Is the relationship to the patient, or are the consequential legal duties, altered if instead of a one-to-one relationship, the doctor is under a contract with a third party to provide care to a series of named individuals, or to those members of the public who present themselves? How does the doctor choose to whom to devote the limited resources of his time and equipment, other staff, etc., or is it indeed the doctor who chooses at all, and if not who does? How does any third party choose to which doctors to make available such resources?

- All these questions assume some specific meaning to the term 'doctor'. But is there indeed some such (even legal) meaning, and if so what is it?

It is important here to note that these questions are posed at a variety of levels. Some are legal, some not; but also some are legal only in part. To take the questions relating to medical records by way of example, what can be made of the idea of 'my medical record'? Factually, it consists of reports which over time I have given to my doctors concerning what I and they have perceived as their business, of observations which they have made including their diagnosis and prognosis, and of reports given to them by pathologists, radiographers, and others. In law it is arguable that I can control the use of the information I have given. But the legal fate of the other parts is less certain. In practice, not I, as a patient, nor the doctors nor any of the members of whatever bureaucracy handles the record have much doubt that all the information is subjected to a duty of confidentiality: whatever the source of the information, the duty allows it to be passed within the medical circle but prevents it from going outside. Thus to ask only this sort of question is to miss the target. That is what is the nature of the duty, what is its cause, and what are its application and effect.

The function of law and of the other methods of regulation are seen in a new light when answers are attempted to the broader and sometimes prior questions. In the concluding part of this work, therefore, I suggest that the beginnings at solutions regarding the regulation of medicine cast doubts over conventional ideas of the function of law, and of regulation, and even more widely over the social forms with which they are concerned.

The method and the argument

This book is not so much concerned with functions and structures of social forms as with the way in which they are seen by those who make regulations. The present and historical data are commonly but not always the same. Moreover, since my actors are real people, as often as not, they misread the reality of the forms they regulate: they come to the business of regulation armed with preconceptions, ideals (here I use the word in its two senses: that is, both as the essence of an idea and a political objective). My study is therefore a plea for the understanding of 'irrational idealism', and the recognition of its importance in the creation of the forms of regulation. My concern lies in the ideal world of imagination and in that no man's land of external rules occupied by lawyers.

My method, then, is to examine images of reality rather than anything that is empirically assessed. For, however rules are made, they are not made on the basis of empirical, still less objective, realities but rather of mental images – ideals is, as I suggest, a good enough word. It is a tool used to describe categories about which it is possible to generalize. In this sense it does not describe actualities nor aspirations. I use it to describe the thinking of the makers of rules. It follows that because this study is concerned with the images of their minds, the emphasis is on historical explanation rather than modern empiricism. Of course, without that it cannot be certain in its conclusions, but just as clearly the assumptions which must precede empirical enquiry need to be organized..

It is important not to confuse the tool with a reality. Popper's strictures[17] concerning the difficulties of metaphysical essentialism are beside the point. His critique of 'methodological essentialism' in the social sciences as opposed to the physical is based on the assertion that these last ask 'how does this piece of matter behave?'. This assumption is false, as can be seen by looking at laws such as Newton's Law of Gravity (which presupposes the absence of resistance) or Mendel's Law of Heredity (which presupposes the absence of mutation). Laws such as these look to how matter would behave in ideal conditions.

In his *Professional Powers*,[18] Freidson sought to explore the application of what he calls the 'formal knowledge' of the professions. In some ways his task is similar to mine. He describes this knowledge as characterized by[19] 'rationalization [consisting] in the pervasive use of reason, sustained where possible by measurement, to gain the end of functional efficiency ... it is élite knowledge'. This far, it is much the same as Popper's 'third world', the world of objective contents of thought:[20] knowledge exists not only in minds but in libraries. But Freidson argues:[21]

> Some of the formal knowledge of any discipline is often expressed as alternative opinions or theories.... This means that formal knowledge can be applied to human affairs and practical action only by making arbitrary and selective decisions.... Guided in part ... by firsthand experience ... practitioners are inclined to follow their own individual situational judgment even when it may contradict received opinion and practice.

And,[22] 'Formal Knowledge ... lives only through its agents'. It is transformed in two ways. First, within an institutional structure, it is simplified by administrative choice. Secondly,[23] 'it is employed inconsistently and informally'. Thus, he says, it is necessary to locate knowledge (included in which are the images of which I write) not in some 'grand scheme' but in concrete individuals. It is in the execution of this that it is most obvious that he has not succeeded: he has not distinguished his knowledgeable concrete individuals from the statistical aggregates of which they form part. Despite his caveats, he has stayed with the measurable and the rational: as I shall insist there is always a danger in reducing men and women to ciphers and so stripping them of humanity.

A part of the knowledge possessed by medical practitioners consists precisely in its informality. Their cultural and occupational experience as individuals equips them to know a great deal that is not explicable to those without that background. At least at times, knowledge is not available to be transformed. It is not visible outside the discourse. It does not exist in libraries. Often, these times are characterized by moral choice; by that area defined by procedure (ways of doing) rather than substance (what should be done). That is, this invisible area is susceptible to rules, themselves created and understandable only from the inside.

The use and limits of history

Law and regulation generally are largely understandable only from a viewpoint grounded in a wider social and political understanding of the past.[24] Quite simply, history will not go away. It is for this reason that I offer some empirical evidence of the past. But it is not necessary (and no attempt is made) to offer a full account of the history even of medical practice: 'all description is necessarily selective'.[25] For ease of exposition, occasionally, I have adopted the quaint, but not always old-fashioned, habit of personalizing historical change.[26] Despite this I have not assumed a consistent progress of history: on the contrary continuity and discontinuity go hand in hand, but, to apply a metaphor, it is not always possible to say which is the substance and which the shadow. Nevertheless, we need something to work on.

My treatment covers many centuries in a few pages and much is taken from perhaps rather conventional, sometimes populist, secondary sources. This work is not a history and some of the detail which I mention may give way to more recent disclosures. It is included because there is a tendency in the literature which wants to say something modern to draw on history from only the beginning of the nineteenth century. My emphasis is over a longer period. My concern is to show what happens if the organizing categories of that century are not applied on a wider time scale: and, I have added a novel interpretation.

My history emphasizes three periods, each characterized by decisive changes both in the organization (and regulation) of medical practice and by such changes in society that their names are standard yardsticks of historians: the Renaissance, the Industrial, and Post-Industrial Revolutions. 'Renaissance' is used to describe, as Mandrou puts it,[27] 'the specific character of the change which was experienced during the century between 1450 and 1550 and which gave the clergy and part of Europe's high society, a new vision of the world'. He argues that the early part of the period was characterized by a heavy emphasis among scholars on philology. It saw the publication for the first time of authentic texts of the learning of antiquity. I have used the term 'Industrial Revolution' to describe that change in political and economic arrangements which was associated with mechanization and which began in the latter part of the eighteenth century. It is emphasized by methods of production. Change in the intellectual environment at the same time is called the 'Enlightenment'. By 'Post-Industrial Revolution' I have referred to those changes in society which have arisen out of the development of various forms of communication (including inter-continental travel and information technologies), the application of science to birth control, and also forms of 'anti-communication', exemplified by nuclear weapons. It is characterized by changes in social intercourse.

The feature these periods have in common is that marked technological, intellectual, and social change (or, now, rate of change) takes place within rather than across generations. When it occurs there is both excitement and disorientation – conditions which because these spheres are not coincident are likely to precipitate enquiry into established values. One of the crucial problems is that each individual not only has to cope with the inevitable changes in himself, but also with changes in his social environment. These are fundamental problems of modernity.[28]

Interesting as it would be to go further, it would upset the balance of the book. I am concerned with describing and explaining existing institutions, ideas, relations. My concern with the past is to the extent that it helps that explanation. But the past is not to be viewed in the terms of the present.[29] As Montesquieu said,

> To apply the ideas of the present time to distant ages, is the most fruitful source of error. To those who want to modernize all the ancient ages, I shall say what the Egyptian priests said to Solon, 'O Athenians, you are mere children'.

It would be to roam too far to enter a general debate as to how far there are such things as lessons or laws of history which can be valid for the future.[30] Churchill once remarked:[31] 'The longer you can look back, the further you can look forward'. The point is true but only so long as the looking back enables organizing categories to be established. If, on the contrary, we use the categories of the present to understand the past, then, by definition, it can tell us nothing. Although the past is not explained by the present, the present may be by the past.

In this book I am not much concerned by way either of prediction or of prescription, with a time beyond the present. Explanations disclosed by history are sometimes the only alternative to a declaration that all is arbitrary. To put it another way, I have devoted such space on history as I have only because the mores, and hence the regulation, of modern medicine are inexplicable without it: traditions live on after their causes are forgotten. When there is an endeavour to establish, or to maintain, an older order it can be reborn. Almost certainly the circumstances in which it operates will be different, and its effects differ; but this is not to deny the intent to relive the past. I am not concerned to trace the life of traditions but rather to discover the manifestations of their causes.

It is clear that the importance of history varies between cultures; even between those of the modern western world. Although the individuals in the New World are the same, to those of the Old, they are emigrants rather than immigrants. In part, the former word emphasizes cultural aspects and the latter economic. To take one simplified example, since the past is less obvious, the frontier and emigrant culture and philosophy of the New World is likely to place less emphasis on historical justification and explanation (as contrasted with sentiment and investigation) than does the culture of the Old. It is more concerned with the individual and the self. Hawthorn[32] makes a similar point considering the reception of Locke in the United States. He suggests that he was misread because his argument for individualism was against a background of social institutions which comprised only property and the State. It did not have the European estates nor an established Church. And,

> Unable to flee into any institution and thereby pass to it responsibility for his beliefs or actions, a man is ... forced to examine himself as an individual alone, to a degree that he is not in any more highly structured society.

It is however not only in an intellectual sense that the past is always more present in the Old. Physically, and particularly architecturally, the past is more there. To take an example, most British towns have graveyards wherein the most visible headstones are commonly of the order of more than a hundred years old. It is not that people have not died since then; rather, since that time more hygienic and sanitary methods of disposal of the dead have been adopted.[33] In some ways, therefore, our everyday consciousness does not see death as having occurred during the last hundred years; modern death is now literally a journey away. Typically, our society now segregates the dying. It removes them from the everyday and places them in isolation in the ascetic 'futuristic' world of the modern hospital.[34] *Per contra*, people living in towns created after that time, as many of those in the New World have been, have less of a sense of continuity with the past.

These factors help to explain the cultural emphasis of the New World on those periods when life is most vital, on the need for choice to be both individualized and simple or simplified, and on extremities of experience.[35] It also suggests a reason for their search for, and the articulation and re-affirmation of, national and community identity: those, as in the Old World, who have them do not look; they can be taken for granted. This explains why this book, whose subject matter is never far removed from health, and therefore from death, treats material written in the cultural milieu of the New World somewhat differently from that created in the Old. The New World is not always a reliable guide to what happens in Europe or even in England. My concern is largely with a profession, the medical. As Freidson says,[36] having discussed a history of the word 'profession', 'it is a historically and nationally specific "folk concept"'.

In seeking to describe the historical sources of the authority of the medical profession over its members and over society it is important to be aware of a major difficulty in understanding historical data: terms change their meanings. As Bevan put it:[37]

> The student . . . must be on his guard against the old words, for the words persist when the reality that lay behind them has changed. It is inherent in our intellectual activity that we seek to imprison reality in our description of it. Soon, long before we realize it, it is we who become the prisoners of the description.

The meaning of terms such as 'disease', 'health', 'medicine', 'illness', 'cure', 'death', and the conceptions of their aetiology are not fixed in eternity. As they have varied over time and between societies, the effect of traditions developed at one point has often been transformed by the tradition adopted in another. I shall have occasion, for example, to discuss some of the problems within our society associated with large modern differences in the meanings of 'medicine' and 'health'. What is immediately important is not so much the change in understanding as the continuity in the traditions which the understandings at any point of time create. To take one instance. Behaviour might originate in response to a religious cause (for example, consent to medical treatment): as that cause fades, it might become justified by secular reasons.

If instead of thinking of medicine and its associated ideas as having definitive meanings, we recognize that they are culturally determined in time and space, it is, I believe, easier to isolate those traditions which have been imported. By the recognition of the possibility of developments elsewhere affecting what happens in one place, it becomes possible to explain existing forms more satisfactorily.

Take for example 'cure'. The question of its meaning can be reformulated as: Why have people always consulted doctors although for most of recorded time the doctor's therapies have not been effective in our modern understanding of the word?[38] The question is fundamental to understanding why patients entered and enter relationships with doctors. It is, of course, their disposition to do so which has allowed doctors to develop the profession and its traditions. The conventional answer places its emphasis on belief and stops short of examining the nature of that belief.[39] If cure always had its modern meaning, the belief can be regarded as mistaken view of reality.[40] But if cure has changed its meaning and its causes are differently understood, belief in it may have been as rational or irrational in the Middle Ages as it is now.

The meaning is closely bound with the history of the aetiology of disease. It too has been transformed. For example, Cartwright explains[41] that a theory of four indivisible elements was proposed for all natural substances. They were earth, air, fire, and water.

> The nature of the four elements suggested four qualities: dry, cold, hot, and moist. The four elements shared these four qualities: hot + dry = fire, hot + moist = air, cold + dry = earth, cold + moist = water. Applied to medicine, the four elements became four humours, formed as follows: hot + moist = blood, cold + moist = phlegm, hot + dry = yellow bile, cold + dry = black bile.

Since it was held that disease was an imbalance of the humours, cure could be affected by the prescription of substances to restore the equilibrium.[42] The triumph of the Hippocratic corpus[43] was that all disease was seen to be natural and not supernatural. It says for example of epilepsy:

> it is my opinion that those who first called this disease 'sacred' were the sort of people we now call witch-doctors, faith-healers, quacks and charlatans. These are exactly the people who pretend to be very pious and to be particularly wise.

It was a feature of the Renaissance that the idea of the natural basis of disease was re-adopted and, still later, out of the technologies of the Industrial and post-Industrial Revolutions – of the Enlightenment – came the idea that cure could be natural. From technical advances by the surgeons and the apothecaries came the idea that cure could be artificially induced. From science came the idea of measurable, predictable cause and effect. From the emergence of science as a rival to ecclesiastical authority came the idea that men could master disease.

But why and in what ways has the concept of cure itself been transformed? Finucane[44] points to some of the changes. He argues:[45]

> Posthumous miracles are events arising not in the presumed actions of the saint – now dead – but in the needs of the people . . . .
>
> [P]ractically nothing was known about health or illness in the 'scientific' sense. Though this is commonly admitted, sometimes the implications are not fully appreciated. The point to note is that the degree of illness in any particular case was only vaguely understood, and the extent of recovered health, or what was assumed to be recovered health, was, likewise, only vaguely understood. In such circumstances, the idea of a 'cure' could only be a social generalization and our own appreciation of the words 'he is cured' has very little application to medieval conditions.

And he adds:[46]

> on many occasions medieval folk were unable to distinguish the dead from the living . . . . William of Canterbury inadvertently illuminated this state of affairs when he calmly wrote that revival from the dead after two or three days was not uncommon in England, though revival after seven days was, he must admit, somewhat unusual.

He then examines the records to show[47] (a) 'the time element was immaterial in attribution of a miraculous cure', (b) '[P]artial or incomplete cures are far from uncommon in all lists of post-humous miracles', and (c) the cures 'need not be permanent'. Support for this different view of cure appears in amongst other sources. For example, Cellini[48] speaks of a doctor who treated people with the plague but who, since 'not many months later' all those he cured fell ill again, would have been blamed for the failure. So also in the early nineteenth century, a law reporter[49] speaks confidently of 'recovery' after surgical intervention for cancer of the breast.

Finucane concludes:[50]

> The power of faith to make the believer feel better, whether 'cured' or not, was as true at Aesculapian temples and medieval shrines as it is today in hospital ward and GP's surgery. Furthermore, a single cure was worth well over a hundred failures, was enough to give a boost to what people desperately wanted to believe. Indeed, there were no failures, since ultimately medieval folk believed that it was the worthiness of the pilgrim, and the capricious will of God, which decided who should be cured.

Finucane perhaps takes too scientific a view of cure in the modern world. However his work clearly shows the change in the conception of its aetiology.

A critique and justification

It is as well to be clear now why some will find my enterprise unsatisfactory. It is unfashionable: in concentrating its attention on what is, I have sought also to avoid stating what it ought to be. I reject Rousseau's dictum that[51] 'he who is to judge wisely in actual government ... must know what ought to be in order to judge what is': I do not seek to aid those who judge, or would like to judge, those 'in actual government'. However, the effect of seeking only to describe or explain a reality may not only be seen to be itself value-laden, but also, because it refuses to criticize the practitioners of its subject – in this case biomedicine – may be seen to judge those who do and specifically to be critical of lawyers and other would-be makers of policy. In short, by describing the modes and forms of regulation of medicine, I may be seen to be defensive of traditional medical ideology. In so far as I place an emphasis on a mysticism in medical practice, I may be seen to be attempting a re-mystification of medicine.

Both these mistake my purpose. It is similar in one respect to that of Foucault in his *The Birth of the Clinic*.[52] My book, like his, 'has not been written in favour of one kind of medicine as against another kind of medicine, or against medicine and in favour of an absence of medicine'. His was a structural study; mine is directly a study of the regulation of medicine in particular and indirectly of regulation by groups in general. It follows from my approach that much of the contemporary literature and debate in biomedicine is not directed at the matters with which I deal.

I have another point to make. Often those other authors seem to offer important arguments based on assumptions which this book doubts. My description challenges a number of commonly articulated ideas which some members of both of the professions with which it is concerned may find novel or strange: I seek discomfort for prejudice. To be brief here, the book does not accept a 'scientific' theory of medicine. The book does not even accept that the practice of medicine is fundamentally concerned with health. It does not accept that professional 'codes of ethics' have much to do with ethics or morality. It does not organize social forms by economic categories.

So also, whether infused by the interaction between doctor and patient, or by health, some have sought to appropriate the term 'biomedical ethics' (or 'bioethics') to describe value aspects of the biomedical discourse. Some may find this study unsatisfactory (or, if they are kind, surprising) because this element of my concerns is not discussed except that it is regarded as a separate but subsidiary debate. This book, I repeat, is not concerned with what ought to be but only with what is. It does not give consideration to how the individual practitioner's own rules of ethics are made and the extent to which they are applied because such debates are commonly concerned with how people ought to want to behave. For example, I shall argue that to science the unknowable is not worth knowing. The consequence is that to applied science, the unattainable is not worth pursuing. As medicine became imbued with science, so the limits of its endeavour have changed.[53] To take one particular, biotechnology is developing the means to alter genes, so medical practice is becoming involved in gene selection. The intervention is new and as yet medicine has no traditions to guide its practitioners.[54]

Accordingly, what I have not done is to seek to impose on medicine an application of some external or purportedly universal moral philosophy. Thus there is no express discussion of many issues enjoying current fashionable interest: in addition to genetic engineering they include abortion, the societal dimensions of transplant technology, drug therapy, experimentation, and the nature of death. My argument does not rely much upon particular forms of distress (for example, terminal illness) nor upon particular patients (for example, women or the young or the old), nor upon particular regimes of intended therapy (for example, surgery or drugs with or without placebos), nor does it enter into what is a 'normal' treatment and what a 'trial'. And in each of these omissions my reasons are the same: these debates arise out of concern for patients, my work is directed at practice.

There is yet another reason why perhaps lawyers particularly will find the book unsatisfactory. The approach is somewhat theoretical and many of the sources it uses are to be found in sociology and philosophy. It almost entirely ignores the contribution of legal theorists. Whether their writings are textbooks or monographs, at best and with few exceptions, it appears artificial to seek to apply their thinking outside the confines of a strictly legal and academic discourse, that is, outside the rather narrow confines of the work of appellate courts. In other words, the substance of the criticism of what Jerome Frank in *Courts on Trial* called 'rule-skeptics' – that they were concerned with appellate rather than fact-finding tribunals – can be applied to most pre- and post-realist writers (as they are known to jurisprudence) who are concerned with the nature of law. By 'legal theorists', I mean those authors who, in the main, write within and for the occupants of law faculties. It does not seem too unkind to say: '"What is truth?" said jurisprudence, and did not stay for an answer'.

It is important to be clear as to the role of theories in both the natural and social sciences. I do not know what else it can be, except to give to facts a significance or a meaning other than their existence; it is to provide the organizing categories by which we can understand our world: to have no theory is to have no questions. To say of individuals or groups that they have a common understanding of reality is to say they have a common organizing theory. The task of the theoretician is to articulate it, its assumptions, and its consequences. It is because the organizing of legal facts is ordinarily so unproblematic that the recourse to express theory is commonly unnecessary.

I regard as uninteresting that type of theoretical debate which is no more than a kind of mental gymnastics. This is all the more so where the gymnastics are confined to the gymnasium – a closed set of *a priori* principles. Godel's Theorem says that no system has the capacity, within its own theoretical assumptions, to offer the means of its own critique because it includes propositions which in its own terms it cannot prove. This theorem applies to law as a discipline although not as a practice: that is, it applies to law as a structure but, in the practical world of lawyers, rules are asserted, not 'proved'.[55] It may be that I have missed some meaning in jurisprudence but I do not merely fail to see how it does, but I do not see how it can, organize the kind of experience with which this book is concerned.

Not only will some find this book unsatisfactory, it is also incomplete, and for several reasons. The first relates to my treatment of history. The second is that one of its purposes is to act as an agenda for the study of regulation. Such answers as any one proposes (and I do not exempt myself) must be inadequate for some purposes. The nature of the idea of biomedicine itself prevents it being treated as a closed discipline: as an object of thought, it is a device for focusing ideas. In seeking to locate its regulations, it ventures into many areas of scholarship. Because they are focused the effects and implications of the learning of many disciplines on each other are more easily disclosed.

To adopt an analogy from the world of sport:[56] Is a bowler in cricket similar to a baseball pitcher, or a batsman, or a fielder? His technique is comparable to (but not the same as) that of the pitcher. He has the same ethic as the batsman and the fielder, but not the pitcher. He has the same end as the fielder, but not the batsman. It is of course possible to isolate the bowler as possessing a separate discipline but we are not much informed about it by a description of the art or the science which does not place them in a context. To locate the activity of bowling, these comparisons (or others like them) can usefully be made. So it is with this book: the law is not described in isolation as a separate discipline, but rather other activities, other discourses, are used to locate it and thus to describe it more fully. One of the purposes is to indicate how the work of scholars in more discrete fields can be used to create new understandings of my subject, and it of theirs.

The field sometimes known as 'biomedicine' thus draws on many disciplines and, even leaving aside applied moral philosophy, the literature which informs it is immense. By early 1982, the Bioethics Library at the Kennedy Institute held over 27,000 articles and 7,000 books.[57] Articles are appearing at over 200 a month.[58] Giesen says[59] that court decisions in the United States 'can now scarcely be assimilated'. And, because of the transnational links between the members of the medical profession, consideration of its regulation cannot be confined to one nation state. So it is that a few scholars can be as informative as a selection from the many. In consequence, in parts, this book rests heavily on those few.

Support for the book's method is gained from the belief that, between disciplines and beyond, ideas are transmitted at the points of social contact between specialists and rarely by scholarship alone. This is, in part, the purpose of multi-faculty centres for higher education and research. It is of some importance for the current study that lawyers gain their knowledge of policy at these points of contact.[60] More generally, in the course of interdisciplinary work, in order to know how one discipline affects others, it is normally sufficient that there be an understanding of its knowledge. To use an analogy, to study the composition *of* light it is commonly necessary to use a primary source; secondary or reflected sources may seriously distort its purity. There is one reservation: to the extent that the effects of the distortion are known, it is possible to reconstruct the purity of the primary source. However, to study *by* light, it is sufficient that there be enough of it, whether its source be primary, artificial, or secondary.

To say, for example as this book says, that medical theory is reflected in law, is not to say that lawyers have been informed about it, or deliberately applied it, but merely that seeking an understanding of such a theory helps to clarify the intuitive rationale of the law. Where material from different cultures is used, it is necessary to be aware of the distorting influence, either obviously where there is a translation from one language to another, or, less obviously, where the symbols are used in a different and often unarticulated philosophical environment.

Some will object that very little is said about mental disablement. That too, however, mistakes my purpose. True, it is often impossible to avoid touching on mental, emotional, psychological aspects of illness (and acts which may threaten health) but these are incidental to the main discussion. Mental disablement is omitted because the focus of the book is on the mode and form, not the subject, of medical practice. The focus is concerned with who does things and how they get done, not to whom they are done nor what is done nor really why. As I will argue, the mainstream of medical practice is concerned with the secondary care of acute illness. Nevertheless the omission begs some questions: it assumes an objective reality to both physical and mental disability and also that they can be distinguished. But these issues are not central to the prime interest. To an extent, these assumptions are problematic but to raise them here would distort the balance of the work without affecting the central ideas. It would be to write a different book.

Readers of this book will notice one other stark contrast with contemporary writing. It is almost wholly uninformed by the new learnings concerning the role of women. Still the reason is the same. The emphasis on practice, not the subject, gives the clue. I have sought to expose the history, the tradition, and habits of mind of practitioners. I have been concerned with a world, albeit a narrow and limited (we might say partial) world, dominated by men and not by women.[61] The modern forms adopted by these practitioners are the heirs of their history. Women have a small part in my description because they have played a small part in what I am describing. No doubt they will continue to increase their influence in the world of practice. But I have not chosen to write about the future.

There is one other general point which ought to be made. This book does not deny either the importance of reason in seeking to expound the laws of nature or mankind's need to seek, as far as they can be reconciled, both perfection and attainable goals. Rationality has a place in intellectual thought, but there are few grounds for supposing that either the aetiology, or the consequence, of all nature can be understood by reason and fewer still that they are immutable or eternal. The corollary is also true: there are limits to reason. Without either reviewing theories of epistemology or attempting my own, it seems clear that some things will always be beyond reason, that perfection is impossible, and that some goals are worth having despite being manifestly unattainable. This proposition is supported, but only in part, by the difficulty amounting to practical impossibility for any scholar fully to comprehend all the disciplines and their developments in even the social sciences (natural scientists have long since abandoned the attempt), and consequently a corresponding impossibility of observing any particular phenomena from all viewpoints. The practice of medicine itself provides sufficient examples of all these.

This book presents a programme, not conclusions: it seeks engagement not agreement. It describes regulation in order to aid the understanding of the relationship of groups to society, and the society of which they form part. It argues bluntly something which is not novel but not always accepted: individualism, and the liberty which is associated with it, is valuable but is inherently destructive of the self: human values can only be enhanced by the recognition of common humanity. It is at this point that I depart descriptive intent and become prescriptive. At its widest, this book seeks a reconstruction of the role of rules outside the fences built by eighteenth- and nineteenth-century economic theory. It is this rebuilding, itself based in our cultural inheritance, which can give freedom new meaning.

2

Medical practice

A topography

Within the context of his wider social theory, Talcot Parsons offered an idealized description of modern medical practice.[1] For my current purpose its convenience is precisely that it is a simplified representation of the way in which modern western society conceptualizes medicine. It is possible to confine the present description to this model alone and to leave aside Parsons' own attempt to relate it to his wider theory. In Parsons, the model was an attempt at a balanced (reciprocal) example of a mechanism for coping with deviance. Here, this aspect, crucial in him, is left aside. I am concerned with doctors' practices, not with their reciprocity with patients; my emphasis is on only one party to the relationship. So also, it does not matter for my purpose that the model is flawed: for the most part, it offers sufficient insight into practice and, more importantly, into the way society views it.

To this two reservations must be made.[2] First, Parsons' model is expressly confined to the 'therapeutic functional context'.[3] As will be seen later, medicine is not confined to therapy. Secondly, he says that society has 'an optimistic bias'.[4] Thus in his discussion of death, society, he says, deals with it by way of ritual rather than reality; and in his discussion of technical innovations, there is a tendency to use them even where their advisability may be doubted.[5] This optimism infects him as well. It leads him to regard illness as transient. But the truth is, of course, that health, and indeed life, as well as illness are temporary. To emphasize one feature of these correlations, distorts the whole.[6]

In its simplest terms Parsons' model suggests that a patient perceives himself as ill and accordingly presents himself to his doctor. His doctor is skilled having been trained in scientific medicine. The doctor on making his diagnosis will prescribe a course of treatment to which the patient, and those in a social relation to him, will unhesitatingly consent. There is an expectation on both sides that the patient's health will improve. Parsons' general social theory is concerned with reciprocal relationships and, although he discusses the involvement of a bureaucracy, his paradigm is where the patient directly pays the doctor for the services. He continues by describing the functions of illness, its effects on society,[7] and the roles of the patient and of the doctor. He says that disturbance of health is sickness or illness – deviancy. Too high an incidence of illness is dysfunctional. So far as it is controllable, it is in the 'functional' interest of society to minimize it. Further, although many illnesses are a natural phenomenon, others are either caused, or may be treated, by motivational factors. He says:[8]

> Illness is a state of disturbance in the normal functioning of the total human individual, including both the state of the organism as a biological system and of his personal and social adjustments. Participation in the social system is always potentially relevant to the state of illness, to its aetiology and to the conditions of successful therapy, as well as to other things.

In recognition of these social facts:[9] (1) the sick person is given relief from 'normal social responsibilities' (and the 'physician often serves as a court of appeal as well as a direct legitimizing agent'); (2) the sick person has to be taken care of; (3) the sick person has an obligation to seek competent help. So long as he remains a sick person, he is characterized by helplessness, technical incompetence and emotional involvement. Although Parsons recognizes the place of psychology for both the patient and the doctor he says that sickness is contingent, the subject of objective criteria, and, as already indicated, temporary. He says despite the objective nature of illness,[10]

> Psychotherapy to the militantly organic anti-psychiatric physician is like theory to the militantly anti-theoretical empirical scientist. In both cases he practices it whether he knows it or wants to or not. He may indeed do it very effectively just as one can use a language well without even knowing it has a grammatical structure.

His observation that typically the patient overestimates the seriousness of his illness and underestimates the time for recovery is of particular importance to my later discussion of the patient's consent to medical procedures and self-determination. Of medical practice he says it[11] 'is a "mechanism" in the social system for coping with illnesses of its members . . . . Modern medical practice is organized about the application of scientific knowledge to the problems of illness and health, to the control of disease.' However, in contrast to some other commentators, he recognizes that the application of science is recent and other traditions live on. Among these other traditions, and closely connected with what he characterizes as the 'optimistic bias' is the application of 'pseudo-science'. This he describes as a form of magic. At this point he follows Malinowski: 'The basic function of magic is to bolster the self-confidence of actors in situations where energy and skill do make a difference but where because of uncertainty factors, out-comes cannot be guaranteed'. Belief by the patient aids recovery and, the physician having recognized this, requires that the patient has confidence in him.

It is important to note that to Parsons the physician has a high technical competence which implies a specificity of function and precludes comparable expertise in other fields. This in turn leads to 'specificity of competence' and 'scope of concern'.[12] Thus the privileges accorded within this limited field must not be abused sexually or otherwise. I shall suggest an alternative explanation lies in physicians accepting Pythagorean asceticism. To Parsons the patient receives 'neutrality of regard'. This means that the ten-dency for the relationship between patient and doctor to become personal is resisted by the 'specificity of function' and the affective neutrality.[13] Further, he says the ideology of the profession places stress on the 'collectivity-orientation',[14] and the welfare of the patient: it contrasts men as 'heartless egoists' and medical men as 'altruists'.[15] We shall see that my suggestion of a 'Pythagorean' dimension in professional practice offers some explanation for this last.

Parsons argues that the universalistic characteristics which in-clude the professional ideology are bolstered by the links via the universities with the world of science,[16] and also by the fact that 'modern medical practice' is organized about the application of 'scientific knowledge by technically competent trained personnel'. This has the effect that selection (even for qualification but more so for promotion) is by performance criteria and this helps to focus ambition and loyalties.

In accord with Parsons' general social theory, the 'collectivity-orientation' of the physician is reciprocal with the object of his work, the patient. As regards that relationship it is the main authority for the doctor's obedience to norms and the patient's obedience to the doctor. He says:[17]

> Reliance on informal methods, even though greater formalization would be more logical, may have its functional significance. Formalization inevitably gives a prominent role to the technicalities of definition . . . . Undoubtedly a certain amount of abuse does 'get by' in the present situation which 'ought not to' and would not in a well-run formal system of control. But it is at least possible that the strong reliance on informal controls helps give the physician confidence.

Or as Freidson[18] puts it more control is possible than occurs. It is a key feature of Parsons' model (one might say it is an essential precondition for it) that the patient, recognizing that he is ill, will present himself to the doctor.[19] The questions that arise are whether patients are in fact capable of recognizing their need for help and if so whether they seek medical aid. In so far as the answers are in the negative, at best the Parsonean model presents a partial picture of health care.

Apple suggests[20] that to the layman two factors are important: the recency of the experience and the degree to which it interferes with ordinary activities. Freidson adds:[21] 'what the layman recognizes as a symptom or illness is in part a function of deviation from the culturally and historically variable standard of normality established by everyday experience'. After a survey of the literature, Zola concludes:[22] 'the more intensive the investigation, the higher the prevalence of clinically serious but previously undiagnosed disorders' there appears to be. Even more important from the point of view of the patient as a free moral agent is what Zola says about the effect of culture on health and on the desire to seek help for sickness. Thus, he suggests, in a distinct sub-culture (and one which many readers will recognize) which emphasized the importance of hard work

> tiredness, rather than being an indication of something being wrong, was instead positive proof that its members were doing right. If they tired, it must be because they had been working hard . . . . On the other hand, where arduous work is not gratifying in and of itself, tiredness would be more likely to be a matter for concern and perhaps medical attention.

Thus cultural differences are a major determinant among those people presenting themselves to a doctor and also in the symptoms, including reactions to pain, that they mention when they get there.[23] To put the matter in commonplace terms, consider the following conversation which many of us have had: 'ıst person: "I have a headache". 2nd person: "Oh, I am sorry". ıst person: "I drank too much last night". 2nd person: "I am not sorry, it's your fault"'. There is a moral content in being ill. Not only, as Parsons says, is there an obligation to seek help but there is also, in varying degrees, a moral obligation both to avoid illness, and, if it comes, to be brave.

The medical clinic

At what we may call the outset of the modern era, Descartes had postulated a metaphysical dualism of mind and body. In doing so, he created what has been regarded as the necessary precondition for the extensive study of the laws of nature governing material things. Generally since then the natural sciences have been devoted to the endeavour to find these laws. In the medical context implicit in such a search is the idea that the body is a machine affected by its chemistry as well as its physics. The Black Report said:[24]

> To the extent that a mechanistic model of health holds sway, the health care services will give priority to such matters as surgery, the immunological response to transplanted organs, chemotherapy and the molecular basis of inheritance. Medicine comes to be structured according to a scale of values associated with such a model. The most sought-after posts will be those at the heart of the model, and medical education and careers are similarly influenced.

At this point it is convenient to describe two distinctions commonly made in health care. They both describe general ideas; they do not have exact or technical meanings and they are not terms of art. First, acute disease or illness is to be distinguished from chronic disease or illness. Broadly, the acute malady is coming to, or is at, a crisis; the chronic is lasting or lingering. There is a link between acute illness, and the optimistic bias and functional therapeutic context described by Parsons. They all stand on one side as representing the side of hope, of the achievable. On the other, lies the lingering, the chronic, illness which by definition cannot be cured with any speed if at all. In the short term, it may be possible to relieve some of its symptoms but because it cannot be the subject of a near miraculous cure and because, for the doctor as well as the patient, the work has to be seen over comparatively long periods, it is not an attractive professional subject.

The second distinction commonly made in health care is between *primary*, *secondary*, and *tertiary* care. As ordinarily used, these correspond to the type of care ordinarily dispensed by the general practitioner, by the general ward in a hospital, and by an intensive care unit, sometimes including all life-saving occasions. It is to be observed that this distinction isolates the work of the general practitioner, whose practice of medicine is complicated by the larger expression of the patient's will (for example, the patient can more obviously choose whether to attend or to take what is prescribed) and by the involvement of some apparently 'less medical' matters such as form filling for other bureaucracies. A later chapter will note the rise of the English teaching hospital and the way in which its activities became the paradigm of medical practice both in theory and as an objective to which for a time almost all doctors aspired. (To judge by results, similar factors worked on developments in other countries.) Because primary care is less concerned with acute illness, it is in secondary and tertiary care, that is, in the hospital, where 'medicine' finds its purest expression.[25]

Accordingly, we must turn to the teaching hospital in order to understand medicine as it is practised. Michel Foucault provides[26] an examination of the clinic (such as a hospital) in which medical science is taught and learnt. Broadly, Foucault's analysis is concerned with the period 1780–1830. The ideal model I sketch from him is an early one, perhaps indeed only relearnt from Hippocrates. In the latter part of Foucault's period, the ideal became more complex: disease was given a chronological place by pathological anatomy. He argues that the modern would-be doctor comes to the clinic with a scientific background, but it is at the clinic that he learns the medical implications of his science.[27] Sydenham is reported to have advised:[28] 'Anatomy, botany, nonsense. No, young man, go to the bedside; there alone can you learn disease.' To Foucault, the ideal clinic possesses five characteristics. It is neither open to all nor completely specialized. The patient's admission depends upon the prospective advantage to the clinician (and his students) of the patient's malaise. In the clinic it is the disease and not the patient which matters, since the disease 'serves as the text'. The patient is not so much examined as his symptoms are deciphered. The teacher, faced then with the disease in front of him, indicates to his pupils the order in which objects must be observed so that they might be seen and remembered more easily. Anything said by the teacher is capable of being tested by experience. In 1825 Corvisart said:[29]

> Theory falls silent or almost always vanishes at the patient's bedside to be replaced by observation and experience; for on what are observation and experience based if not on the relation of our senses? And where would they be without these faithful guides?

Foucault comments:[30]

> The whole dimension of analysis is deployed only at the level of an aesthetic. But this aesthetic not only defines the original form of all truth, it prescribes rules of exercise, and it becomes, at a secondary level, aesthetic in that it prescribes the norms of an art.

No doubt there could be other ways of organizing knowledge of diseases; generally in western medicine, however, they are not used.[31] The process of the clinical experience is the way in which the modern doctor learns. And, central to it is the idea that he is concerned to devote his sensibility to the signs and symptoms of disease.[32] It is precisely this idea which dominates his attitudes to the norms, legal and other, which in turn control his reactions to his sensibility. The method of learning, itself lifelong since facts which have been learnt can always be invalidated by experience, conditions the doctor to look at the disease and not the patient. There can be no surprise that in England even as the clinic was being established, the teaching of anatomy was in effect legalized by the Act of 1832.[33]

The clinic reinforces what Parsons but not Foucault calls 'affective neutrality' and is itself reinforced by it. Further, because the doctor's sensibility is both acquired and esoteric, it is to be expected that his views of the norms of biomedicine (including their development) will also be esoteric. As Foucault puts it,[34]

> The most important moral problem raised by the idea of the clinic was the following: by what right can one transform into an object of clinical observation a patient whose poverty has compelled him to seek assistance at the hospital? Furthermore ... the clinic was also carrying out research; and this search for the new exposed it to a certain amount of risk.

And a little later he gives the answer:[35]

> Since disease can be cured only if others intervene with their knowledge, their resources, their pity, since a patient can be cured only in society, it is just that the illnesses of some should be transformed into the experience of others.... And in accordance with a structure of reciprocity, there emerges for the rich man the utility of offering help to the hospitalized poor: by paying for them to be treated, he is, by the same token, making possible a greater knowledge of the illnesses with which he himself may be affected....

These, then, were the terms of the contract by which rich and poor participated in the organization of clinical experience.... The doctor's gaze is a very small saving in the calculated exchanges of a liberal world.

But is it right to regard 'affective neutrality' as a link between Parsons and Foucault? After all, there is, on one view, a conflict between the doctor's 'affective neutrality' in Parsons and his 'pity' in Foucault. But neutrality is not necessarily the same as indifference. We may take it that the 'pity', although depersonalized, is a part of the motor of the relationship, the reason for it. Without it the doctor is less of a physician and more of a biologist; the 'affective neutrality' is a part of the work the motor does, the way of working. It is 'affected' because, whether real or apparent (that is, 'put on') a neutrality is a precondition to the practice of medicine.

Scientific and Hippocratic medicine

Views of medical practice can be classified into three types: scientific, participatory, and Hippocratic or classical.[36] Even within the modern western world it is possible to find expression of each of them. Each influences the techniques of regulation affecting medicine. This section is primarily concerned to define the scientific and to contrast it with the Hippocratic; the next will distinguish the participatory and classical forms. The scientific mode, then, addresses itself to a mechanistic and secular view of medical practice. It adopts the Cartesian duality of mind and body, and says that medicine is only concerned with the functioning of the body as a machine. It treats the doctor as a biotechnician. In this mode medicine is susceptible to economic and democratic theory. It indicates the possibility of a large measure of legal control, particularly by 'informed consent' theory.

The participatory mode, by contrast, stresses the joint search for the expression of the values of both physician and patient. It can be rested on the Kantian idea of each individual having an unconditional worth, itself derived from the categorical imperative, namely, 'Act as if the maxim of your action were to become through your will a general natural law'. Just as there are surface similarities between the Christian ethic, 'Love your neighbour', the utilitarian ethic of the maximization of happiness and the categorical imperative, so also the participatory theory in its various formulations is available for the construction of regulatory systems. However, having an emphasis on co-operation between individuals, it exists, at best unhappily, with the coarser mechanisms of regulation found in law.

The classical theory of medicine starts its analysis at a different place. Unlike the scientific mode, it does not treat the body as a machine. Unlike the participatory theory it does not give equal importance to both doctor and patient. It starts in the mysticism of the doctor's activity. Essential to it, but secondary, are the contributions of science and the values of the patient. In this theory, mind and body are not separate: the question 'whose body is it?' is without meaning.[37] Medicine is seen as a closed discipline whose practitioners regard their subject – the enduring war against particular forms of suffering – dispassionately and over a longer time scale than do externals (including patients). It is not susceptible to outside regulation, whether moral or legal or bureaucratic.

Scientific medicine

Later I shall describe the rise of medicine and of science as imperatives and the impact of the 'Enlightenment'. Here I consider medicine as a science. It can hardly be doubted that in its modern western form it is, at least in part, such an enterprise. Sherwood Taylor offered a description of natural science as:[38]

> the grouping of well-tested observations into an ordered and intelligible scheme, based on general Principles or Laws, discovered from such observations and capable of being used to predict future phenomena.

Since then, Popper has argued[39] that although the objective of the scientist may be to find a true explanation of observable facts, normally all his experiments can do is to show that a particular theory is false. Indeed a century earlier Darwin remarked:[40] 'Never trust in science to the principle of exclusion'. The laws of science are, then, those predictions which have not been shown to be false. More importantly, as Sherwood Taylor said,[41]

The world of science is an intelligible and self-consistent view of the universe, but its intelligibility is due to the fact that we exclude from science all data which are not expressible in terms of mass, length and time.

All else, as we shall see Hume saying, should be committed to the flames. The nineteenth-century French doctor, Bernard put it:[42] 'Systems do not exist in nature.... What we know may interfere with our learning about what we do not know.' The scientist starts with facts and tests their significance against an hypothesis but not against a theory. Science rejects philosophical metaphysics and thence, irrationally, moral philosophy and the humanities generally. For example, the Royal Society, that creation of the Restoration (it was founded in 1662) and British base of the natural sciences, specifically excluded metaphysics, divinity, morals, grammar, rhetoric, and logic from its concerns.

Joining his science to his view of religion, T.H. Huxley wrote:[43]

Positively the principle may be expressed, in matters of the intellect, follow your reason as far as it will take you, without any regard to any other consideration. And negatively: in matters of the intellect do not pretend that conclusions are certain which are not demonstrated or demonstrable. That I take to be the agnostic faith, which if a man keep whole and undefiled he shall not be ashamed to look at the universe in the face, whatever the future may have in store for him.

In another vein he, at least, also recognized:[44] 'man is not a rational animal'. The rise of science and of the tolerant rationalism expressed in Huxley's principle have obscured these other aspects of humanity. And it is these other aspects which are crucial. To reject religion as a basis for personal belief and action is one thing; to reject it as the basis of other people's is quite another.

It is convenient here to adopt much of Bertrand Russell's conclusion regarding the nature of science:[45]

The authority of science ... is intellectual not governmental .... It prevails solely by its intrinsic appeal to reason.... It pronounces only on whatever at the time appears to have been scientifically ascertained, which is a small island in an ocean of nescience. There is yet another difference from ecclesiastical authority, which declares its pronouncements to be absolutely certain and eternally unalterable: the pronouncements of science are made tentatively, on a basis of probability, and are regarded as liable to modification. . . .

Emancipation from the authority of the Church led to the growth of individualism, even to the point of anarchy. . . . Modern philosophy ... has retained, for the most part, an individualistic and subjective tendency. . . . Unlike religion, it is ethically neutral.

The contrast between ecclesiastical authority and natural science was important for Russell's purposes. For the current discussion it is not necessary to consider his allegations of the absolute and eternal nature of the former. Later I shall return both to the historical *modus vivendi* between ecclesiastical and medical authority and to a religious and secular distinction between the different contributions of the patient. It suffices here to observe we are reasonably accustomed to a trinity: God, society and the natural sciences. What we can understand less is that until the last hundred years or so, no one separated their investigation even if they specialized.[46] It may be remarked, although this at least is one mistake of which Russell is less guilty than some, that the creation of intellectual pigeon holes is only recent – accounts of histories of ideas in one of these which fail to reflect the others fail also to describe the thinkers. Still more recently, and here Russell was at fault, was God put in one of these pigeon holes. It may be infantile to regard as dead that which has merely been put away but English positivism has so marginalized God as to have done just that. From theology, we get to the sociology of theology and hence, via that positivism, our ability to assert its irrelevance.

It is more important, however, to refute Russell's unfortunate assertion that science is ethically 'neutral'. Science is both an end and a method. It is ethically ambiguous, but this does not make it 'neutral'. It can be accepted that the purpose of science is the search for truth and, for all it matters, that truth is ethically neutral: although what the meaning or significance of such a statement is, is obscure. It probably means that facts have nothing to do with ethics. What cannot, without more debate, be accepted is that the means of ascertaining the truth are ethically or morally neutral.[47] Science, like other methods of thinking, can be both prescriptive as well as descriptive. As an imperative, science (and its derivative, technology) says that even if the utility of an experiment is not apparent, it should be proceeded with because the utility might appear later. A variant of the same is that even if the experiment appears to conflict with some ethical statement, as for example in some types of investigation of the embryo, the possibility of a later utility justifies the current procedures. The example of the pioneers of science in challenging the accepted values of their time is held out as validation of current experimental design. (At this point it is as well to offer a caveat. There are times, and this is one of them, when a commentator on human thinking is compelled by the object of his study to relate as received reason that which lacks reason.) The challenge of those pioneers to the use of law to regulate investigation is used to show that any such limitation is an abuse of power and an obstacle to progress.

Medicine, in part, adopts the aims and methods of the natural sciences: it seeks to understand physical processes; and, it insists upon proper experimental design, validity of observation and method, correct logic and verifiable conclusions. They share something of the same motivational force. In this sense medicine is a science. But this sense does not relate the science (which so described is no more than a branch of biology) to any of the purposes of medicine, for example, the restoration of health. However, it does no violence to language to add to this meaning, the application of the science to aid cure by way of using the 'laws' so discovered. Applied science is commonly, though not necessarily, based upon a technology of one sort or another (for example, the chlorination of the nation's water supplies or more accurate diagnosis through chemical analysis of tissue). In this additional sense, medicine is still properly regarded as 'scientific'. But medicine, I argue, has also a more fundamental purpose than cure. Simply put, it is no less than a part of man's endeavour to combat brute nature. Only in so far as it uses the methods of applied science in the pursuit of this objective, medicine is scientific.

The distinctions between the scientific mode of medicine and the participatory or classical modes do not lie in such considerations. In so far as medicine defines the area of nature it seeks to control, it is not applying science as a method. In the definition of its own goals, it must, like other sciences, have recourse to an ascientific philosophy. It follows that, like other sciences, scientific medicine can never be complete. One difference between the modes of medicine lies in what it is that is to be cured. Is it the disease or the patient or both? In so far as it is proper to regard the disease as an entity of its own, as something apart from the patient, the essential difference between the application of technology to destroy it and the application of technologies in other fields of endeavour is diminished. On the other hand, in so far as the disease is not an independent 'it',[48] but is necessarily connected with the patient, then medicine is not merely an applied natural science.[49] On such a basis, 'patient', 'disease', 'cure' are not separate although related concepts: they are symptoms of one whole. The competent practitioner has no choice but to relate to that whole. Where they are separated, the psychological involvement of the practitioner may vary between them; where they are one it cannot.

One way of expressing the problem is, adopting the Cartesian distinction of mind and body, to ask how far medicine is only concerned with the body. As the Black Report said:[50]

> This philosophy of the body conceived as a machine and the body controlled as a machine provided an impetus for scientific experiment and a stream of practical outcomes which for an increasing proportion of the population seemed to validate a mechanistic perspective.
>
> There can be no doubt about the success with which such an 'engineering' approach has been applied.

But this success does not by itself 'prove' the ultimate truth of Descartes' hypothesis; the fact that a hypothesis works some of the time, and in some circumstances, does not make it 'true'.[51] On the basis of the validity of the distinction, it is often held that medicine is a science and, with Russell, that it is ethically neutral. If this were so, there would be no special need to examine its regulation except at the level of unimpeded technical exposition. Once more it is important to note the lack of reason. Even assuming that pure sciences are in some sense neutral, it does not follow that the application of their derivative technologies is. A knowledge of poisons is one thing; to poison is another.

It is not however necessary for those who hold the scientific view of medicine, to deny that doctors do have to make ethical decisions. It can be argued that the ethical realm is external to medicine. Further, this thinking can be expanded to say that all the normative systems which regulate medicine are independently validated: they can only be examined in relation to medicine as applied versions of their own more general discourses. The approach of such 'medical positivists' – Pellegrino and Thomasma call them 'medical reductionists' – confines the role of the doctor *qua* doctor to the technician. As such it finds a way to assert a role for others in fixing the objectives of these technicians.

In this book I am not so much concerned with whether medicine is a value-free science as whether such a science is possible. I am concerned in particular, on the basis that it is not value-free, with what are the modes of regulation that express its values. I have already noted that central to the idea of western medicine is the clinic. At once further dimensions are added. Medicine is not only about science or technology but also about an interaction between human beings in a particular setting. It is therefore necessary to observe the ways in which these added dimensions correct and amplify the idea of medicine as a science.

Hippocratic medicine

Very largely I have assumed that the school of medicine which is dominant in modern western, or at least British, practice is that derived from the classical Greek physician, Hippocrates.[52] One may speculate why the influence of these teachings should have survived[53] and indeed, to justify this assumption it is necessary for me to sketch some of their history. I do so later: there is a strangeness in applying an historical continuity over so long a time. However, I do not believe I have stretched the evidence in accepting the proposition.[54]

It is convenient here to anticipate one reason for the need to look at the Hippocratic corpus: at the decisive point in the organization of medicine (in the early sixteenth century) the men who were involved were overtly inspired by that school. For the moment however it is important to note that it is from it that the following modern ideas can be traced (or, if the continuity is not accepted, the following are held in common with it):[55]

(1) The idea that medical science can be developed by observation at the bedside. Medicine could be the object of empirical study rather than merely thought about, that there were natural rather than supernatural causes of disease, and that the way forward was to systematize the available knowledge and collect more.

(2) The ideas:[56]

> Life is short and the Art long; the occasion fleeting; experience fallacious and judgement difficult. The physician must not only be prepared to do what is right himself, but also to make the patient, the attendants and the externals co-operate

and the physician is the servant of his art.[57] These are central parts of the professional manifesto. They show themselves in regard to the management of the particular sick patient. Thus Hughes has suggested:[58] 'The professional mind ... appears as a perversion of the common sense of what is urgent and what less urgent' and:[59] 'to the layman the technique of an occupation should be pure instrument, pure means to an end, while to the people who practice it, every occupation tends to become an art'. The manifesto also shows itself in the physician's relations with related professions.[60]

(3) The Hippocratic Oath[61] (which is set out as Appendix to this book). Today the Oath as such is rarely sworn but much of its ideology still rules. The ideas derived from it are:[62]

(4) The Oath is sworn by symbolic gods – 'Apollo, the Physician, Aesculapius, Hygeia and Panacea'. Although essentially pagan in that it rests on several gods, the school suggests a compromise or balance between competing but discrete strategies. Apollo, among his other attributes, was the god of medicine and, in mythology, the father of Pythagoras. Aesculapius was a Greek doctor (in fact or myth) who practised on the basis of self-help.[63] In his teachings therefore there is much of what I shall call the 'radical critique of medicine'. Hygeia was goddess of cleanliness and may be taken as an early affirmation of the importance of public health. Panacea is more difficult to attribute but may be taken to be the forerunner of modern alternative medicine.

(5) Teachers are as parents and other practitioners are as brothers. Implicit in this, but of some importance to general Pythagorean teaching was the idea of community of property. It would seem that now confined to the professional sphere it includes both tangible and intellectual property. Herein in part lie the seeds of the links with the teacher-researcher of the university and with the brotherhood characteristic not only of medicine but also generally of professions in contradistinction to trades.

(6) The learning is confined not to an individual practitioner but to a closed circle. Modern 'democratic egalitarianism' and commercialism has sought to obscure the import of this ideal but it still looms large. If the objects (that is, the client/patient) of the profession can understand all, the professional is reduced to an artisan, a trader; if only the practitioner can understand, he is a professional.

(7) The injunction to professional confidence. It is wider than information required in the course of treatment; it recognizes and exploits the fact that professionals are entrusted with personal information as general confidants.

(8) The purpose of the practice is the healing of the sick and the

alleviation of suffering. Exploitation is forbidden. There are consequences in relation to the idea of professional altruism and the role of the market.

And (9) The injunction on the Hippocratic physician not 'to cut for stone' but to withdraw in favour of those who did this kind of work. It is best interpreted as a prohibition, in particular, against lithotomy rather than surgery generally[64] and, more widely against procedures where the risks outweigh the possible benefits to the individual patient. After all, as we shall see, a successful part of the Hippocratic method was the use of the facilities we now associate with the health resort – a strict regime of diet, exercise, rest, and bathing; that is, it was non-interventionist. Seen in this light this prohibition reinforces professional altruism and enjoins the practitioner from doing things beyond his competence. It is secular in that it is not directed to a theological objective. It rejects procedures aimed at enhancing the reputation of the practitioner unless they are for the benefit of the patient.

The Hippocratic ideal is therefore broad enough to encompass ideas of experimental science, patient-centred but doctor-directed medicine, a guild approach to practice and knowledge, and in large measure each of the modern approaches to health care. The ideal is not broad enough to include other ways of organizing activity about disease. In particular, it cannot encompass either a patient- or society-dominated approach or even an equal partnership. It is indeed true as Pellegrino and Thomasma say that 'the patient has a richer, more personal knowledge of the disorder'[65] than the doctor. But Hippocratic medicine *qua* medicine is not directly concerned with the patient's method or extent of gaining knowledge of the disorder. As an activity once commenced, it is concerned with the doctor's knowledge gained as it were at the bedside in the clinic.

The Hippocratic corpus appears to be a mixture of philosophies and the Oath in particular appears to have come from Pythagoras.[66] The elements of his ideas which have dominated western medicine for more than two millennia include not only asceticism, strict sexual mores, the keeping of confidences, and the relationship of father-teacher to son-student, but also mysticism, passionate sympathetic contemplation, ecstatic revelation in understanding Nature, and a consequent reluctance fully to accept the authority of other religions.[67] The link between these factors shows itself in his mathematics. Pythagoras began with a reality based in numbers. His most famous achievement, known to generations of schoolchildren, was to show that, in a right-angled triangle, the square on the hypotenuse is the sum of the squares on the other two sides. This led to the discovery of 'incommensurables'; numbers which have no common measure except unity. Russell explains:[68]

> Let us suppose each side is an inch long; then how long is the hypotenuse? Let us suppose its length is m/n inches. Then m^2/n^2 = 2. If m and n have a common factor, divide it out, then either m or n must be odd. Now $m^2 = 2n^2$, therefore m^2 is even, therefore m is even, therefore n is odd. Suppose m = 2p. Then $4p^2 = 2n^2$, therefore $n^2 = 2p^2$ and therefore n is even, *contra hyp*.

It followed that 'whatever unit of length we may adopt, there are lengths which bear no exact numerical relation to the unit'. For Pythagoras, and also for many of those who since his day have used some part of his teaching, the real world of arithmetic was not reflected in the ideal world of geometry. Hence there could be a search for an ideal, separate from, but informed by, the real. Thus mysticism, contemplation and understanding Nature are linked.

The Shorter Oxford English Dictionary defines 'mysticism' as 'belief in the possibility of union with the Divine by means of ecstatic contemplation'. Weber argued[69] that in some types of psycho-physical processes, 'action which is meaningful and so understandable is not to be found at all, in others the meaning can only be understood by specialists'. He used the term mysticism where there were 'experiences which cannot be adequately expressed in words' and which 'are not fully understandable by those not attuned to them'. This mysticism is linked to another aspect of the Pythagorean nature of medical practice. By 1772, Gregory was urging[70] medicine as 'a liberal profession whose object is the life and health of the human species, a profession to be exercised by gentlemen of honour and ingenuous manners'. Later I shall note the way in which gentlemanly honour and manners became generally attainable virtues. But as regards medicine the idea of the gentleman embraces this but is also more specific. It rests in the Oath which, as I have said, is Pythagorean. But also within that philosophy (or cult) is the idea that contemplation is the highest activity of man.[71] It is thus, as I shall show, directly linked to the idea of the gentleman.

In so far as there is any truth in this it is less than fully accurate to regard the satisfaction or motivation of the doctor as being confined to commerce. Of course not all doctors share or act out the purpose of the ideal. Whether the expression of the (unceasing) pursuit of ultimate values is regarded as having a connection with a Divinity, it does not seem unreasonable to regard it as a mysticism. Further, even where the Divinity is recognized, its character as I shall show has never been wholly dictated by ecclesiastical authority. It is accordingly more appropriate to use the term 'mystical' than 'religious' to describe it. Today the mysticism of medicine is twofold. It maintains the elements of gentlemanly behaviour and it is centred on the clinic and the body which is exposed there. For this reason, in their different ways, Parsons and Foucault reflect ancient beliefs in focusing their analysis on the doctor–patient relationship and the clinic where they meet.

3

Theories of medicine

Participatory and classical medicine

Thus far I have discussed some of the insights of Parsons and of Foucault which are relevant to the doctor and patient relationship but which are merely illustrative of other ideas in their works. It remains to examine a philosophical construct based on the facts of that duality. In considering what may be regarded as medicine's moment of truth, I turn to Pellegrino and Thomasma. Unlike both Parsons and Foucault, they are wholly concerned with medicine. Because it is so full and because it is defined by a perception of what is, I relate their reasoning at some length. It should be said that I see in their work an ambiguity and it is this which lets me use it as explanatory of both participatory and classical theories of medicine. The ambiguity is caused by the fact that on the one hand Pellegrino and Thomasma are purposeful. They seek to show that medicine and philosophy ought to learn from each other. On the other hand they are descriptive. Thus they say:[1]

a philosophy of medicine is called for by our cultural crisis. But ... a philosophy of medicine divorced from the realities of theory and practice in medicine would be as useless to culture as it would be emaciating to both philosophy and medicine.

Later they argue:[2]

Those who take the trouble to teach and function at the bedside emerge with a deepened respect for the complexities of the physician's moral choices. But ethicists without these insights have generated an unfortunate backlash which hinders precisely the critical engagement of the moral issues in clinical decisions contemporary medicine needs.

Addressing what I have asserted is a critical question – whether the scientific theory of medicine is sufficient – they argue,[3] 'medicine itself represents a tension between therapeutic aims and explanatory theory' but,[4] 'medicine, even as science must encompass the special complexities of *man as subject* interacting with *man as object* ... medicine *qua* medicine cannot deal with general scientific laws as such, but must locate them in a time, place, and person'. So far the argument appears to say that medicine is scientific, but crucially to Pellegrino and Thomasma:[5] 'Medical science ... becomes medicine only when it is modulated and constrained in unique ways by the humanity of physician and patient'.

In an endeavour to understand medicine, they seek a philosophical method in Aristotle's distinction of *praxis* and *theoria*.[6] '[A] philosophy of medicine must be an ontology of practice, a search for meaning in the practice of medicine, and specific applications of the results of this search.' (It may be added that in this book I seek the specific modes and forms of the imperative norms disclosed by this search.) They say that theory is not sufficient because account must be taken of 'the world of the street'.[7] Their starting point, then, is 'the possibility of a cure in the real world of practice'.[8] This reality is conditioned by the value factors of the 'lifeworld', and it corrects theoretical postulates of practice; the practical world is seen to be the 'logically prior setting in which and out of which ideas are born'. It is to be noted that since tertiary care involves sophisticated technology its use is more likely to give society 'pleasure' than the everyday use of primary or secondary care; later I shall assess a contrast made by Hirschman between 'pleasure' and 'comfort'.

Thus armed with a method, Pellegrino and Thomasma ask 'What is Medicine?' Its main concepts are health and disease. Like Parsons and many of the other sociologists of medicine, they recognize that these are both biologically and culturally defined. They also follow them as regarding the 'clinical interaction'[9] as the unifying factor in medicine as a discipline. As a relationship it is necessarily imbalanced: responsibilities arise[10] 'from an ethic of survival in a complex and specialized society'. Ominously for those whose concern is only with legal regulation:[11]

Mutual responsibility is an essential mode of the clinical relationship because it involves a deeper human and moral obligation than adherence to rules, guidelines, or [codes of conduct].

The relationship is cemented by trust born of the physician's curative intent and the comparatively, in everyday life, rare emotions of tension, fear, anxiety, resignation, and patience. They cite Seneca on the patient's responsibility:[12]

> Why then, are we so much indebted to these men [physicians and teachers]? Not because what they have sold us is worth more than what we paid for it, but because they have contributed something to us personally.

Medicine is thus seen to be an inter-human event of mutual consent, a craftsmanship of healing within the imbalanced relationship, and a didactic relationship to eliminate physical suffering. Central, then, to the idea of medicine, is 'the body'. This however is more complex than the Cartesian duality of body and soul. It includes[13] the creation and presentation in symbols of that experience of our body which cannot be objectified, its creation and presentation, as well as the organization of a field of perception on a preconscious level.

They go on to argue[14] that the disease can then become a theoretical concept which can be regarded as apart from the patient, as an 'it'. 'Yet even this objectification cannot hide the fact that disease is a conceptualization of a disorganization of a patient's whole world, with implications for the patient's self-image and position as a person.' They follow Ruthschuh[15] in saying:

> The ill person enters three relations – one to the self, another to the physician, and still another to society and environment – all of which are governed by need for the help. The physician also enters three relations – one of responsibility to the sick person, another to the disease (what is the cause? what to do?), and another to society. Society is also involved with individual good for the patient, the common good, and a relationship of aid, prevention, and research on the causes and effects of disease.

This analysis re-enforces Parsons' ideas of disease as a social dysfunction. That was an attempt to answer the question 'why medicine?' Pellegrino and Thomasma take the argument a stage further. They seek to understand[16] 'how theoretical knowledge can be applied to concrete, individual body-persons with therapeutic results'. In part, the answer lies in scientific knowledge of the necessary connections between symptoms and disease and in part, following Plato's proto-love between physician and patient and Aristotle's rhetoric,[17] it is 'a cognitive art which must concretize and individualize its knowledge'.[18] It is an art similar to teaching and law in being directed to the person and unlike engineering which is directed to techniques. It is not a fine art which is directed to the aesthetic.

But what are therapeutic results? Pellegrino and Thomasma cite Canguilhem:[19]

> It is life itself, and not medical judgement, which makes the biological normal a concept of value and not a concept of statistical reality.... Those who themselves tried most vigorously to give 'normal' only the value of a fact have simply valorized the fact of their need for a limited meaning.

Thus the clue to establishing the normal in medicine[20] 'derives from both the realm of scientific models of disease and the life of patients in their social milieu'. In this context, then, they discuss the scientific link to the individual. It implies the causal agents of disease are real; there is a capacity to objectify ourselves, and that which is objectified is not unique; but also, the more specific medicine becomes, the more the uniqueness of the body becomes important. It follows,[21] clinical judgement must be a complex process of perceiving individual uniqueness in the midst of common objectivities. This enables a distinction to be made between primary, secondary, and tertiary care: as active bodily engagement is diminished, so too is the self. Consequently, in tertiary care the body is treated more as an object because the self is diminished or even threatened. Whereas, at the other extreme, in primary care the self is relatively more engaged. It is to be observed that this connection between the 'lifeworld', the individual, and tertiary care can thus be seen to alter the doctor–patient relationship. It suffices here to say that it illumines a result which commentators have not doubted but have been unable to explain: how it is that, in order to save life, the doctor can legally impose treatment without any consent.[22]

Pellegrino and Thomasma say:[23]

> The ... threefold aspect of clinical judgement – diagnosis, prognosis, and therapy – depends upon reference to the body.... Clinical judgement is governed by therapeutic necessity because the medical event is constituted by a need for physical help, health being one of the foundational needs of man. Therapeutic necessity is the ground of the legal and moral nature of clinical interaction.... But therapy cannot be viewed as scientifically predictable and secure. And because the values of patients and

society enter into all stages of the clinical interaction, therapy is inherently value-laden.

They quote Cassirer:[24]

It would be a naïve sort of dogmatism to assume that there exists an absolute reality of things which is the same for all living beings. Reality is not a unique and homogeneous thing; it is immensely diversified, having as many different schemes and patterns as there are different organisms.

Nevertheless,[25] '[t]he condition of possibility of cure ... is that bodies organize themselves in a common manner, although the extent and degree varies'. Despite the shared world of real objects and a commonality of language, there is 'an insight into concrete singulars' depending on compassion 'which might be described as a pre-articulated shared awareness of bodies regarding the human condition' conveyed by the body to other bodies without necessarily using intervening language. They conclude that medical morality can be derived from the medical act rather than 'older ethical theories or in cultural relativism'.

In their analysis, they go on to look at the nature and scope of clinical decisions. Before considering this it is convenient to summarize what they say about the moral basis of medicine. As I have indicated they seek to locate it in the act of medicine and not in some externality. They reject also the confusion that the achievements of technology have caused between what can be done and what should be done. For Pellegrino and Thomasma it does not matter whether science is value-free because medicine, unlike any science, is based on[26] 'a relationship of healing promoted by need, which works in, with, and through the body'. There is therefore no such thing as value-free medicine. It is bound by the relationship of healing. On this basis, medical ethics are not merely applied ethics.[27]

Medicine involves values in three ways:[28] it combines knowledge and skill about healing; its theory is a structure of principles about practice; and, it is intrinsically linked to human purposes. They contend that it is possible to construct axioms out of the same source as medicine – the ontological basis of medicine – and by relating them to medicine, arrive at medical ethics. Thus, leaving aside what they say about the patient's corresponding moral duties, the first axiom is based on the foundational good of health. It is: that the doctor should 'help or at least do no harm'.[29]

Secondly, that individuals have an intrinsic value leads to the axiom that 'Care must be taken for the susceptible individual'. This implies[30] that care for individual precedes the physician's attention to the common good. Being based upon the living body in need, the axiom moves beyond comradeship, contract, or legal or cultural expectations. The third axiom they deduce is that[31] 'the common good as it affects medicine should not clash with the common structures of living bodies'.

Curious as it may seem to lawyers, Pellegrino and Thomasma state that these axioms are descriptive and not prescriptive. They only become prescriptive when health becomes a primary good. As they say,[32] in ethics and morality, the basic opposition more often than not arises between two apparent but mutually exclusive goods than between good and evil. One of the principal problems is the identifying of values and placing them in an order of priority. Health is a foundational good, but not the only one; and it is open to value-laden cultural interpretation.

They argue:[33] that it is the 'special dimension of anguish in illness' based upon the fact that[34] it is the perception of an altered state of existence (which may or may not be associated with demonstrable pathology) which distinguishes healing from other relationships involving inequality of knowledge and skill. In what I call the classical theory the physician shoulders this anguish.[35] This explains why professionals are not content to do their best with available tools; why they search for better; and why in times of economic recession they complain about the lack of resources to do the job they think they ought to do. I would argue that it is this at least as much as the cynical suggestion[36] that physicians use more sophisticated services because they have a higher financial yield.

Pellegrino and Thomasma say:[37]

> Without denying the possible analogy with, let us say, the lawyer–client relationship, it would be difficult to argue that the degree of injury to our humanity and the kind of injury we suffer in litigation are identical in their existential consequences to being ill.

They are right, but not always. As trial lawyers know, litigation is sometimes the illness and sometimes the therapy.

The physician as a member of a profession has professed that its members have special knowledge and skills, which they will use in the patient's interest and not their own. That is the act of profession. It is a promise. Common education, standards, and ethics are accidental to it. The central act of medicine is therefore the act leading to its end, the right healing action for a particular patient. Departing from the rigour of their analysis and betraying the cultural bias of North America with its emphasis on the individual, they suggest:[38]

> A patient in need who consults a physician wants to know what *is* wrong, what *can* be done about it, and what *should* be done about it ... The patient's moral agency is at risk, and a special obligation of the act of profession is to protect that moral agency while treating the patient.

This is all possibly so, but not necessarily. The fact that values of physician and patient may differ does not mean that in the physicians' act of profession, in their promise, they have not said other than they will help only on their terms. It is only on certain cultural views that the individual rather than the doctor or society is allowed to define what is for the individual's good. It is here therefore that the participatory and classical theories of medicine part. In the classical theory, the moral agency of the patient is suspended for the duration of the relationship, although at least in non-serious illness, he can also judge if and when to end it. In serious illness, where the living body is confined or threatened, as we have seen, even Pellegrino and Thomasma concede that that agency is diminished and the physician becomes paramount.

In this connection Pellegrino and Thomasma discuss the line of 'codes of ethics' from Hippocrates to the current one of the American Medical Association.[39] I quote them at some length:[40]

> That ethos, which is still the dominant influence on how physicians see themselves, is that of the benign, authoritarian, dedicated, and competent craftsman who acts in the interest of his patient out of motives as practical as a good reputation and as lofty as love of mankind. The transaction is, with minor exceptions however, unilateral. It centers in what the physician does for the patient, who is in the main a passive recipient, one who cannot penetrate the mysteries of what is happening to him, and whose illness would be adversely affected if he knew the truth about his condition. There is no sense of accountability to the patient, only to the physician's own conscience; no opportunity for valid consent; no sense of responsibilities to society or to other health professions; no sense of the corporate obligation of the profession for quality of care, accessibility, and the like; and

no sense of the obligation of the patient, as member of the human race ... to participate in medical work which may benefit only future generations.

If, in this, a more modest, a secondary, role for the patient is substituted for their hyberbolical 'no's', a more accurate description of the ethos engendered by the classical theory emerges. It can be conceded that it is an ethos and not an ethical theory. Pellegrino and Thomasma do not see it, but such a theory is, with the points of departure I have noted, provided elsewhere in their own analysis.

The insights opened by their work do not, however, stop here. If the central act of medicine is the act of profession, it becomes necessary to examine the way in which the promise can be and is fulfilled. In terms reminiscent of Parsons, they say,[41] usually the relationship begins when the patient consults the physician because an event has occurred which exceeds the patient's threshold of tolerance. Each of them (both patient and physician), the classical theory would argue sequentially, brings a series of (sometimes prior determined) values to the relationship. They say, espousing the participatory theory again in terms which repeat its point of departure from the classical theory:[42]

> It is important to interject here that the term 'patient' does not necessarily imply a passive restoration in which the physician is the sole agent. The patient ideally also participates in the restoration. He or she is seen as bearing a burden of illness which requires some action or decision mutually arrived at for cure to take place. The patient can yield this moral agency to the physician only by direct mandate.

The imposition of an ideal as an account of the real based upon 'the world of the street' is not appropriate. Nor is it clear what they mean by 'direct mandate'. It is possible to argue from within the classical theory that the mandate is given by the patient entrusting himself to the physician's care, and so long as he maintains that 'entrusting' the physician is mandated.

To return to Pellegrino and Thomasma's analysis, they suggest, as we have seen, that clinical judgement consists of three questions: What can be wrong? What can be done? What should be done for this patient? In their discussion they fail expressly, although perhaps they succeed within the interstices of their answers to the first two questions, to articulate a fourth question:

What will happen? Despite this, their description of clinical judgement is invaluable in explaining the various types of reasoning adopted by the doctor in his work. As regards 'what can be wrong' they argue that:[43] 'this part of the process most closely fits the scientific paradigm and under ideal conditions can yield a diagnostic conclusion with a high degree of certitude'; but that, since it is based on probabilistic logic and medicine is individualized,[44] 'the diagnostic conclusions are still open to question'. They say that the establishment of a working or 'differential' diagnosis is more akin to a dialectic than to a scientific hypothesis. Turning to 'what can be done', they say[45] that, particularly where the therapeutic manoeuvres are not radical or where a specific treatment does not demonstrably alter the natural history of the disease, the scientific element of decision is even more reduced.

The last question, 'what should be done', is also the end for medicine. They argue:[46] 'Scientific, personal, and professional values intersect each other ... the categories of *must not, must, should,* and *may* can all shift, depending upon myriad factors in the patient's life situation'. Thus informed, they ask whether medicine is a science, art, or virtue, and conclude it is all three.[47] Of science, it has deductive, inductive and retroductive inference originated by hypothesis. Of art, it has craftsmanship. Of art and virtue it has 'the bedside manner, "Aesculapian power"'.

Having determined the essence of clinical judgement they are in a position to examine the discretionary space in which it operates. Importantly for legal policy-makers, they insist:[48] 'If medicine cannot entirely be classed as a science, then its mode of reasoning cannot be completely scrutinized and controlled through institutional and political policy'. Because the ends of medicine are fixed by its own internal discourse, and are informed by insights obtained at the bedside in the clinic (which I categorized earlier as a mysticism) those external to it, whether in the health care bureaucracy or the legislature or wherever, cannot also define them without taking away medicine's unifying essential characteristic. Indeed in some degree this is true of the sciences, both natural and social, but they lack the extent of medicine's unity. External regulation can therefore more easily be imposed on them.

The classical theory of medicine goes the one stage further and says that since this is true, and since also external control cannot be complete, being a patient is merely to produce the conditions required for the doctor to exercise his medicine rather than necessarily to take part in the act of medicine: medicine's mode of reasoning cannot be completely scrutinized or controlled by a mutuality in the relationship. The concept of discretionary space is therefore of even more use in defining the scope for the operation of the classical theory than it is for Pellegrino and Thomasma's participatory theory.

They say that the more society has a homogeneous value system, the wider can be the discretionary space accorded to the physician. Thus in pre-Hippocratic societies the medicine-man could intervene with nature on behalf of society as well as the individual. It was the Hippocratic invention of the freedom from magico-religious constraints which privatized medicine and led to the physician becoming the benign, paternalistic figure retaining his hieratic and rational capabilities. In the modern age the discretionary space is being narrowed by a variety of forces:[49] the democratic ideal has challenged the claims of any group to special privileges; health takes a lot of resources; there is awareness of abuse of power, economic insensitivity, and over-zealous pursuit of self-interest; there has been a rise in the use of 'rational' legal forms and in pluralistic and relativistic value systems; value and technical decisions have become confused; and, medical imperialism has expanded beyond disease to many aspects of life.

These forces, they say, are having radical effects on physician relationships. Thus[50] the law is challenging the sacred – the mystical – character of medicine; the emergence of team medicine is crowding the professional space; the complexity of the modern hospital is bringing in the exercise of legal, moral, and social responsibility of lay managers; and the physician is in part, providing as a quasi-public utility, a technical expert for policy decisions.

Be this as it may, it is useful here to re-emphasize the main point of departure between the participatory and classical theories. It is that the classical theory doubts the idea that patients want, or can reasonably be allowed, to fulfil any expectation that they will be primary agents in the treatment. One is reminded that the Hippocratic doctor is also a Pythagorean gentleman with a patrician's sense of superiority. Not only chronologically, the classical theory pre-dates Kant's Categorical Imperative and is not informed by it. The participatory theory in turn doubts the inherent paternalism of the classical. It is precisely this point of departure which I argue takes it into the realm of 'ought'. If this part of my argument is not accepted, then the classical theory is seen as irrational. Paternalistic or irrational (indeed possibly, both) as it may be, I shall also argue that it is the classical theory which has been the dominating influence on the regulation of medicine.

Rival health-based theories

The previous section showed that 'the central act of medicine' can be seen as the 'act leading to its end, the right healing action for a particular patient'. Such a view is based on clinical interaction. In his *The Role of Medicine: Dream, Mirage or Nemesis*[51] Thomas McKeown provides a radically different starting point for medical practice. It is, he says:[52] 'To assist us to come safely into the world and comfortably out of it, and during life to protect the well and care for the sick and disabled'. He regards the definition of 'health' in WHO's Constitution – 'a state of complete physical, mental, and social well-being and not merely the absence of disease or infirmity' – as too broad. It requires subjective evaluation and, because of its emphasis on 'well-being',[53] 'the concept goes far beyond the responsibilities of health services'. For McKeown 'the task of medicine is not to create happiness, but so far as possible to remove a major source of unhappiness, that which results from illness and early death'.

In discussing the causative factors of these sources of unhappiness, McKeown comes to the conclusion that the reduction in mortality and morbidity over the last three hundred years has been influenced hardly at all by clinical medicine.[54] All the major diseases, including those which killed, showed steep declines before therapeutic measures were taken.[55] Thus leprosy in Europe was virtually extinct by the early or middle fifteenth century and bubonic plague at the middle of the seventeenth. The causes for this included the achievement of[56] 'a state of relative equilibrium' between microbes and the 'ever-varying state of the immunological constitution of the herd'. On this basis 'the trend of mortality from infectious diseases was essentially independent of both medical intervention and the vast economic and social developments of the past three centuries'.

McKeown argues that where a population is undernourished disease is more likely both to occur and to spread. As regards the comparatively affluent West, he says:[57] 'if a choice must be made, free school meals are more important for the health of poor children than immunization programmes, and both are more effective than hospital beds'. It has been changes in the environment which have lowered death rates. He concedes that in England, the changes were introduced as health measures and that a few doctors were involved in establishing the medical arguments for public health legislation. However, the supposed causes were largely mistaken and the local government authorities which carried out the scheme called not only on the professional help of district medical officers of health but also on the expertise of others, including civil engineers. The third major determinant for health, says McKeown, is behaviour, of which in the past the most influential change has been in reproductive habits:[58] 'The decline of the birth-rate was very significant, since it ensured that the improvement in health brought about by other means was not reversed by rising numbers.'

This analysis leads McKeown to the conclusion that the determinants of health are nutritional, environmental, behavioural, and finally, and least, clinical. He says:[59] 'It is not easy for doctors to accept that medicine is not vitally concerned with the major determinants of health'. On the basis of this analysis he seeks to find a new role for doctors. He suggests that there is an essential place in environmental planning for those concerned with disease. He implies that they should also have a role in behavioural planning. Since, he says, one of the major causes of disease in modern society is smoking, doctors should seek as far as possible to restrict the habit. Generalizing, he says that the habit starts before people are old enough to choose and that, since it is a drug of addiction, when they are old enough they are not able to. Apparently not noticing the insertion of his own values he says that smoking does not improve the quality of life. Mackenzie, for example, confessing that his knowledge of the cigarette was limited, argued that[60], 'tolerance is one of the virtues that tobacco inculcates' and that[61] 'It is certainly true that the great majority of men of letters have been smokers, whether they were poets or dramatists, philosophers or historians, essayists or novelists'. And more generally Elias has discussed the shifting of taboos.[62] In particular, and to put his argument briefly, he says that the tendency is that instinctual gratification should more and more be done in private, and if not in private at least be socially restrained. The explanation for the change is often based in health, but the reason would seem to be more aesthetic. To all of which I add that the 'private' has expanded its scope so that gratification can be less and less a source of socially displayed joy. Elias's point gives an alternative, and more satisfactory, reason for the current attacks on social smoking.

McKeown's conception of the role of the doctor is traditional enough for him to include the clinic. But even here, however, he departs from orthodoxy. He cites McDermott:[63] 'Today's often repeated cliché that what the physician does has relatively little influence on health is more correctly stated that what the physician does has relatively little influence on those indicators of health that are largely irrelevant to what he does'. And,

> the great difference between measuring quality in the public health system, in which it can be reckoned by changes in disease pattern, and in the personal – encounter – physician system, in which it is a matter of the appropriateness of a human act: so-called 'outcome' results are obtainable in the former, but as a practical matter are seldom helpful in the latter.

McKeown comments:[64]

> When clinical procedures are not evaluated scientifically, they are evaluated intuitively; each practitioner makes up his own mind about the usefulness of, say, radical mastectomy, tonsillectomy, cervical cytology and prolonged rest after myocardial infarction. The benefits of intervention and the associated technology are frequently overestimated, and this may result in the neglect of patients after the acute phase of illness, or of those (such as the subnormal) who provide no scope for active measures.

McKeown thus seeks a greater emphasis on the non-acute patient. The tasks he sets the clinician are:[65] reassurance; treatment of an acute emergency; cure of conditions (other than acute) which threaten the duration or quality of life; and, care and comfort. He argues that the problem with the clinician is that much of his emphasis is on acute emergency. The reason is that his teaching and his teachers have been imbued with the mechanistic aetiology of disease. He points out that the most successful medicine-men today are the accident surgeons, the dentists, and the obstetricians: all of whom deal[66] 'mainly with healthy people'.

Earlier I looked at the Parsonean model of medical practice. Two themes were seen to run through it: that it is disease-related and that there is a reciprocity in the relationship between doctor and patient. McKeown's analysis accepts the first but not the second of these. The reason for medicine's relation to disease is of considerable importance. In part, no doubt, it is concerned with both possibilities of cure and, as McKeown says, with prevention.

But, at this point, the explanation stops too short. As Parsons argues, it is in society's functional interest to minimize illness. Its instrument is medicine. It cannot be concluded from this that, on the one hand, society does everything it can to achieve this purpose; plainly it does not. It has other functional interests. Nor, on the other hand, can it be concluded that the minimization of illness is medicine's only purpose. Illness which threatens well-being or the existence of life is but one example of brute nature oppressing man both as an individual and in society. Medicine's contribution is to limit that oppression. Here lies the root of its power. It is this which gives rise to what Pellegrino and Thomasma call its 'discretionary space'. Within that space there is iatrocracy. And, as with any other system of government, it is simpler, although not always wiser, for those with power not to consult the governed.

So also when medicine is seen as opposing brute nature on behalf of society, a more ready explanation can be found for the order of priorities society allows it to have. Nature is more violent in the acute stages of illness;[67] it is administratively easier to control these stages by isolating them within the hospital. Further, where scientific medicine can control brute nature, medicine gives society hope. It is for this reason that society permits, and wants, medicine to devote extraordinary resources to dealing with extraordinary manifestations of illness. The resources, for example, committed to organ transplants are out of all proportion to any other benefit society gains. This argument is important not only as an explanation of resource allocation but also because it tends to redefine the purpose of medicine as being in something other than health. By redefining the purpose in this way, it offers a separation, if not a divorce, between medicine and health.

The second element in the Parsonean theory – the reciprocity – has been considered by Bloor and Horobin.[68] They argue that his ideal expects the impossible. The patient in his scheme is supposed only to seek medical advice when he is ill; that is, up to the point of seeking the advice, he is to be a fully rational (and informed) moral agent. Once in the doctor's hands he is expected to defer, to abandon, or suspend his agency. It is, they say, a 'double bind'. Parsons' position is however more justifiable if we add to it two limiting factors: first, the idea that it is the doctors, not the patients, who behave on the basis of medical theories; and, secondly we rid ourselves of an exaggerated view of the importance of medicine. On such a basis we can propose other ways in which doctors might behave (but we cannot be sure how these other ways would affect the totality of their work). Such a basis does not imply that patients must accept the application of doctors' theories, although it is more convenient for doctors if they do so. Bloor and Horobin's critique accepts medicine's own assessment of its external worth and criticizes its internal values. The limiting factors here reverse this view: they question medicine's own assessment of its contribution to society but accept its internal values.

Other versions of 'the radical critique'[69] not only begin with 'health' but also with the individual as the primary moral agent. Szasz says:[70]

> For millennia, men and women escaped from responsibility by theologizing morals. Now they escape from it by medicalizing morals. Then, if God approved a particular conduct, it was good; and if He disapproved it, it was bad. How did people know what God approved and disapproved? The Bible – that is to say, the biblical experts, called priests – told them so. Today, if Medicine approves a particular conduct, it is good; and if it disapproves it, it is bad. And how do people know what Medicine approves or disapproves? Medicine – that is to say, the medical experts, called physicians – tells them so.

These versions of the critique provide attacks not only on esoteric expertise in the clinic but also on optimism. Thus, although Szasz does not mention Erasmus, he says in terms which recall the latter's satire in *Praise of Folly*,[71] 'It is well known that all human affairs ... have two completely opposite faces':[72]

> Human life – that is, a life of consciousness and self-awareness – is unimaginable without suffering. Without pain and sorrow, there could be no pleasure and joy; just as without death, there could be no life, without illness, no health; without ugliness, no beauty.

Szasz goes on:[73]

> All our exertions – moral and medical, political and personal – are directed toward minimizing undesirable experiences and maximizing desirable ones.... What complicates it ... is the fact that many of the things we regard as desirable are opposed by, or can be secured only at the cost of, others that also we regard as desirable.... This is, quite simply, why the pursuit of relief from suffering, reasonable though it may seem, cannot be an unqualified personal or political goal. And if we make it such

a goal, it is certain to result in more, not less, suffering. In the past, the greatest unhappiness for the greatest number was thus created by precisely those political programs whose goal was the most radical relief of suffering for the greatest number of human beings.

So also Dubos argued:[74]

It is a dangerous error to believe that disease and suffering can be wiped out altogether by raising still further the standards of living, increasing our mastery of the environment, and developing new therapeutic procedures. The less pleasant reality is that, since the world is ever changing, each period and each type of civilization will continue to have its burden of diseases created by the unavoidable failure of biological and social adaptation to counter new environmental threats.

McKeown's view is that this thesis is not fully demonstrated as regards developments in the last three hundred years except that, for example, the trend to fewer and later pregnancies possibly has led to an increase in cancer of the breast.

Illich joins the polemical radical critique. He too is opposed to what he sees as medicine's false optimism.[75] In effect he argues:[76] that Hippocratic mystical medicine degrades the patient; that it does more harm than good; that it causes demands for its services and a socio-economic system which generates ill-health; and that it seriously diminishes the capacity of the individual to deal with his own health problems.

Kennedy[77] voices concern at the way society appears to allow doctors to give authority to, and specifically to give legal effect to, their views of health and sickness. He points to various examples of where the doctor's say so determines the status of the individual. Is pregnancy an illness? Does a doctor's opinion make any difference to whether a man is fit for work or whether homosexuality is an illness? Kennedy goes further in drawing attention to the way in which society, having let doctors legitimate findings of illness, also lets or requires them to use therapeutic measures to deal with problems that could (he says should) be dealt with by other means. Thus psychotropic drugs are used on a massive scale to deal with housing or domestic or employment or educational issues. Medicine is thus seen to support the socio-economic system.

This is a particular instance of the radical critique of professionalism. Generally, it stresses the impotence of clients, the control of clients by professionals, and the distortion involved in reconceiving issues in the discourse of a particular profession. Johnson, for example, defines[78] professionals as those who define both the needs of consumers and how those needs should be met. Cain has argued, regarding solicitors[79] (and much of her argument is applicable to doctors, particularly in primary care), that the role of the professional is as a translator of clients' problems into a language or a discourse which they create; that they therefore are conceptive idealologists. Implicitly applying this type of thinking, in a recent paper,[80] Kennedy attacks the English courts' reluctance to validate the patient's decision-making in the doctor–patient relationship. He argues that the need to recognize the importance of the patient 'flows from the Kantian imperative of respect for others'. He suggests a programme based upon aspects of the transatlantic doctrine of informed consent, which he says the courts could and should adopt.

To Berlinguer:[81]

> the present doctor–patient relationship ... is self-involved and exhausted at the individual level. At best, the doctor prescribes what the patient must do, personally and effectively, to fight against disease. But that disease may be the visual expression – at the personal level – of a phenomenon having a social impact. A doctor–patient relationship of a merely individual character ... fails to convey a signal to society or to serve as a springboard for changes in morbific social relations.

For example:[82]

> a chemical war has broken out and ravages continuously in polluted air, water, food, and working environment, i.e. the forced intoxications to which we are all exposed; other so-called 'voluntary' intoxications may be added as, in reality, they too are effects of being subjected to conditioning, pressures, sometimes too, compulsory behavior, and are called drug abuse, alcohol abuse, tobacco consumption, or drug addiction.

In all this these exponents of the radical critique are presenting a fundamental challenge to medicine and its regulation. Briefly, if McKeown is right, we ought to follow Berlinguer and include a health imperative at every level of social and economic planning. If Illich and Kennedy are right then not only should that imperative apply but also we should be wary of accepting the opinions of these medical experts. If, on the other hand, the proponents of the participatory or classical schools are more accurate in their description of what medicine is about, then the law has a lesser place in regulating the doctor; and the doctor a lesser place in regulating society. To put it another way, if the doctor is a limited specialist then he can be left to specialize within limited bounds. What is important about this in a description of the regulation as it is and not as it might be, is the way this debate affects the exposition and interpretation of the law: in this field, as in some others, it is easier to state what ought to be rather than what is. Partly because of this greater ease, the 'ought' helps to define the perception of the 'is'.

In *The Birth of the Clinic*, Foucault argues that up to the end of the eighteenth century:[83]

> medicine related much more to health than to normality . . . . To this extent, medical practice could accord an important place to regimen and diet . . . . This . . . involved the possibility of being one's own physician. Nineteenth-century medicine, on the other hand, was regulated more in accordance with normality than with health.

There can be no doubt about the modern attraction of 'being one's own physician'. The bewildering excesses of technological medicine functioning mainly in the limited sphere of acute secondary care are taking place in a consumer and individual based community. Even Parsons' model presupposes that the patient will seek help: unless and until he does, the physician is powerless.

Two of the problems facing the modern health care professions are 'self-medication' and the cult (or cults) of 'alternative medicine'. These terms are best regarded as parts of a continuum rather than a contrast to each other. They are distinguished by their orthodoxy or by how common they are. 'Self-medication' itself may be divided into (a) the use, for therapeutic purposes, of materials which have other purposes, and (b) the use of those which are only for health. In the first class there is a whisky toddy[84] for the common cold and in the second aspirin. Further, we may note that some substances change from one class to another. Thus tobacco won its initial popularity by reason of its suppo. ed therapeutic effects.[85] This benefit was proclaimed by Jean Nicot, French Ambassador to Portugal 1559–61, and via him tobacco became fashionable at the court of Louis XIII. The English smoked for both social and medicinal reasons. That it was not universally popular is shown by James I's authorship of *The Counterblast to Tobacco* in 1604. Part of the unpopularity was due to the King's dislike of Raleigh and part to problems associated with the apothecaries' claims to monopolies over the sale of medicinal herbs. Somewhat similar histories could be written of opium[86] and alcohol.[87]

Self-medication is itself largely regulated at the point of sale.[88] The modern chemist or pharmacist who is himself professionally registered deals in products whose sale is licensed. This dual method of control is supplemented, in certain cases, by auxiliary rules of law. For example, the Venereal Diseases Act (1917) and the Cancer Act (1939) prohibited the advertising or sale of remedies purporting to cure those diseases except under a doctor's prescription. (The control is further supplemented by rules of the Institute of Advertising, the Independent Broadcasting Authority, etc., prohibiting the promotion of certain products or controlling the manner of promotion of others.) It is probably true that there are more prescriptionless but therapeutic-intended contacts between pharmacists and customers than contacts between doctor and patient.

For reasons that are not entirely clear, the Anglo-American world has taken one response to the regulation of alternative medicine and the European mainland another. It suffices here to say that the term 'alternative medicine' is clear in its negative sense – it is alternative to the medicine of the medical profession. Positively, the term is ambiguous. It embraces a range of praxis and theory some of which is contradictory, some of which is compatible with orthodox western medicine. Stanway[89] argues that modern medicine is organized about a mechanistic – 'plumbing' – concept of the body. It ignores the 'mind, soul and the spirit'. Much of alternative medicine at the level of theory is devoted to this 'supersensible world'; and at the level of praxis, to regimen and diet.

In this way alternative medicine in particular presents orthodox medicine with a second and related fundamental challenge. It is both theoretical and practical. In both it joins the radical critique. It aids its theory by providing alternatives commonly heavily emphasizing self-help. In this there are more than shades of Illich, Kennedy, and Szasz. In restoring a role to regimen and diet there are more than shades of McKeown. However, in seeking to combat 'medical imperialism' it uses 'health imperatives' as its weapons. I argue, however, that man has to live his life under many normative regimes. Among them are: law, morality, ethics, aesthetics, instinct, emotion, habit, economics, science, biology, and medicine. His freedom comes of his choosing and judging between competing rules. When one of these systems, as here, is raised to a primacy, freedom is imperilled.

In some ways Szasz is right to say 'many of the things we regard as desirable are opposed by, or can be secured only at the cost of, others we also regard as desirable'. And he is right too to place this view in the context of medical imperatives and the volition of the free moral agent. Medicine is the science most immediate to our existence. Its imperatives govern more effectively than any police-state because our bodies are the informers.[90] Yet medicine is not merely applied biology. Medicine is more, and even if we make the facile (and even ridiculous) assumption that one day biology might be fully understood, we would still be faced with medicine as an interaction between humans. For this reason, among others, it is not foreseeably right to regard the doctor as merely an expert whose professional existence can be bought by the state, institutions, or individuals. It is necessary in this field, as in others, to draw a distinction between 'formal' and 'substantive' rationality. The formal rationality of medicine as defined by its own internal values is not to be confused with the substantive rationality of healing.

For the planner, legislator, doctor, and patient the potentiality of this confusion is increased by the expansion of biological and medical imperatives from the self-categorized and recognizably sick to the healthy. The confusion does not go away by denying that medicine has internal values nor by pointing to the element of lay control which has been imposed.[91] Later, when I seek an answer to the question of what is meant by saying that the practice of medicine is a profession and what is the internal form of regulation, I shall return to the point.

A caveat must be made. On some views, biomedicine can be all embracing.[92] Health can be accorded a higher priority than materialism or production – we eat to be healthy, we work in order to eat. Not only can the dictates of 'health' be seen to rule over our every conduct, but also its metaphors dominate large areas of language and hence thinking. Freud's link between things of the mind and medicine has greatly expanded the influence of health metaphors.[93] Childress[94] argues 'Metaphors highlight and hide features of the principal subject ... by their system of associated commonplaces ...' but 'A single metaphor may not structure the whole pattern of thought, experience, and action'.

And so also too, history, architecture, and politics, to name but three separate activities, can be reinterpreted in terms of 'health'.[95] Is it not possible to say that a distinction should be made between the basic health care structure of any society, constituted by the conditions of its delivery taken as whole, and the superstructure of laws, institutions, and ideas? That history has unfolded through a series of stages each determined by the prevailing conditions for the delivery of health care? That the motor for this development from era to era is provided by the 'class struggle', classes themselves being determined by the relationships of particular groups to the conditions for the provision of health care? The bourgeoisie, for example, provide, and are the main users of the means of, that form of medicine that developed in Europe and America in the nineteenth century? And finally, that when the stage is reached where the demand for health care comes into conflict with the existing conditions there begins 'an epoch of social revolution'?

If we remember McKeown's suggestion that the main determinants of health are nutrition, environment, behaviour, and the clinic, can we not provide a 'health' (not 'medical') rather than material explanation for every revolution in history? And through it should we not see why, although some doctors have often played a part in them, the medical establishment has often opposed major changes in the system of health care? Does not all this explain why the medical establishment, being part of the delivery of health care at any point in time, always has appeared to oppose its restructuring even where they might be emancipated by it? Is this not the lesson of Lloyd George and of Bevan in terms of technical medicine, of Allende in terms of the provision of basic primary care or of the 'successes' of the Russian and Chinese revolutions at the level of nutrition? Further, if we remember Zola's findings that different cultures have different medical expectations and desires do we not find an explanation for different patterns of revolutionary behaviour?

The problem with this argument is that by saying all, it says too much. In effect it observes that health is a precondition to life and concludes that therefore life is functionally organized about it. What it fails to see is that human existence as we know it has other preconditions and preoccupations. By giving primacy to one, it reduces the importance of others. It is difficult to accept the diminution of all other values in man. Thus in considering wider aspects of biomedicine, we must be especially careful not to give them an importance they do not have. This book is concerned with medicine's regulation. It can therefore accept its internal values. It is not helpful here or elsewhere to accept its external valuation without question or reservation.

An explanation

The radical critique is contemporary. It recognizes the social and psychological importance of science. It rejects mysticism. It recognizes the consumer as the dominant partner in the doctor–patient relationship, but regards the citizen as subservient to the consumer democratic state. In all this it is plausible to the modern mind. It is not fruitful to attempt to set out the contradictions in this amalgam of approaches. Nor is it necessary. It is more interesting to consider how and why such ideas have gained in popularity. Implicit in such explanations is a description of the transformation of the perspective in which the regulation of biomedicine is received.

Let there be no mistake. Although, as I argue, the form of the phenomena expressed in the radical critique is new, in other forms, at least, aspects of it have had a lengthy history. There is for example nothing new in the idea that the citizen has a duty enforceable by the criminal law to seek to maintain his own health for the good of the State. What is new is the metamorphosis of that idea into one which almost argues for the criminalization of tobacco and, at the same time, for the legalization of cannabis.

A clue to the essence of this transformation lies in its two roots – the diffidence shown to the ideas of self and of consumerism. It is no great surprise therefore that to find this essence it is necessary to turn to psychology, to utilitarian philosophy, and to economics. I shall return later to these points as I discuss what amounts to the law's reaction to the modes of medicine set out in an earlier chapter, and if not to the radical critique, at least the same phenomena which inspired it.

There is an initial point to be made. Considerable parts of public debate are conducted in dynamic language. We describe a great deal of economic and public life with words which describe rates of change; and at times, in a way which appears to suggest that it is these rates of change which are the constants. In economics there are words such as 'inflation', 'deflation', 'expansion', 'recession'. In politics 'swing' is used to describe the fortunes of political parties. In health, by striking contrast, static language is used as a deliberate understatement. Thus words such as 'comfortable', 'satisfactory', 'stable' are used in relation to the sick rather than the fit.

The reassurance of the use of the static is required precisely because of the concern about the direction of change. We rarely
think of a healthy body for whom nothing need be done. In all
other areas of life we think and talk of 'trends', comparing the past
with the present or the present with the future. I argue that this
reflects a general conceptualization of movement, of change, of
instability, in human life. The consequences of this mode of thinking are as yet ill-explored. Tentatively I would suggest that it is an
integral part of our relation with the world and change. When,
however, we deal in health and life we know that change leads on
to death: there is, after all, nothing more natural than decay.

It is convenient here to anticipate a part of an argument in a later
chapter concerning patients and their self-determination. There, I
closely follow Burt, *Taking Care of Strangers*, and adopt what he
calls the 'Rule of Opposites'.[96] Whether the Rule is a description
of a psychological truth or a metaphysical construction is beside
the point. What is important is that it provides a means to explain
the variability that each individual has in his relations with other
people.

Briefly, the Rule says that 'each critical organizing principle is
rational and irrational thinking – distinguishing between or compounding self and other, reality and fantasy, causes and effect, and
the like – rests on the implicit premise that the diametrically
opposed principle is more desirable, more satisfying'. In the words
of the once popular song: 'The other man's grass is always green-
er'. There is therefore in each individual an oscillation between
polarities, for example, conceiving ourselves[97] as separate or
boundless, as choicemaking or choiceless. I show how this dynamic conception challenges the static ideas of the free adult upon
which conventional theories of liberty, including those of J.S. Mill,
are based.

It is important here to note that, by this argument, as medicine
has become scientific so the previously subjective doctor–patient
relationship also has been rendered objective. That is, whereas in
past times the doctor's healing power (such as it was) was as much
based upon 'Aesculapian power' (Burt does not use the term but
compares the older power to the modern placebo effect), it is now
based upon the objectivities of pharmacology and physiology. One
doctor's therapy should be the same as the next. New methods are
only to be approved after statistical analysis of 'double blind' tests
– clinical trials should not only be based on the efficacy of the
therapy that is responsible for the effects, they should be adminis-

tered in such a way that neither the doctor not the patient knows
for certain that it is being used.

It is not only that the doctor's gaze has transformed his patient
into a carrier of a disease but also, particularly in this century, that
under the influence of the scientific ideology, the doctor's oscillation between his polarities of self and other, choicemaking
and choiceless, has changed from encompassing his patient (even as
the carrier of disease) to his science. The rise in scientific, in
bureaucratic, and, above all, in impersonal medicine has broken
the psychological link between doctor and patient. Burt argues
that the inevitable consequence has been that patients too have
sought an objectivity in the relationship. In the United States, at
least, they are achieving that objectivity by asserting a claim to
self-determination through the courts and by the doctrine of informed consent.

This much begins to explain not only that new doctrine but also
those features of the radical critique which challenge the unfettered
authority of doctors. However, so far the explanation is still in
terms of the traditional, although now modified, doctor–patient
relationship. To explain other aspects of the critique it is necessary
to have regard to its underlying economic theory; that is, to the
phenomenon of the modern consumer and the relationship of the
citizen to the democratic consumer state. Albert Hirschman in
Shifting Involvements[98] has begun such an explanation.

Although, as will appear, Hirschman writes of a public-private
cycle, he is not fully convinced as to regularity of the processes he
describes. His is not so much an account of their history as of their
existence. His work is important for its critique of conventional
consumption theory and its understanding of aspects of collective
action. Through his analysis, it is possible to understand more of
the effects of power at the levels of both the individual and society.

In coming to conclusions very similar to those of Burt, Hirschman offers an examination of the role of disappointment as the
motor for the oscillation he perceives. The shift from private to
public and back again is modern. Whereas the ancients acknowledged a shift from *vita activa* to *vita contemplativa*,[99] the oscillation with which Hirschman is concerned is between a life
concerned with public affairs and a life concerned with primarily
increased material welfare. Just as with Burt the oscillation is
propelled by normal psychological forces, so with Hirschman
disappointment is a normal and indeed essential feature not only of
humanity but also of human thought.

He notes that before actually engaging in any activity 'people formulate the *project* to do so'. This includes that of consumption, (and, in the context of health care, to which Hirschman does not specifically refer, the seeking of help from a doctor):[100]

> Part of this project are certain mental images or *expectations* about its nature and about the kind and degree of satisfaction it will yield. The independent existence of the project with its expectations implies that it may differ considerably from reality as it is experienced when the project is executed, that is, when consumption actually takes place. Hence the possibility of ... disappointment.

Hirschman deals with two possible objections to giving disappointment such a high role.[101] First, he answers those who argue that disappointment does not arise because once a choice is made the individual goes to considerable lengths to maintain 'cognitive consistency' by suppressing contrary evidence.[102] He accepts this view but argues:[103] 'Disappointment frequently will have to pass a certain threshold before it is consciously avowed'. Secondly, he gives a much larger role to the concept than is usual in economic assumptions about rational behaviour.

He goes on to argue that the assumption of perfect knowledge is that people are suppposed to calibrate their purchases and time-uses by matching their preferences, which are fully known to them, against the equally well-known world of consumption experiences. But Hirschman argues that preferences can be altered by previous expression of preference and furthermore the extent of the alteration of preferences varies between different types of purchases. The language is of economic theory but already it can be seen how inapplicable this consumer orientation is to health care. It is difficult to see a convincing argument that a theory based upon 'perfect knowledge' can have any application to choices within medicine.

Further, the endeavour to bring all behaviour within the ambit of neo-classical economics often asserts[104] that 'income-producing or consumption activities' can be compared with 'nonmonetary wants'.[105] However this assumes that: 'the consumer carries within himself a universe of wants of known intensity that he matches against prices'.[106] But 'We never operate in terms of a comprehensive hierarchy of wants ... but at any one point in our real existence ... we pursue *some* goals which then get replaced by others'.[107] Once again consumer theory can be seen to have little relevance to medicine: in the former choices are between competing goods; in the latter, for the patient, they are most often between therapy or no therapy. So also, because goods and services have similar economic effects, the economist equates them. But to a supplier they are not the same: after selling goods he no longer has them; after selling services he is what he was before. Consumerism in the provision of services is an economic not a sociological construction of reality: it is not only as Freidson says[108] the 'differences between professionally controlled service ... and the use of a commercial product ... stem from the status of the profession'.

Hirschman's beginning leads him to consider varieties of consumer disappointment. The consideration builds upon Simmel's distinction between money and other consumer goods in that all except money 'harbour either surprises or disappointments' that are experienced in the course of use.[109] Scitovsky[110] saw discomfort as being either unsatisfied wants or boredom. It is relieved in either case by various consumption activities. Crucially, Hirschman defines his terms:[111]

> Pleasure is the experience of travelling from discomfort to comfort while the latter is achieved at the point of arrival. Hence a contradiction between pleasure and comfort: for pleasure to be experienced, comfort must be sacrificed temporarily.

Since therefore pleasure and comfort are incompatible, it follows, argues Hirschman, that the least disappointment (that is, the least absence of pleasure) is to be obtained from those things which are consumed in the act of pleasure, for example food: except for the memory of them, they leave nothing upon which to focus lingering disappointment. By contrast, classic consumer durables such as refrigerators afford the minimum of pleasure so long as they provide the comfort for which they are intended. Thus he argues:[112]

> Actually when we say that we take certain of these permanently comfort-yielding durable goods for granted, we may well address a reproach not only to ourselves, but to the goods in question. We fault them precisely for being all comfort and hardly any pleasure.... Hence, the drastic change in the *balance of pleasure and comfort* that comes with durables is unforeseen and the small amount of pleasure they yield is initially disconcerting.

It is to be noted that this argument can be applied with equal force to health. Bad health, like a bad refrigerator, is a source of discomfort; good health, like a good refrigerator, is a source of comfort, but not pleasure. It is perhaps this which explains why individuals in modern western society who are predominately more healthy than those in any previous society are so concerned not merely to maintain their level of health but to seek the pleasure of improving it. I would argue that this is true both at the level of society through preventative and primary health care and at the level of the individual through 'keep-fit' and certain dietary regimes, and some aspects of alternative medicine. So also the publishing world produces books, with great apparent profit (they are written for those who can afford them and who, for that reason, do not generally include the lame or the chronic sick), in an almost endless supply, which deal with diet, fitness, and sex – a fair proportion of which are directed not at pleasure but at therapy. The argument explains the paradox that Hippocrates noted when he observed:[113]

> In the case of athletes too a condition of health is treacherous if it be an extreme state; for it cannot quietly stay as it is, and therefore, since it cannot change for the better, can only change for the worse.

Further, in so far as disease can be regarded as an 'it', the transformation from its presence to its absence is pleasure. And, as noted above, if we expect certain actions to be easier than reality turns out to be, we will be disappointed. Because there is not much that does not take longer and cost more than we expect, it follows that we are potentially always likely to be disappointed twice over with physician's therapies: both the cure and the manner of its achievement are likely to cause disappointment. The reality of perceived disappointment is limited by whether the threshold between real and acknowledged disappointment has been passed.

One further point can be made: all this begins to explain Zola's findings that cultural differences are a major determinant in those people who present themselves to a doctor and what they say when they get there. It is a cultural difference based at least in part upon the particular threshold of disappointment. As the individual acquires more experience of doctors, so the threshold moves. However, a substantial part of the threshold is supported by professional mysticism. I will argue that this in turn is supported by an emphasis on social rather than individual perspectives. As the mysticism is increasingly doubted i.1 our individualized, rationalized, scientific age, so the threshold of disappointment in the doctor–patient relationship is reduced. It is to be noted that this argument reinforces Burt's conclusion that medicine's turn to science broke the psychological link between the patient and the doctor. It is not merely a matter of the breaking of a psychological link, it is also a matter of the withering of the social connection. The radical critique is a consequence of much broader phenomena.

To return to Hirschman: he proceeds from his argument that pleasure and comfort are incompatible, to press the reasoning by subdividing consumer durables into those which provide comfort, those which provide pleasure, and those which form a hybrid class. The hybrid is expanded by the addition of non-utilitarian, sometimes personalized, features to an otherwise merely comfort-producing object. It applies to, for example, readjusting the home by way of its furniture and decorations and to the curious practice of polishing motor cars. Once again the application to health is apparent. The consumer is learning that in order to receive pleasure, there has to be a personalization of the comfort-producing goods or services. As we shall see, the way this is achieved in the face of bureaucratized and impersonal medical care is through the expression of the individual's claim to self–determination.

Hirschman argues that there is an essential difference between goods and services. The number of the former may be increased or decreased but it is finite. In the case of services, such as education or health care, the initial new demand for them is likely to produce increases in the number of suppliers who, by reason of their relative inexperience, are likely to produce a worse service. Consequently the consumer disappointment observed in the case of durables is likely to be accentuated in the case of services. There is a second distinction which he might have pointed to. It lies in the differences of our responses to consumer durables and services.[114] He goes on to suggest that the reason why publicly provided services (that is, services paid for indirectly through taxation) are more prone to criticism than those which are bought directly lies not in a fact that the latter are better but in the fact that because the consumer has used cash to purchase them, he has a psychological stake in not criticizing them.

From this he argues that where a large number of 'goods' are suddenly made available to a whole population then there will be mass movements of pleasure to comfort and consequent disappointment.[115] Somewhat tentatively, despite calling upon evidence from Adam Smith (who spoke of 'trinkets and baubles fitter to be the play-things of children than the serious pursuits of men')[116] and Rousseau (who used the word *conifichet* to describe a frivolous object of little utility, of poor taste, desired out of vanity and social rivalry), he suggests 'antagonism toward material culture comes to the fore in periods of economic expansion when consumer goods, frequently of a new kind, become more widely diffused'.

Consequently,[117] 'the recoil from "consumerism" is by no means an invention or a monopoly of the nineteen-sixties'. And,[118]

> New material wealth is ... placed in a double bind: if it filters down to the masses, the conservatives are aroused because it threatens the social order. If it does not filter down, the progressives are appalled by the widening disparity in consumption standards. And since the evidence is never unambiguous, new products and wealth can be and often have been accused and accursed on both counts.

There is, however, a second double bind to which new products are subjected. On the one hand they excite expectations and hopes which turn out to give only transitory pleasure. This is similar to my suggestions above that there are epochs when excitement and disorientation are prevailing feelings and that medicine is an expression of man's desire to control brute nature. On the other hand, says Hirschman:[119]

> In a remarkable reversal, the things which man invents and produces are suddenly turning from frivolous and trifling to extraordinarily threatening and sacrilegious.... A modern version of the ancient concept of forbidden knowledge is very much with us, in the guise of the negative and noxious side effects of various, initially much-hailed, mass-produced novelty products.... Here is a modern, 'scientific' way of reverting to the ancient thought ... that dire consequences will follow if man's quest for knowledge proceeds unchecked.

Once more the relevance to health care and the radical critique can be noted. First, this view explains the ambiguities in a rejection of modern mass-marketed foods in favour of a return to older, less processed varieties. Second, and quite separately, it casts further light on our ambiguous attitudes to new advances in acute medicine and pharmacology: despite the lives that are saved, and the anguish relieved, at the mundane level of unknown side-effects, are the resources they demand worth it or are they indeed sacrilegious?[120]

It is necessary at this point to follow Hirschman's general argument; I shall relate it to medicine later. He insists that it is not only the will-o'-the-wisp quality of these new products which is the cause of disappointment, rather in some cases, it may be their availability. It may be noted *en passant* that this has some similarity with Hirsch's idea of 'positional goods'[121] – goods which because of their rarity or other qualities cannot be universally enjoyed (as are, for example, the beaches at Rimini and Benidorm) – and so are confined to an élite in society. It would seem also to apply to the high status of some professions. Of course because disappointment has different effects on different people and in respect of different products, it is not thereby possible to conclude a macro scale shift from private to public:[122] 'Disappointments are diffuse and inchoate, and turn into general frustration and perhaps depression.'

In order to explain how it is that there are large shifts over time in both directions, Hirschman examines limits on conventional economic theory and what he sees as the prevailing ideology[123] which 'proclaims self-interested behaviour as a social duty'. Conventional theory is built around primary choices – Frankfurt[124] called them first-order desires. It says nothing about opportunities and choices to change life-styles, which are second-order desires. Those who are capable only of first-order desires are 'impoverished nonpersons'. Hirschman adopts Frankfurt's term `wanton' and says:[125] 'It turns out, then, that consumption theory, one of the most sophisticated branches of economics, has so far dealt exclusively with those infrahuman wantons!'

Of course, some aspects of conventional theory allow for changes in taste but by no means as satisfactorily as does the use of these two levels of preferences. Thus, I may wish to give up smoking (a second-order desire) but my actions may show only a choice between brands – my conscience is not always master. Hirschman argues that whether a second-order preference will be allowed to express itself will depend not so much on the severity of the disappointment with a first-order choice but upon any disappointment combined with some other precondition.

Margolis his suggested[126] a theory of choice which endeavours to expand the neo-classical idea of rational economic man deciding his best interests for himself in the market place of private goods.

He postulates two selves within each individual – the self who values only his inner being and the self with a perception of group-interest. In this way the self-interest of the neo-classicist may be interest in self or kin or group. But I suspect that both traditional neo-classical writing and Margolis fall prey to the complexities of the everyday. Here there are oscillations between self, kin, group, society, and each of their sub-divisions. Rational economic man cannot exist in this world.

Hirschman tries to explain[127] 'the periodic outbreaks of mass participation in public affairs and of collective action in general'. Olson[128] showed that even where the benefit to rational economic man of certain objectives which are attainable through public action exceeds the cost to him of his involvement, he is nevertheless unlikely to participate; even if he does not, he may well have a 'free-ride' to the benefit.

This, however, argues Hirschman, depends upon a disregard for the individual's past experience and its 'rebound effect'. In classical theory, in considering future conduct, the past should be ignored – the cost of future conduct should be less than the prospective benefit. However, reality suggests a sometimes disproportionate adherence to past policy followed by the adoption of its opposite.[129]

> Another way of expressing the matter in the economist's language is to say that once a transaction that one has entered into has turned out badly, a transaction with opposite characteristics may have negative transaction costs .... The transaction will in effect be subsidized by none other than the transactor himself.

Thus, where the worker sees a public interest in, and public result from, his work, to that extent his work is a part of the benefit accruing to him. Moreover, the public benefit is one of self-perception: it is not necessarily linked to societal rewards.[130] This is stating in abstract terms what health care workers believe the health care bureaucracy thinks in fixing the cash remuneration for their efforts. To put it another way, although for example nurses consider themselves underpaid commonly they are constrained from doing anything about it by reason of the public involvement of their work.

Hirschman goes on:[131]

> Once this essential characteristic of participation in collective action for the public good is understood, the severe limitations

of the 'economic' view about such participation, and about the obstacles to it, come immediately into view. The implication of the confusion between striving and attaining is that the net distinction between costs and benefits of action in the public interest vanishes, since striving, which should be entered on the cost side, turns out to be part of the benefit ... the only way in which an individual can raise the benefit accruing to him from the collective action is by stepping up *his own input*, his effort on behalf of the public policy he espouses.

This is most clearly seen in relation to religious pilgrimages and in the satisfaction of the sports supporter for both of whom the journey is an important part of the benefit of the exercise.

It is for example shown in what is or was supposed to be the characteristic of the British attitude to participation in sport: viz. it is better to have played and lost, than never to have played at all. Sport, I shall suggest, is the preparation for action. It is an attitude which in other terms expresses the 'gentleman's' approach. I shall suggest that W.G. Grace had an influence on this but more important in terms of establishing the ideology, although not the reality, was Lord Byron. It is significant that he was also a leader of the 'Romantics' who, as a group, opposed the materialism of empirical science.[132] The gentleman, as I will also argue, is not new to material comfort, he has nothing to prove, except his personal position as a member of society. It is significant that the manner of proving it is not the winning but the expression of participation. It is also significant that the ideology of playing has been modified by the advent of those who need, and receive, material rewards (that is the athletic equivalent of the parvenu bourgeoisie) into sport at its highest levels.

Once more, assuming I am right to expand Hirschman's use of 'public', the relevance to health care can be seen. One of the effects of the scientism and bureaucratization of medicine has been that more health care is conducted by teams. Generally this is regarded as an unfortunate but inevitable development. However, team medicine brings its own rewards to its practitioners. As Hirschman says, particularly where the purpose is some perceived public good, there is pleasure to be gained by individuals both in the striving and in the co-operation from uncompleted attempts at impossible objectives by teams of which they are part.

As team medicine is increasingly practised, the very involvement of others renders the objective more obviously public, thus increasing the pleasure to be obtained from this form of participation. Although, as I argue, the patient's role has been reduced by the appearance first of the clinic and then of scientific medicine (which ought to have privatized the pleasures of physicians), the use of the health care team has provided a counterbalance, and in institutions and busy practices, superior compensation. Large numbers of individuals can be the object of doctors' concerns but they cannot be its subject. They can only know large numbers of clients from the issues they bring to them: with fewer, practitioners can join with those clients in seeking to define the issues with which their expertise may be able to help.

Hirschman is concerned to establish waves or shifts of involvement. He argues that the outcome of public action does not determine the extent either of dissatisfaction or of withdrawal. What does is the way that it is actually experienced. Although the public activity may be pleasurable, it commonly uses more time than has been allocated for it. He says that there are a number of reasons why people should continually underestimate the time needed to accomplish their objectives.[133] There is an

> illusion that [the activity] can be accommodated rather easily, without neglecting or sacrificing any of one's usual duties, occupations and pleasures. Another illusion under which people often labor is that their own point of view makes unique common sense and will easily carry the day. The strength of opposing interests and opinions comes as a surprise.

These illusions are added to that already noted that the objective is likely to be Utopian and so be more time-absorbing than expected.

In addition to 'time overruns', the quality of the experience of public action is often unpredictable.[134]

> [T]he political activist will rediscover for himself the maxims Machiavelli proposed in *The Prince* and the dilemmas Max Weber analyzed in 'Politics as a Vocation' and Jean-Paul Sartre in *Dirty Hands*. In the process he may well violate the prevailing ethical code to a far greater extent than he ever dreamt of doing when he was merely pursuing his own personal gain and private consumption goals.
>
> This experience can, of course, be so dismaying and so contrary to expectations as to produce an immediate withdrawal from public life. But the opposite reaction is also possible and perhaps more common: a heady feeling of excitement is generated when the consciousness of selflessly acting for the public

good is combined with the sensation of being free to overstep the traditional boundaries of moral conduct, a sensation that is closely related to power.

On the basis that medicine is in some respects a public act, this analysis goes some way to explaining paternalism in health care, and why it is that those without the 'insights of the bedside' are so ill-equipped to deal with it. Even on the assumption that paternalism is to be condemned within the private moral code, that is to say in our dealings with each other, the precept is not so readily applied in the public professional act of medicine.

And, as I have argued, as medicine becomes objectified and bureaucratized so its public character is more apparent to those who participate because of their consciousness of team membership. There is a dual effect: the patient is reduced in importance and at the same time the potentiality of paternalism is increased. The point is more applicable in those systems where there is a greater divorce between work and reward, that is, where the practitioner can behave more like the ideal-typical professional I shall describe.

In order to complete his story of the private to public to private cycle, Hirschman reconsiders the meaning of public and private. He argues that the normality of private virtue is modern. It has replaced the Renaissance emphasis on civic virtue. He notes that a private man 'used to be found at the lowest end of the social scale' and that the opposite was true of women.[135] There is nothing in what he says to indicate that his analysis is not applicable to the extended meaning I have given to 'public'. Indeed I suggested that the very transformation he notes is itself reflected in the existence of the radical critique. In its early forms, in the hands of Ouida and G.B. Shaw[136] it amounted to a refutation of the public benefit of medical science and practice.

Hirschman considers the shift back from public to private. He says:[137]

> The greatest asset of public action is its ability to satisfy vaguely felt needs for higher purpose and meaning in the lives of men and women, specially of course in an age in which religious fervour is at a low ebb in many countries.

Hirschman argues that just as public action becomes attractive because its real costs were seen as benefits, so, if disappointment is enough, they will be translated back into perceived costs. If public action is sufficiently publicly debunked, disappointment will set in, and that this happened in 'The Demolition of the Hero'[138] in the seventeenth century and in the allegation of 'ego-trips' against public activists in the 1960s. The point is not dissimilar to one made by Foucault:[139] 'the passage from the epic to the novel, from the noble deed to the secret singularity ... is also inscribed in the formation of a disciplinary society'.

I have argued that medical practice is not merely functional but also, in origin and in residue, mystical or religious. If I am right in this it is to be expected that the debunking of it by scientism and by the radical critique is likely to result in a loss in the attractions of medicine as a public act. In concrete terms, the effect of malpractice litigation in respect of medically untoward occurrences, particularly in the United States in the early 1970s has, by reason of the disappointment they have engendered, privatized the attractions of medical practice. So also one could point to the self-righteous frustration with which much of the medical profession greeted Ian Kennedy's Reith Lectures and their subsequent publication. I would conclude that such attacks, particularly when made in the manner either of political debate or of *realpolitik*, amount to no more than self-fulfilling prophecies.

Indeed, perhaps at the core of my concern are: the radical critique, malpractice actions, an a priori and apparently unjustified universalization of a right to self-determination and an ill-informed application of consumer ideology. All these are most likely to shift medical practice from a mode which is, by and large, tolerable to one which is not, and which moreover would require very different forms of regulation. At their extreme, nothing would remain except a private capacity to enrich its practitioners at the cost of those who are, by definition, most in need and capable of being helped.

In Hirschman's argument there is a contrast:[140] 'a public motive and purpose can be credibly introduced as topping off a basically self-serving action, while the opposite operation is impossible. The claim to be doing good by doing well is acceptable and even plausible, whereas the inverse claim is not'. And,[141]

> the idea that the public happiness is best served by everyone pursuing private gains may have served not so much a self-glorifying function for the new class of capitalists: it also fulfilled the more pressing need to relieve acute guilt feelings experienced by many a so-called 'conquering bourgeois' who actually had long been exposed to a non-bourgeois moral code.

He continues:[142]

> once public man reels under the accusation of hypocrisy – the
> charge, that is, that public action is essentially self-serving – the
> turn to the private life can be viewed as a move toward reality,
> sincerity, and even humility. Just as the public life comes as a
> relief from the boredom of the private life, so does the latter
> provide a refuge from the paroxysm and futility of public en-
> deavours. More generally, to be concerned only with looking
> after one's private needs, to 'cultivate our garden', is to give up
> the twin illusory and hubris-laden pretenses of improving the
> world (*vita activa*) and of understanding its laws and secrets
> (*vita contemplativa*), and to attend instead to matters that have
> an immediate, down-to-earth usefulness and practicality.

The reference to cultivating the garden and thus to Voltaire's
Candide is well chosen. But more potent still is the reminder of
Omar Khayyám's *Rubáiyát*. Khayyám is sometimes credited with
the discovery of algebra. He wrote:[143]

> Myself when young did eagerly frequent
> Doctor and Saint, and heard great Argument
>   About it and about: but evermore
> Came out by that same Door as in I went.

> With them the Seed of Wisdom did I sow,
> And with my own hand labour'd it to grow:
>   And this was all the Harvest that I reap'd –
> I came like Water, and like Wind I go.

It is difficult to conceive of a greater expression of the futility of
the *vita activa* (the Doctor) and, assuming the accuracy of the
attribution, especially of the *vita contemplativa* (the Saint). And
yet, could Khayyám have felt, or told us about, the pleasures of
the 'pot' if he had not done what he did when young? Can we
understand his solace without also having frequented 'with Doctor
and Saint'?

Some history: the scientific imperative and medical science

In law,[144] and in science,[145] positivism dates from the sixteenth
century and the beginning of the seventeenth with St Germain and
Coke,[146] and with Descartes and Bacon.[147] Associated with this is

the introduction of inductive methods into both disciplines: in law, the drawing of generalized principles from cases in law reports; in science, the rationalizing of empirically assessed data. This is so despite the fact that, of course, earlier phenomena which could be translated into these terms can be found. One example is Hippocratic medicine itself. My point relates, not to the purposes of empiricism, but its function in the formation of ideas.

Two centuries later, at the end of the eighteenth or the beginning of the nineteenth century these ideas were consolidated in the Enlightenment. That is, in that period which considered science to be universal and autonomous, art to be an objective judgement, and morals to consist in the self-legislation of universal laws by autonomous individuals. With the first general applications of technology utility became the touchstone – the alchemists' dream – in the natural sciences. Of course there were technological concerns and innovation prior to that time; the point is that only from the turn of the nineteenth century did they qualitatively affect everyday life, and, moreover, at the same time change itself became an everyday occurrence. And with the Utilitarians, and with Saint-Simon and Comte,[148] the same measure was applied in the new social sciences. The dogma of the Enlightenment was confirmed – if the cause of something is unknown, it must be found out; if something is possible, it must be done; and, if something is unknowable, it can be ignored. The unknowable was largely defined by reference to an inherent impossibility of its being expressed in terms of mass, length, and time. As Hume said:[149]

> If we take into our hands any volume ... let us ask: Does it contain any abstract reasoning concerning quantity and number? No. Does it contain any experimental reasoning concerning matters of fact and existence? No. Commit them to the flames: for it can contain nothing but sophistry and illusion.

Those who did not ignore the unknowable were dismissed by practical men as 'Romantics'. They, in turn, cherished the description.[150] It scarcely occurred to either side that there are some things which must be only dimly understood, or that for human life to operate at all it is necessary most of the time to proceed on the basis of but limited comprehension. The Romantic vision of superior reality was placed first in contrast and then in rivalry to the imagination of the worldly. Shelley put it:[151]

> Whilst the mechanist abridges, and the political economist combines, labour, let them beware that their speculations, for want

of correspondence with those first principles which belong to the imagination do not tend, as they have in modern England, to exasperate at once the extremes of luxury and want.... Such are the effects which must ever flow from unmitigated exercise of the calculating faculty.

In retrospect, it is enormously hard for even the 'non-scientific' or 'non-technical' minds of our age to appreciate the novelty of the emphasis on mass, length, and time. It is no less difficult to understand that once that idea had been absorbed it was still necessary for man to realize that some of these general principles might have practical applications. Our vision is obscured by the Industrial Revolution – the application of the artificial extension of man's physical power. It is possible for us to realize that some commonplace ideas of today were once heresies (although perhaps we do not understand how they could have been so designated). It is far harder to realize that many more were regarded as eccentricities.

In the context of the approach of medical men to their activity and of society to them, it was Foucault's argument[152] that the investigation moved from what for simplicity can perhaps be called the mystical to the knowable, but also in looking for the knowable it displaced the patient's role. It may help briefly to recall a number of the scientific and technical developments both in medicine and more widely between the Renaissance and the Industrial Revolution.[153] I am concerned with the sociological not technological effects of these discoveries. To generalize, the lesson which mankind was learning was put by Newton:[154] 'If I have seen further it is by standing on the shoulders of giants'. That is, science and technology could develop by teamwork between generations. But it is a generalization whose importance was only recognized later.

Thus, Harvey discovered the circulation of the blood in 1628 but it appears that it lacked practical application until the middle of the nineteenth century.[155] Gilbert's *De Magnete* (1600) was an introduction to magnetism, but it was not until more than a century later that Franklin invented the lightning conductor. It was even later before Galvani and Volta managed to produce any usable electricity. The connection between magnetism and electricity was not apparent until Faraday showed it well into the Industrial Revolution in 1831. Galileo and Newton had used telescopes, and the latter had advanced knowledge of the refraction of light.

But it was only much later in 1850 that J.B.L. Foucault demonstrated that light was not material. So also heat was supposed to be an element until 1848, when Lord Kelvin provided an alternative explanation.

In chemistry, there has long been a belief in basic elements out of which all matter was composed, but since they were such as earth, fire, water, and air, there was not (so it now seems to us) an empirical base to these ideas. Chemistry as an orthodox science not only had to shed from itself the mysticism of alchemy but had to await the technology for isolating gases. This was not effectively accomplished until the second half of the eighteenth century when some were separated and identified, in particular by Priestley and Lavoisier. It was the latter who established the idea that an element was the limit of chemical analysis – a substance which could not be further decomposed. Dalton built upon this idea in his *New System of Chemical Philosophy* (1808–10); and it was only after this theory had been worked through that it became possible to study organic (or bio-) chemistry. Apart from their long-term effects on chemotherapy, the importance, from the point of view of the current work, is that chemistry and biochemistry teach us that at least some organic compounds are made up of non-vital components. Life is material and, taken with the emergence of the scientific imperative, materialism was justified by the laboratory.

Perhaps the three sciences which have most changed the way in which man thinks about himself are astronomy, geology, and biology. This change, in turn, affected the purpose, and the possibility, of medicine. It is, I would argue, mainly dated in the early to middle years of the nineteenth century. In astronomy, the vision of an earth-centred universe gave way to the idea that the earth, and man, were but a minute part of the cosmos.[156] It is of course possible to reconcile both schemes with a Deity, but they do not provide either the same view of God or of man's place. Geology showed that mountains had been made of sea-beds.[157] The examination of fossils showing extinct life forms challenged the orthodoxy of the Biblical story of creation and theology's contribution to the estimated age of the earth. The effect was to cast doubt on the authority of the Church and churchmen.

Biology was largely confined to natural observation and systematic data collection until the development of optics meant that microscopic structures, including the complexity of insect anatomy, the cells of the amoeba, and the capillaries and nerves of animal tissue could be seen for the first time. As such the science did nothing to disturb orthodoxy in metaphysical or religious ideas. It was the nineteenth century which saw the fundamental developments in the biological sciences which themselves, together with the knowledge of geology and the doubts created by astronomy, successfully challenged the old ideas. (The success of this was enhanced by advances in applied technologies.)

Virchow published his cell-theory – that the body is a 'cell-state in which every cell is a citizen' – in 1858.[158] It challenged the ideas of the body as a single entity or a simple collection of tissues.[159] In 1857, Pasteur began the research which led to his germ theory. Once more, conventional ideas were under attack. Disease was not caused by miasma or bad air but by germs; and, germs could grow. As Pasteur put it, 'Life is a Germ and Germ is Life'. At around the same time Darwin published his *Origin of Species* (1859) and *The Descent of Man* (1871). These too challenged older comforting ideas.[160] The combination of Virchow, Pasteur, and Darwin not merely affected medical science, it provided a substitute for the authority of the Church and of God. That substitute not only gave an alternative explanation for life but it also cast doubt on the source and expression of ethical norms. These authors, with Bernard,[161] cleared the way for 'scientism' – the idea that science is value-free. This is not to suggest that they suddenly altered man's perception. Darwin himself said:[162]

> It has sometimes been said that the success of the Origin proved 'that the subject was in the air' or 'that men's minds were prepared for it'. I do not think that this is strictly true, for I occasionally sounded out a few naturalists, and never happened to come across a single one who seemed to doubt about the permanence of the species.... What I believe is strictly true is that innumerable well-observed facts were stored in the minds of naturalists, ready to take their proper places as soon as any theory which would receive them was sufficiently explained.

His granddaughter, Nora Barlow,[163] appeared puzzled by this passage and its contrast with, for example, Coleridge's description of *Zoonomia* by Erasmus Darwin, Charles's grandfather. Coleridge had called that work 'the Orang Outang theory of the human race'. To Mrs Barlow, the crucial difference between Erasmus and Charles was that the former offered speculation, the latter 'generalization under the strict control of related observation'. The point for us is that Virchow, and after him Pasteur, offered a theory which opened up new avenues for medical scientists to investigate. Darwin's area of study was, and was seen to be, available to wider social and political theory.[164]

Each of them, Virchow, Pasteur, and Darwin, spoke to a community which was not yet scientific. It was the newly acquired prestige of science and the pre-jargon mode of discourse it used at that time that made their work accessible to the larger audience. However much it is true that the theory of evolution was the creation of Darwin's unique qualities (a matter which is now generally doubted), and whatever the direct influence of the one on the other, what is clear is that the general idea was 'in the air'. Darwin and Spencer both used the word 'evolution'. The debate still lingers. Should we ride with nature or assert our control over our destiny by opposing it? Hawthorn describes[165] T.H. Huxley's sympathy for Spencer and the crucial qualification he put on Spencer's ideas of socially encouraging natural selection. There were links, he says, by way of reaction, to Booth (founder of the Salvation Army) and to the Webbs ('founders' of Fabian socialism). All kept the science, and the positivism.

As regards medicine in particular, by showing that man was organically similar to animals, Darwin appeared to cast doubt on the relevance of the soul. It was a demonstration of the Cartesian mechanistic model of the body. All laws of nature, including those concerning the causes of disease, were discoverable by those who had the patience. In part, mysticism was taken out of religion and religion out of medicine. As medicine became imbued with 'scientism' and objectivity in diagnosis, less reliance was placed on the patient's description of his own symptoms, and correspondingly more importance was placed on the medical man's evaluation of the physical signs of disease. The practice shifted from the ancient dogmas of Hippocrates and Galen to the lessons of science: it remained esoteric.[166]

At the practical level, the passage of the Anatomy Act 1832 was as important as these developments in theory. It made possible a sufficient supply of cadavers for the advancement of science and education. It formalized the clinic. Prior to the Act, the only lawful supply of cadavers that medical men, and medical students, had was a small number of bodies of executed criminals. The Act gave them access to three new sorts of supply: the bodies of those who died in hospitals and Poor Law institutions who were unclaimed by their relatives; the bodies of those who had agreed *inter vivos* to dissection; and, the bodies of those whose executors agreed to it. It was said:[167] 'The object was two-fold – namely, to facilitate science and to prevent crime.' Scientific it may have been but it prohibited a dissection within forty-eight hours of the death. In part, the Act was a reflection of ideas similar to the increasingly fashionable theories of political economy. The increased supply was required, said Southwood-Smith,[168] to make available to 'the lowest practitioners of the medical art – that is, to persons who are at present lamentably deficient, and into whose hands the great bulk of the poor fall' the same source of knowledge as had the physicians and surgeons of the rich.

Most likely, however, the prevention of crime was a necessary condition for the Act. The Preamble expressly mentions that murder had been committed to provide bodies to be sold illicitly to the Schools of Anatomy.[169] More remarkable still was the letter from the Royal College of Surgeons to the Home Secretary.[170] It confessed that its rule requiring those who presented themselves for examination to have studied 'Practical Anatomy' had led to 'The large prices which have of late been given for Anatomical Subjects [which] have operated as a premium for murder'. Nor, for the sake of the public, was it willing to abandon the rule. Opposition to the Act was concerned with injured feelings (by way of religion, association with murderers and otherwise) and derived from the fact that[171] 'There was already a prejudice amongst the poor, that the rich had no sympathy for their sufferings, and this...would tend materially to increase that prejudice' by enabling the bodies of deceased relatives to be sold.

This is a history but it can perhaps be noted that today with almost all the formal objection gone, there is surely still an uneasiness in the use of cadavers. But no longer can this be articulated as a matter of religion or class or association with crime. The benefits are apparent and rational; the disadvantages are less clear. Perhaps they can be described as a pit-in-the-stomach feeling about medical mysticism and power, about unease in the face of external imperatives. Have we moved so far that we fail to understand the description of the dissection, against the background of a thunderstorm, of Jeremy Bentham's corpse by Dr Southwood-Smith (a friend and eventually his taxidermist) at the Webb School of Anatomy[172] in 1832? He said:[173] 'Never did ... funeral obsequies chanted by stoled and mitred priests in Gothic aisles, excite such emotions as the stern simplicity of that hour at which the principle of utility triumphed over the imagination and the heart'.

4

The profession of medicine: Some more history

Earlier, I asserted the modern legacy of the Hippocratic tradition. Hippocrates himself lived in the fifth century BC in the so-called Golden Age of Greece. The tradition is linked to our age in a variety of ways. Since the paterfamilias was responsible for health care, the Roman view, for example as advanced by the elder Pliny, was that[1] there was 'no need of physicians'. As Daremberg remarked[2] they were 'sans medecins, mais non pas sans medecine'. Certainly, the Romans knew of legal actions for medical expenses,[3] and hence we may presume of medical men's fees. Despite Pliny there were those kept Greek medical learning alive in that more prosaic regime. To us the most important of these was Galen (AD 131–201) whose influence, as we shall see, continued to beyond the Renaissance and Dioscorides whose description of herbs was to puzzle that age.[4]

For a millennium neither Rome nor Christianity was prepared to adopt ideas of experimental science, nevertheless the prescriptions if not the methods of Galen took hold. And it was his writings, with their links to Hippocrates, that were used (and glossed) in Arabia and in Europe in the Middle Ages, in monastic medicine, and in the later part of that time in universities in Italy and France.[5] Of particular significance was the group which settled at Salerno in around AD 900.[6] For reasons not (yet) understood, the Salerno School became both international and inter-denominational. Its heyday was the eleventh and twelfth centuries. The School practised both physic and surgery. It was a teaching school and it was the first to confer doctorates on medical men. When the influence of Salerno waned (also for reasons not yet understood) much of its learning and methods passed to the multi-faculty universities including eventually Padua, Bologna, Montpellier, Paris, and those of Oxford and Cambridge.

When there was a change from belief in gods who were not interested in man to a God that was, the way was opened for a clerically led interventionist form of medicine.[7] One of the achievements of the Judeo-Christian tradition is that disease was seen to be caused by His wrath or by His imposition of a test. The link is shown in the medieval practice of naming diseases after saints.[8] Erasmus, reacting in the early Renaissance out of his evangelical humanism, condemned the practice as a 'sea of superstition' which attributed more to Saints than to Christ.[9]

In the Middle Ages the Church was the principal seat of learning and the centre of an authoritarian regime. It did not encourage, and at times discouraged, free thinking. Such scholars as there were spent most of their energy writing commentaries on a limited number of texts. Physicians displayed a distinctly ambivalent attitude towards the Church. On the one hand, they were themselves educated which meant that in most cases if they were not in Holy Orders, they had received their schooling from clerics. On the other hand, they preferred the authority of Galen, Hippocrates, and Dioscorides to that of the Bible.[10] Thus the medieval proverb: *Ubi tres medici duo athei* (Where there are three doctors, there are two atheists). In part, as we have seen, this was a reflection of their Pythagorean ethic.

Since, however, disease was caused by divine displeasure and moreover since those who practised medicine and theology (and we might add the law) were virtually the only lettered classes, the links between the Church and medicine were strong. In the thirteenth century the Pope decreed '*ecclesia abhorret a sanguine*'. As far as medicine was concerned, this confirmed the style of the contemplative physician content with only diagnosis and prognosis. It prevented the priest-medicine man from himself taking part in any procedure which drew blood. It thus confirmed the breach between scholastic learning and the practical craft of surgery and reinforced the position of others, including apothecaries, who could do so.[11]

All this was not a deliberate division of labour, still less medical specialization in a modern sense: with the exception of some supervision by physicians over the quality of drugs, inter- or infrafraternal co-operation was unknown. The nearest that the practitioners came to acknowledging these others was by way of rivalry, but here not so much in an economic sense but in a

religious one. There was no more a division of labour than between the ministers of one religion and another. In the main, the
activities of the others were irrelevant to the physician and his
work. Despite the Hippocratic recognition of surgery, the modern
functional link between it and physic was not on anybody's agenda. The divide was a matter of theory, practice, mode, and extent
of education, as well as of status. It does not surprise the modern
mind that over the years there has been a merger. It could not have
occurred to medieval man, and thus for perfectly good reasons
each succeeding step toward the currently held view was opposed
in its time. As Freidson points out:[12] 'A profession attains and
maintains its position by virtue of the protection and patronage of
some élite segment of society ...' and[13] 'There were many types
of healer; the ones we know most about served the élite'.

The new vision of the Renaissance was not only a time of return
to the learning of antiquity; other trends were as significant.
Whether or not by way of a link with this return, the authority
and authoritarianism of the Church were questioned by Martin
Luther and by Erasmus and the 'evangelical humanists', among
whom in England we may include More and Colet. It is important
that these men considered themselves conservative not revolutionary; their reaction to events of their time might have 'changed the
world', but this was certainly not what they intended.

Amongst the ancient writers, the 'humanism' of Cicero proved
important. It was probably from him that the Renaissance re-
established the central place of the individual. Durkheim argued:[14]

At the time of the Renaissance, the individual begins to become
conscious of himself; he is no longer, at least in enlightened
regions, a simple aliquot fraction of a whole, he is already a
whole in a sense, a person with his own physiognomy, who has
and who experiences at the very least the need to develop his
own ways of thinking and feeling.

Once this was achieved it became open for both protestantism and
scientism, in their different ways, to develop their recognizably
modern forms.

For a variety of reasons, the Renaissance was also the time at
which there was a renewed emphasis on the social graces. Men
could establish their position in society by their manners; the older
aristocracy made room not only for the *nouveau riche* but also the
gentleman. And, as is discussed in a later chapter, it was possible
to learn and cultivate his behaviour, his thinking, his being. What-

ever the causes, the opportunity thus afforded to the 'self-made' was itself a precondition for the re-establishment of the Hippo-cratic (Pythagorean) gentleman-physician.

Hippocrates and Galen had developed their medicine by observation. When their ideas were readopted, it seems that their method of understanding by observation was at least as attractive as their ethical and normative ideas. Their legacy to the Middle Ages was facts which, as it turned out, were often wrong.[15] Galen's experience of anatomy was based on the dissection of pigs: religious considerations of his age prevented the cutting of the human cadaver. Vesalius, for example, in *The Structure of the Human Body*, 1543, was so committed to Galen that he believed that human anatomy must have changed between Imperial Rome and the Renaissance. The legacy of Hippocrates and Galen to the later Renaissance was a methodology of practice and of research. It is notable that many of the artists of Renaissance Florence, includ-ing Michelangelo, were members of the *Arte dei Medici, Speziali e Merciai* (the medical guild) in order to study anatomy and in order to gain access to druggists' pigments.[16]

In the field of specifically medical practice, although there were writings during the Middle Ages,[17] for the most part, enquiry was by way of philology. To some in the later Renaissance this was not however sufficient. A new breed of doctor, sometimes known as the *neoterici*, was becoming pronounced. Specifically, in the field of surgery, gunpowder created a new type of war-wound. And from recently discovered lands, new plants (notably, as we have seen, tobacco) and new diseases were imported and no record of them could be found in Dioscorides. One of the most striking examples of the rejection of the past learnings was the burning of the works of Galen by Paracelsus: Pagel[18] observes that 'opposi-tion to the sources extant at his time is most prominent in all his writings'. Paracelsus himself was notable for his knowledge of late medieval alchemy[19] and the occult. He is best known to some as the founder of chemotherapy.[20]

Over the longer term, the renewed emphasis on the individual and scientism in medicine introduced a dilemma from which medi-cine has not recovered. If the basic unit of science is the individual (atom, plant, animal, etc) and if medicine is in part scientific what becomes of either the social fact of the medical act or its mystic-ism? The early conditions which produced the pre-eminence of the gentleman-physician, in the longer term also led to the expansion in the numbers of doctors, a growth in scientism, and the dilution in the quality of its ideal. This conjunction of trends – particularly in a society whose institutional forms were medieval but whose modes were infused with individualism coupled with the new spirit of scientific adventure – enabled (or caused) the profession to mould its regulation into a form which is recognizably modern. The foundation of the separate colleges or guilds or companies for medicine expresses this reality.

It needs however be appreciated that for a King, Council, Parliament, City to grant a monopoly or privilege, even with penal regulations for its infringement, did not (and does not still) mean instant obedience. In days when society was less integrated and its various policing powers were by our standards weak, there was an even more obvious gap between the pronouncement of a rule and the achievement of its purpose. The point, although perhaps obvious, is apt to be forgotten in discussing the development of regulatory schemes. Certainly the history of medical regulation illustrates it. So also the mere fact that an occupational group was given 'enforceable' privileges, powers, and duties and perhaps called itself a guild did not mean that it immediately acquired all the characteristics implied by that term. They include, as I shall argue, a corporate morality. On the other hand, the fact that this last in particular is lacking may be a fatal flaw.

At the outset of the Renaissance (the later part of the fifteenth century) the Church still controlled important areas of medicine and it had the relevant powers to license practitioners in exorcism. The grant of such licences was not confined to University men; indeed only a very few of the licencees possessed the degree. In 1511–12, Henry VIII instigated the first Medical Act.[21] It made it an offence to practise physic or surgery without either a degree or a bishop's licence. Such a licence could be granted in London by its Bishop or the Dean of St Paul's and outside London either by an ordinary bishop or by the Pope (after 1534, the Archbishop of Canterbury). Cartwright says[22] that this was in consequence of the weakening of ecclesiastical prestige. By contrast, Copeman suggests[23] that the introduction of the licence was an attempt by the Church to regain control over medicine. The Act is silent as to these matters. It does say it was needed because a number of ignorant persons were practising. It lists smiths, weavers, and women.

Whatever the effect of the 1511 Act, in 1518 the Company of Physicians was formed by charter which was confirmed in 1523 by an Act of Parliament.[24] In 1551 it became the Royal College of

Physicians of London. The 'Practice of physic was reserved only to those persons that be profound, sad and discreet, groundedly learned, and deeply studied', that is, University men. Such persons were exempt from various civic duties but enjoined not to engage in trade. It perhaps needs to be re-stressed that at that time, and well into the seventeenth and eighteenth centuries (if not longer) the practice of physic did not involve a great deal of direct physical examination of patients. It had maintained a loyalty to Galen from its foundation until at least well into the seventeenth century.[25] Physicians issued written *concilia*. The Company's original jurisdiction, and until the nineteenth century its principal concern, was London (and seven miles around).[26]

Thomas Linacre was the moving spirit of the foundation of this College of Physicians and its first President.[27] He was associated with Erasmus, More, and Colet – themselves, as we have seen, leaders of early Renaissance England. Linacre himself had spent the years 1487–99 in Italy, receiving his MD at Padua, and for a time enjoying the court of Lorenzo the Magnificent at Florence. In Italy, in accord with the character of the Renaissance, he translated the original Galen from Greek into Latin. In establishing the College of Physicians, Linacre was anxious to set up a deliberately Hippocratic School in England. In intent, it was ancient; in form, medieval; and, in spirit, Renaissance.

At its foundation and since, the College has been an élite. Its powers have rested partly in law, for example, its Charter, and partly on the social connections of its members. In the early days, by insisting on the use of Latin and by embracing the Royal and other court physicians it secured its place in Society. It was however more than an élite. It was organized; and about a particular view of medical practice. This was Hippocratic medicine. It is instructive to compare the original Charter and the early statutes[28] against the main tenets of the Hippocratic tradition.

(1) *Externals must co-operate.* The College had powers over the quality of goods sold by apothecaries and at times sought to prevent any practice except by the order of a physician. Fee splitting between physicians and apothecaries was prohibited.

(2) *The physician is the servant of his art.* The Censors were called '*censores, literatum, morum et medecinarum*'. The practice, morals, and writings of the individual members were to be controlled by officers of the College.

(3) *Practitioners were as brothers.* All Fellows had to attend all

committee, ceremonial, and social meetings of the College and unseemly contention was finable. A physician could not take over the patient of another without recognizing his interests.

(4) *Exploitation is forbidden.* A bargain to restore a patient to health was prohibited; all that was allowed was a moderate fee in proportion to the patient's condition and the physician's own labour. The College reserved a right to correct injustice in relation to fees.

(5) *Holy things are revealed only to holy men.* 'No man is to teach medicaments to the population nor to reveal to them the names of medicines lest the people be injured by their misuse.'

It was otherwise with other medical men. They were 'un-Latined'; their training was by apprenticeship. In the pre-Renaissance period, many occupations were organized about the guild. In England, where by far the largest centre of population was London, these guilds were the companies of its City. By the Middle Ages, they were self-governing confraternities giving mutual aid and protection to their members and furthering their common purpose. They regulated means of unfair competition such as advertising and also such matters as standards and prices for the outside world. They provided their own inspectorates and their own courts.

So far as medicine was concerned the striking thing is that although there were sporadic attempts, it was not separately organized as such. The physicians belonged to the international fraternity of 'Latined' scholars, the so-called *republica literaria*, and, in England, only became guild-like after the foundation of the College of Physicians in 1518. It was not until the later Renaissance that the surgeons became partly free of the Barbers' Company and still later the apothecaries gained independence of the Grocers'. In Tudor times, although physicians could use surgery (or act as an accoucheur) the need for each branch ever to undertake the work of another was contested. It is to be noted that under the early statutes of the College, physicians prescribed, and apothecaries sold, drugs.[29] The different jurisdictions of the several branches of medicine changed over time. Three centuries later, in 1827, the consolidated position was explained by C.J. Best:[30]

For some disorders, relief is sought from medicine, for others, from topical applications.... The first description belongs to the physician and apothecary, the second to the surgeon. The professors of each branch of medicine must sometimes go beyond their proper limits. It may be necessary for the apothecary to use the lancet, and the surgeon, to administer medicines, either to prevent the necessity of an operation, to prepare the patient for it if necessary or to recover him from its effects if performed.

Following Durkheim, I shall argue guilds have an enduring external power. It is perhaps illustrated by the relative failure of an Act of 1542–3,[31] the 'Quacks' Charter'. That Act legalized therapeutic practice (originally, apparently, whether for a fee or not) which involved the external use of herbs, roots, and waters by anyone who had experience by speculation or practice. It hit at aspects of the monopolies of both physicians and surgeons. Potentially it could have expanded to the rest of their activities. That it did not reflects the way in which power is diffused in a differentiated society. According to Clark, in 1625[32] the court held that the Act extended only to gratuitous practice.

In 1540, an Act of Parliament[33] secured a Union of the surgeons' guilds and permission for a member to practise as a surgeon but not a barber.[34] The increase in society's esteem of these 'un-Latined' craftsmen was coincident, and probably connected with, the expression of scholars' interests and ideas in the vernacular. For the two centuries from 1540 to 1745, the practice of surgery was carried out by members of the United Company of Barber-Surgeons.[35] The surgeon members of the United Company still required a Bishop's licence under the terms of the Act of 1511. In 1745 the surgeons left to form a separate company of the City of London. In 1800 they departed from the City, with its overtones of trade, and obtained their Charter from the King to become the College of Surgeons. In 1843 a new Charter was granted and it became in formal terms a Royal College.[36]

Until the early seventeenth century the apothecaries were a part of the Grocers' Company, although their shops were subject to supervision by the College of Physicians. The Company had the monopoly of importation of foreign spices. In 1617 the Society of Apothecaries was separately incorporated as a company of the City of London.[37] This took place for two main reasons. It was an effort to enhance their specialization. Just as important, the physicians were once more concerned with the growth of empirics (that is, people who thought they could practise without theory).[38] The physicians were pleased to be able to keep this jurisdiction under their supervision. The members of the Society of Apothecaries dispensed drugs. They charged for these but were prohibited from levying a fee for any advice by the provisions of the Charter of the Royal College of Physicians. Their shops remained under the nominal supervision of the College and their apprentices were supposed to have gained its President's approval before practising.

As the function of the apothecary changed so did the other estates of medicine. Gradually, by adjusting the price of the drugs they sold to include an element to account for the free advice, they established themselves as the medical advisors to the poor. Clark says:[39] 'One of the unwritten chapters of English social history is the story of the ascent of the apothecaries'. It would seem that the changes were not exclusively English. During the seventeenth century, the apothecaries' practice in Europe (specifically Paris and Rome) as a whole typically reduced the time spent on shopkeeping and increased that on preparing medicines and visiting patients. To an extent (which some books exaggerate) there was also a rise in their standard of education. In England it remained based on apprenticeship, but in some cases Latin became an entrance qualification and there is evidence that some apothecaries attended dissections in the Barbers' Hall.

Late in the century, in London, the College of Physicians began to reassert a concern for the medical care of the deserving poor. After an abortive effort in 1675, a dispensary was established in 1696 and a second in around 1702. Clark, in his exhaustive history of the College,[40] finds no trace of them after 1725. He is at a loss fully to explain why they came or why they went. He suggests a part of the impetus was humanitarian and a part was the unsuccessful attempt to head off the encroachments of the apothecaries. Necessarily, as the College records on the matter fade, he is less clear as to the reasons for closure. He speculates, but doubts, that it might have been due to the complacencies of the age. Although to an extent he takes the point, it seems possible that he has underestimated the consequences of the philanthropic giving.

In 1703 the College sought to impose its statutes on an apothecary who, after the custom of his trade, gave free medical advice but sold his medicines.[41] It argued as regards out-patients that there was a duty on physicians to visit the poor and that the College had 'by a joint stock, erected dispensaries in town where the physicians had given their advice *gratis* and the patients might have their physic prescribed ... at very small expense'. Clark suggests[42] that the court may have been influenced by ideas of treatment of the poor or by the joinder of function of the physician and the apothecary. However that may be, the trend of the previous century was upheld.

At the beginning of the nineteenth century, it was held that an apothecary could charge for advice.[43] Towards the end of that century it was said his role included 'dispensing or mixing medicines, giving medical advice and attending the sick as medical advisor'.[44] Throughout, although it was followed by legal consequences, whether an act was part of the function of an apothecary remained a question of fact rather than of law.[45] By the middle of the century the absence of making-up the prescriptions of others did not prevent a practice being that of an apothecary.[46] The distinguishing features of the apothecary were that he was prepared to visit patients and to give advice and to prescribe on his own initiative even in his own shop.[47] Those who merely dispensed without giving advice were chemists, druggists, or pharmacists. In short, this latter group, which was incorporated as the Pharmaceutical Society in the middle of the century, was doing very similar work to that of the Apothecaries Company at its foundation two centuries earlier. Today, dispensing and the sale of medicines is carried out by or under the supervision of pharmacists.[48]

As regards institutions for the sick, their main foundation occurred in the eighteenth and nineteenth centuries, that is between the Renaissance and into the Industrial Revolution – the few hospitals founded before that time were not then exclusively for the ill. These last included St Bartholomew's in 1123, which began medical education in 1662, and St Thomas's in 1207, which began medical education in 1695.[49] The eighteenth-century hospitals included Westminster (1719), Guy's (1721), St George's (1733), the London (1740), and the Middlesex (1745). Others were established in some provincial towns. Abel-Smith remarks:[50]

> The newer foundations depended largely on current subscriptions to finance their expenditure. The progress of the voluntary hospital movement depended on the willingness of the rich to help the poor, and the money was provided for religious and wider humanitarian reasons. And the scale on which this money was given to hospitals over a period of two centuries indicated a tremendous sense of social duty and responsibility.

He goes on to point out 'Gifts were not, however, disinterested'. The mechanism for the organization of their funding was the 'public trust', more commonly called in lawyer's language, the 'charitable trust'. Donzelot discusses this form of giving:[51]

> [philanthropy] is not to be understood as a naïvely apolitical term signifying a private intervention in the sphere of so-called social problems but must be considered as a deliberately depoliticizing strategy for establishing public services and facilities at a sensitive point midway between private initiative and the state.

He goes on to distinguish philanthropy from charity which[52]

> was alien to this kind of investment; it could only be kindled by the fires of extreme misery, by the sight of spectacular suffering, and then only for the feeling of inflated importance accruing to the giver through the immediate solace his charity brought the sufferer.

Donzelot's contrast between philanthropy and charity is not the same as that of the modern lawyer. To them an almost unprincipled series of specific instances of both his terms are conflated in their concept 'charity'. It seems possible that the expression, 'charitable trust', is a rhetorical device designed to conceal the motivation and effects of this form of public giving. In any event, the law now gives a jargon meaning to the term 'charitable' and there is a special body of rules concerning the administration of these funds.[53]

The Royal Family, the aristocracy, and the social élite were all early subscribers to the hospitals. 'Old governors recruited new governors from their friends and those who wished to be their friends.'[54] Governorship and subscription carried the right to nominate patients and those admitted tended to be those in personal service, that is, in service in the household rather than trading employees, of the governors. They were people to whom a social duty of caring was owed. The principal medical staff, physicians, and surgeons, were recruited from among those the governors consulted privately. Like the governors, these staff were largely unpaid for their hospital work. This honorary work was relevant in maintaining and attracting private clients: willingness to do it demonstrated the individual's attachment to Pythagorean or Hippocratic asceticism. It was this attachment which in turn attracted the private, and paying, client.

At this point I must digress. It is a part of my argument that industrial growth and economic liberalism are linked. Baker[55] is critical of Atiyah's view in *The Rise and Fall of Freedom of*

Contract which I accept. Baker's finding that executory contracts were enforceable in the courts from the sixteenth century is neither surprising nor does it contradict *The Rise and Fall*. I take economic liberalism to be an expression of the cult of individualism. It is not possible here to expand the point or to reflect on other causes: it suffices to remark that as the cult took hold so its economics was reflected in the views of the judges. The cult, as I have argued, in its modern form came from the Renaissance. It was given a renewed emphasis in the Enlightenment: individualism and its economics began in the sixteenth century and gained in intensity at that much later date. History does not move in historians' chapters.

In the early part of the nineteenth century, under the influence of the Enlightenment, and under pressure from this cult, the general law moved not only to consolidate the emerging ideas of freedom of contract but also to lay the foundations for the creation of rights amounting to property in certain types of ideas (at first, at least, confined to those which were commercially exploitable). At the same time the world of science was moving in the opposite direction. There was a greater expectation that scientists should publish. The merchant received his reward in money and through that medium his place in society. The scientist, who at that time almost by definition possessed sufficient funds, gained his place, that is, the esteem of those who mattered to him, by his ideas and not his wealth. True plagiarism occurred, for example, by Lavoissier of Priestley's discovery of oxygen, and, probably also earlier, by either Newton or Leibnitz of the other's discovery of calculus. But it was motivated by pride and not money and was condemned by moral sanction rather than law. The great expansion of scientific knowledge served to strengthen rather than weaken this approach. The basic tenet that a scientific theory was both capable of repeatable experimental validation and could be used as the basis of prediction also served as an incentive to publish, in terms that were intelligible to that community.

However this may be, medicine was distinguished from other forces and events. As early as the end of the seventeenth century the collective secrecy of the College of Physicians was under severe attack from pamphleteers, mainly, but not exclusively, outside its ranks. It led to the abrogation of the College's statute which prohibited the publication of medical skills.[56] This in turn reinforced the openness of the general scientific ethic. But it would seem that medical men as such were and still are unhappy at popularization of their knowledge, and I doubt that this is entirely due to a distrust of simplification. More likely, a part of the desire not to tell is attributable not only to diagnosis being acquired by the 'insights of the bedside' but to prognosis and particularly prescription requiring that form of understanding.[57] I would argue that the reluctance continues to distinguish them from the general run of the scientific community.

Until the beginning of the nineteenth century, medicine in all its branches was substantially unregulated outside London. By then there had been great changes in the distribution and size of the population; although the balance still lent toward London, it was becoming impossible to ignore the provinces. The College of Physicians attempted to extend its monopolies to them but it failed, at least directly.[58] The upward trend in aspiration and status of other medical men continued. As wars have always done, the long wars with the French produced, and satisfied the need for more, and more accomplished, surgeons. Similarly, there was a failed attempt by some of the apothecaries to force the newly emergent chemists and druggists out of the market; they could not carry their fellows. The apothecaries could not preserve their position by looking downwards. The move was translated into a campaign for a general medical qualification. But although the stratification of the estates of medicine was under stress, it could not be easily abandoned.

Following Foucault, I have suggested there was not a linear progression to rationality or to the abandonment of the doctor's privilege in his relationship with his patients. Indeed one consequence of the coming of the clinic was to increase his authority. But times of change are times to rethink and often reassert old values in new ways. Probably the most important attempt in this direction was that of Thomas Percival in *Medical Ethics; or a Code of Institutes and Precepts adapted to the Professional Conduct of Physicians and Surgeons.*

The significance of this work needs to be located. In 1955 Forbes could suggest,[59] 'No later work has modified in any material degree the precepts and practice defined by Percival'. This is, of course, a judgement of retrospect. Included in it is a possibility of one of two things: Percival's work was either a code of ethics or a reflection of a cultural understanding. Although circulated privately for some time, it was first published generally in 1803, with further editions in England in 1827 and 1849. More significant than its purpose was its reception in England and in the United States. In the former its importance is based in its authorship being a provincial practitioner, that is, outside the centres of English medical power; those who knew how to behave to others or even what changes should be implemented did not need it explained.

There seems little doubt that in North America it has been treated as a Code from which all later official formulations have sprung. The work's ready adoption[60] by several of the medical associations of the United States is explained by its backward looking content but futuristic formalism; there with all values in question the stability of the past needed to be codified. It is another example of the former colonies keeping so much of British institutions in metamorphic form. This is not surprising nor does it affect the thesis I shall advance that professional ethics can only be known or cared about by the initiates.

The tone of Percival's work is quickly established. The dedication (to his son) says it will 'soften your manners, expand your affections, and form you to that propriety and dignity of conduct, which are essential to the character of a GENTLEMAN'. And paragraph I: 'Hospital physicians and surgeons ... should study, also, in their deportment, so as to unite *tenderness* with *steadiness*, and *condescension* with *authority* as to inspire the minds of their patients with gratitude, respect and confidence'. So also paragraph II: 'The *choice* of a *physician* or *surgeon* cannot be allowed to hospital patients, consistently with the regular and established succession of medical attendance'. It is against this background that the work discusses the proper relationships between practitioners in the three estates of medicine – when each should be called in and how they should relate to each other. Patients are discussed, but only in terms of how medical men can secure their trust and hence co-operation.

With Percival looking back, in other ways medicine was looking forward. The Apothecaries Act of 1815 was passed.[61] It extended the legal powers of the Society of Apothecaries to the whole of England. Of course the Act failed: the Society did not have the administrative capacity, even if it had the will to enforce it. The Act reinforced the link between apothecaries and the trading ethos by reaffirming their need for an apprenticeship and the controlling influence over the Society's affairs of the College of Physicians. More important, however, in the same year, 1815, the Society imposed: a five year apprenticeship; certificates of attendance at lectures in anatomy, physiology, and the theory and practice of medicine; and a requirement that a candidate must have 'walked the wards' of a recognized hospital for at least six months. This was similar to the rule the College of Surgeons had imposed two years earlier that new members should have been attached to a hospital surgical ward for one year. The effect was that medical students had to spend time in hospitals. There was a growth in the number of hospitals and the beginnings of systematic study. In 1821, Charing Cross Hospital was founded to provide education. It was followed by University and King's Colleges both of which were multi-faculty and included a hospital and associated medical school. In 1836, London University received its Charter and began giving degrees in medicine but it was not until 1854 that they were recognized for licensing purposes. The growing practice of the dual qualification of LSA and MRCS in time led to those holding them being known as general practitioners. The practice produced examinations but no generally organized education.

The growth in the numbers of doctors meant that only a small proportion could reach the ranks of the full honorary physician or surgeon. It became common for posts to be granted by purchase or nepotism and aspiring candidates were exploited and frustrated. Abel-Smith suggests these young doctors had one way in which they could show skill superior to that of their seniors to the profitable private patient. They could specialize: 'specialization was a form of self-advertisement'.[62] On the continent, the trend was even more marked.[63] At any rate in England, specialized hospitals were started and, in contrast to the older hospitals, were controlled by doctors. They were more aggressive in their fund raising and thus diverted resources from the voluntary hospitals. Some of them introduced charges which were in competition with those of the general practitioners. They were accordingly not popular with those in the established centres of medicine.

Quality and status are not always coincident. At the beginning of the Industrial Revolution, the Fellows of the Royal College of Physicians were regarded by the rest of society as the élite. The College was among the last to adopt modern ideas of scientific medicine.[64] At that time, although a notable few (and some its licentiates) had for their own intellectual purposes, rather than for the corporate identity of their College, re-created aspects of both theory and practice, the knowledge and understanding required of the Fellows was still largely based on the classical, particularly Galenic, writings. Since a university degree was required, they were, with exceptions in the form of foreign, Scottish and Irish degrees, in the main graduates of Oxford and Cambridge; and, as such necessarily members of the Church of England.

Having the status of gentlemen, they entered even the houses of the powerful through the front door; other sections of the medical profession used the tradesmen's entrance. For example, in the early nineteenth century, even within the Royal College of Surgeons there was a grievance of its Members concerning the requirement that they should only use the back door to the College itself. The front door was reserved for the governing Fellows. It seems likely that the power of the physicians, their influence, was reinforced by the application of Hippocratic ideas of professional confidence. If they knew little of what is today regarded as of medical value, at least they could act as the confidants of the powerful. Their advice was sought on matters of state as much as of medicine. The trust thus earned was, both individually and collectively, an important part of the source of their influence.

In France, as Foucault shows, there was a similar, but characteristically earlier, greater, and more elaborate use of institutional medical power.[65] In 1776, the Government established the Société Royale de Medicine. According to Foucault, it became responsible for investigation of epidemic movements, for recording treatments and experiments, and for supervision of, and prescription to, doctors in the field. Out of these powers a stage was reached[66] where:

> The Société no longer consisted solely of doctors who devoted themselves to the study of collective pathological phenomena; it had become the official organ of a *collective consciousness* of pathological phenomena, a consciousness that operated at both the level of experience and the level of knowledge, in the international as well as the national space.

In England initially this role was fulfilled by *The Lancet* and the *Provincial Medical and Surgical Journal* (which later became *The British Medical Journal*). Following this argument of Foucault in the next chapter, I shall show such devices are important in developing collective morality.

The conditions (and methods of payment) of work in the first half of the century were in conflict with the classical professional model which presupposes that the professional practitioner is a 'gentleman'. The concept assumes a purposeful existence based upon the lack of want of material needs or desires. Wakley, a leader of the 'medical reform' movement, was much concerned with incomes. But one of the most potent arguments of the professional is dignity, not comparative wages. This ambiguity was partially resolved in 1832 by the formation of the Provincial Medical and Surgical Association. The object of this, in common with some other rank and file organizations, was to improve the conditions of qualified doctors, but also, in contrast with some of the others, to engage in scientific discourse.[67] In 1855 it expanded to become the modern British Medical Association. It is to be emphasized that the Association's origin was the representation of provincial practitioners, that is, practitioners distanced from the professional élite. On the other hand, it rejected a posture of outright opposition to that stratum. Indeed from the first it included not only general practitioners but also hospital physicians and surgeons. The provincial alliance was crucial because the theory, praxis, and reception of medicine were changing so as to blur the functions of the old orders of medicine. The Association was uniquely placed to take advantage of the change.

To anticipate events, the British Medical Association, from having a scientific and social origin, has become involved as a part of the machinery of government. It has for example used both its epidemiological power (by organizing reports from members) and its prestige to extend iatrocracy. One significant example of this was its involvement in the agitation for the Schools Health Service. And so also was its concern in the 1930s over levels of nutrition and more recently the campaigns regarding crash-helmets, seat-belts, and smoking. It not only acts as spokesman for the profession and its members but also is directly and by statute involved in the administration of certain 'health' related Acts of Parliament.[68]

In 1858 the first of the modern Medical Acts was passed.[69] The Act established the General Medical Council to supervise a register of qualified medical people. The Act did not seek to outlaw unqualified or unorthodox practice: it made it an offence for the unqualified to pretend to be qualified. In this, in one way, it followed Adam Smith's idea that demand would determine supply, and in another, Chadwick's that therapeutic medical practice was not very important. Although the Act provided for the General Medical Council to supervise education, it did not seek to impose a single examination. By making provision for an authorized pharmacopoeia, the Act maintained the doctors' control over pharmacy. As a whole the Act disappointed some of its advocates. It failed to place power in the representatives of the general run of qualified men: rather it effected a compromise between what the Royal College of Physicians, the Royal College of Surgeons, and the Society of Apothecaries saw as their interests. Clarke suggests that the Act (or rather the Bill of 1844) was both an example of increased State power and of Parliament being used to ratify decisions taken elsewhere.[70]

However that may be, two things were clear: the settled compromise achieved within the British Medical Association (which by then had included London practitioners) enabled it to influence the balance within the eventual Act and indeed eight out of twenty-three of the first General Medical Council were members of the Association. Secondly, and more surprisingly, the Act compelled a homogeneity.[71] The consequence of this Act was that there was no discrete role left for apothecaries. It confirmed what could have been seen earlier, the encroachment by physicians on them. As physicians rested less on Aesculapian power and began to rely more on science, and chemotherapy in particular, they began doing the apothecaries' work.

The Act succeeded where the 1815 Act failed. Boards of Guardians were no longer able to employ unqualified medical officers. The new breed of doctor brought two characteristics: he had received his medical training in one of the voluntary hospital medical schools and, perhaps in part because he managed to afford to go there, his social status was likely to be higher. Because the Act created a single body to register the qualified, that body was in position to provide sanctions for breaches of medical ethics.

The Amendment Act of 1886[72] provided for all practitioners to be qualified in the then three branches of practice, namely, medicine, surgery, and midwifery. It also made provision for the election of general practitioners. It paved the way for the formal recognition of the general practitioner and consultant hierarchy. Some wished to model this last by comparison with Queen's Counsel and juniors at the Bar.[73] In the long run the general practitioners managed to persuade the profession as a whole to accept the idea of the 'consultant' as a class of doctor better but more specialized than they but who would only see patients when they were referred by a general practitioner.[74] Despite the evident financial interest in this arrangement, it was expressly justified in terms of the dignity and honour of the profession.

At the beginning of the nineteenth century admission to the hospitals themselves, whether as in- or out-patient, depended on the decisions of the governors or often a small group known as 'almoners': the clinic *qua* clinic had not achieved its pre-eminence. In some hospitals, the medical staff could admit accident cases but generally there was lay control. The effect was that most patients were only admitted if they were 'curable': the hospital was for rest rather than treatment. The inmates were poor but not destitute. The relative status of these people was important. We have already seen that as medical technology grew, the doctor could understand the illness from his own observation; authority moved from the patient to the doctor. So also, as the teaching hospital assumed importance and because its inmates were of dependent status, the trend for the shift of authority was more pronounced. Because the inmates were poor[75] 'charitable work became the key to fame and fortune'. And, since after 1813–15 doctors increasingly were taught in these hospitals, the methods they learnt were applied generally. The doctors required a guarantee of interesting cases for research or teaching (which were themselves sources of medical reputations and income) or a quick turnover which might give an indication to potential private patients of the competence of the practitioner.

It was not however until the middle of the century that the doctors there began to assume real responsibility for admissions; began, therefore, to re-apply the Hippocratic tradition of classical medicine. They did this by gradually taking control of the types of cases to be excluded and then, by imposing quotas on categories (for example, medical or surgical) to be included under the system of governors' nominees. Towards the century's end, the hospital was becoming a more effective place for the treatment of illness. Anaesthesia and the introduction of anti- and aseptic techniques by Lister (following Pasteur's germ theory) had begun to make surgery safer. With the new century chronic illness was not treated, and was not seen to be treatable, in hospital; acute illness was.

It was natural that the question of payment for the honorary medical staff should be raised. The objections to payment were the same as before: payment (to either hospital or staff) might affect the appeal work; and as the Cave Committee said:[76] 'although the services of the staff are honorary, they obtain a valuable return in the form of medical and surgical experience and enhanced reputation which accrues to the member of the visiting staff of a great hospital'. That is, honorary status was the foundation of lucrative private practice; and the staff would less easily be able to keep other practitioners out of these places of prestige.

Although for a long time the voluntary hospital with its internal medical hierarchy[77] remained the centre of excellence, and provided the model for aspirations, similar patterns applied to the provision of medical aid for the poor. The Poor Law Amendment

Act 1834 had sought to give outdoor relief to the aged and sick but only workhouse provision for the able-bodied who did not support themselves:[78] the workhouse was intended to provide a standard of amenity less than the poorest paid labourer (it was known as the principle of 'less eligibility'). The scheme was paid for in the main by local traders as ratepayers. It was administered by Boards of Guardians elected by these paymasters.

Despite the 1815 Apothecaries Act, particularly outside London, regulation of the profession was substantially unknown, and the rise in the demand for doctors led to quacks and charlatans. One reason for the increase was that the Poor Law Unions were required to appoint medical officers and most often they did so with little regard for competence; and indeed many Boards employed unqualified people. At least in the case of the Unions, because basic qualifications were largely irrelevant to the pay-master there was a tendency to pay poor wages. There is evidence that there was considerable employment of partially qualified young men who tendered for appointments on the basis of taking the least possible payments. It would seem, however, that this can be only a partial explanation for the increase in unqualified practitioners because the numbers of those in practice considerably exceeded those employed by the Unions.

At the beginning, as with the voluntary hospitals, the patients served by these medical officers were therefore not chosen by them. The officers had it in their legal power to declare anybody to be sick and therefore eligible for outside relief. But domiciliary work intruded on the time available for private practice. It was easier in time, effort, and resources for them, and for the Guardians that outdoor relief should be refused. Further, it was seen to be important to 'prevent medical aid from generating or encouraging pauperism'.[79]

With the advance of technical medicine and with the growth in collective consciousness (precipitated by similar training and by other factors) there was, as we have seen, a consequent growth in the social status of doctors. The newly qualified knew more, expected more, and, what they said carried more weight in, and indeed outside, the Poor Law institutions. The rise of the hospital and particularly the teaching hospital gave institutional reality to the idea in the Hippocratic Oath which required of doctors that there should be reverence for their teachers and that medical knowledge should be shared among them but to the exclusion of others.

So also the Hippocratic injunction that externals should co-operate with physicians was combined with aspirations to upward mobility among the generality of practitioners. From their lower social status, they sought to emulate the political influence of the Royal College of Physicians. By the middle of the century this was manifested in public campaigning. *The Lancet*[80] conducted an influential investigation which opened the way to the passage of the Metropolitan Poor Act 1867. We may note in passing that Abel-Smith suggests, but with some exaggeration,[81] that it was 'an important step in English social history. It was the first explicit acknowledgement that it was the duty of the state to provide hospitals for the poor.' Strictly he is right only as regards hospitals; the point is exaggerated because the State, that is, the governmental authorities, had already assumed responsibilities in health care in respect of vaccination for all those, including the poor, who desired it.

The Act and the associated Poor Law Amendment Act of 1868 required the building of infirmaries for different categories of sick people. These were physically separated from the workhouse and thus more easily fell under medical control. In the early days they did not usually aspire to the standards of the voluntary hospitals, and indeed at times a modified form of the Poor Law restrictions was applied to prevent malingering. Gradually, however, questions of admission became determined by medical superintendents. Apparently for reasons which included professional status, they copied the institutions where they had been trained and admitted only acute cases.[82] The strength of iatrocracy became more than sufficient to undermine the economic acceptability of the principle of 'less eligibility'. Doctors were able to substitute medical for lay judgements. In the limited intellectual and mystical field they claimed as theirs they were able to define who should, and hence who should not, receive their compassion.[83]

5

Professionalism

Professionalism

All this leads a clearer idea of the nature of the occupation in the years of, and preceding, the Industrial Revolution. There is moreover, we may recall, one other fact of which account must be taken in order to understand the nature of the profession: it is not possible to review the history of the doctor–patient relationship without considering the transformation of the meaning of 'cure' discussed in Chapter 1. The function of the relationship has changed.

Social status and incomes were not (and are not yet) dependent merely upon any measurable success. Before the opening of the nineteenth century, there were clear distinctions between the physicians, the surgeons, and the apothecaries. In retrospect, we can see that both the surgeons and the apothecaries were achieving limited success in a modern sense. The former did so by applying to civilian populations the techniques they learnt in war; the latter by the increasingly skilful use of pain-killing drugs, particularly opiates.

Whatever was the position as judged by *success* in the years between the Renaissance and the Industrial Revolution the *mode of organization* of both surgeons and apothecaries became more like that of the Royal College of Physicians.[1] And even that sector of the medical profession which was outside the leadership group, the provincial practitioners, was never unanimous in even attempting to achieve a total autonomy. For example, from the foundation of the Provincial Medical and Surgical Association to that of the modern British Medical Association, the desire was to produce an arena in which those doctors could advance their science amongst themselves as well as jointly seek to enhance their prestige.

This history is my first cause to reconsider the sociologists' view of the nature of the idea of the profession and indeed the rise in professionalization. It is unnecessary to enter into the debate concerning the meaning of these terms. Although he offers a useful account of the various and sometimes contradictory meanings in the word *professional*,[2] Freidson also says:[3]

> Historically, the profession's development ... seems to have required protection from the urgent ignorance of its clientele, the mischief of low-class competitors, and other forces destructive to an infant discipline.... Freed from trade and competition, supported by the state ... it was ... able to develop the capacity to nourish itself.... *While the profession's autonomy seems to have facilitated the improvement of scientific knowledge ... it seems to have impeded the improvement of the social modes of applying that knowledge.*

There are, as I argue, a number of difficulties with this view. In the main, however, it asserts that the occupation was not a profession until it was technically competent, that throughout the nineteenth century it could be described as 'an infant discipline'. Except in a definition which assumes the conclusion and a forced discontinuity in history it runs against the English evidence that either of these is true. Not dissimilar criticisms of the Royal College of Physicians were being voiced at the end of the seventeenth century. By the opening years of the nineteenth Percival's backward looking code of ethics was establishing the occupational mores which have lasted until today. So also, as we shall see, even in the absence of any modern technical competence, the State (via the Privy Council) was increasingly relying on the College. Its authority, far from being 'infant', was if anything patriarchal.

It is this understanding which leads me to doubt two influential types of analysis: first the thesis[4] that *professionalism* in some way began in the nineteenth century and secondly, its economic reinterpretation.[5] The key points in the evidence for the former are: (1) the creation of effective boards to enforce professional ethics; (2) the increasing bureaucratization of professional organization generally; (3) the growth in individual professional incomes; (4) the growth in numbers of practitioners; and (5) the growth in paraprofessions.

Each of these factors has had important consequences. I doubt however that they are sufficient to sustain the thesis that the rise in professionalism is associated with the early part of that century, or its capitalism. The reorganization of the medical profession at that time ran counter to the prevailing ideologies of classical economics. As Foucault shows, the almost contemporaneous attempt to apply those ideologies to medicine failed in post-Revolutionary France. Further, I see the history I have set out as showing that the institutions and structures of medicine pre-date the Industrial Revolution. As regards medical practice, as Holmes shows,[6] these trends were apparent at an earlier period and they were associated with at least some non-capitalist phenomena. To him, the rise was an increase in status and coherence, training was formalized and outside the grammar school and university system, recruits came from higher social strata and their growth in self-esteem and self-confidence was reflected in increasing internal recruitment, that is, sons following fathers.

The growth in scientific medicine (but not yet in scientism) led to large numbers of English doctors seeking the whole or part of their training at Leyden and after 1726 at the Edinburgh Medical School. It may be remarked that the influence of these two schools on English medicine preserved the link between English practice and the Continent, and goes a long way to refuting the suggestion that the Anglo-American profession, in contrast to those in France and Germany, was not linked to the form of the medieval University.[7] The growth of the provincial towns led to formalization of the organization of the medical practitioners; at the same time high social status could be achieved by professional skill rather than land ownership. There is no doubt that this trend appeared after the seventeenth-century trend described by Plumb[8] in which the

> image of a gentleman ... represented ... the triumph of the aristocracy at the expense of the middle class, whose own merits – prudence, reticence, professional education – came to be regarded as either boorish or comic ... the possession of land achieved ... a sanctity in western Europe – it was the way to salvation, the route by which a merchant's children might become gentlemen.

In other words, social status in the provincial cities by way of professionalism is a phenomenon which had begun by at least the eighteenth century. As we shall see, it was not generalized among such practitioners until the early years of the twentieth.

The economic reinterpretation of professionalism requires a number of assumptions for which only some (and, I say, only partial) historical evidence can be supplied. Thus in Berlant's hands:[9] 'Ten of the many aspects of the general process of monopolization seem to stand out'. They are

(1) 'The creation of commodities .... The task is to convince a buyer that the service is a commodity, that it should be sold for a price or fee and that other forms of exchange such as friendship are not legitimate.'

(2) 'The separation of the performance of service from the satisfaction of client interests' – Thus a cure is not guaranteed.

(3) 'The creation of scarcity .... In the case of the medical profession, scarcity has been most effectively achieved by licensing.'

(4) 'The monopolization of supply' – This has been done by 'persuading the state to eliminate competitors' and the professional control of education.

(5) 'Restriction of group membership .... It increases membership loyalty by increasing per capita income within the same market, independently raises prices by decreasing supply relative to demand, and helps make possible noncompetitive relationships among group members.'

(6) 'The elimination of external competition .... Typically, the group claims to supply the only authentic commodity (for example, declares others "quacks")' – It needs legal licensure and ethical claims.

(7) 'The capacity to fix prices above theoretical competitive market value' – Despite anti-trust legislation, price fixing, recast in moral terms, continues to exist.

(8) 'The unification of supplier's – Co-ordination requires the development of a sense of mutual interests, group identification and the creation of a system of group controls to ensure equal pricing.

(9) 'The elimination of internal competition' – Thus there are medical ethics, and prohibitions on price competition, advertising and bargaining.

(10) 'The development of group solidarity and co-operativeness .... Fraternalistic devices constitute some of the major noneconomic means by which internal competition is eliminated.'

Curiously Berlant regards the Hippocratic corpus not in monopolistic terms but as an attempt[10] by a small 'charismatic group of physicians to create a monopoly of virtue'. Although he recognizes the asceticism, it is necessary for his argument that this attitude should be in contrast with economic monopolization. In my argument, as will appear, the latter, if it occurs at all, is a by-product of an ethos.

A more complex interpretation but one still (despite his remark[11] that 'it would be a vulgar mistake to dwell on economic interests alone') rooted in economics is offered by Freidson. He says:[12] 'Many of the powers ascribed to professions by critics cannot be discerned in the activities of everyday practitioners ... we must move outside the workplace and into the broader political economy'. For example, in terms similar to Berlant he says:[13]

> The most impressive form of credentialism works to produce an occupational cartel, which gains and preserves monopolistic control over the supply of a good or service in order to enhance the income of its members by protecting them from competition by others.

Freidson goes on however to distinguish[14] public from private licensing. In the United States the latter is often more important[15] because the Federal government depends on it.

He says:[16]

> So long as the goal of therapy is maintained and physicians are held to know how to achieve it, physicians will maintain a place of privilege and 'authority' by virtue of their expertise quite independently of bureaucratic office, and patients will hold a place of subordination by virtue of their helplessness and ignorance.

He argues:[17] 'A service orientation is not exclusively held by a profession but because of its public perception the profession is given its autonomy'. And he states:[18] 'professionals ... act as gatekeepers of desirable goods and services.... The physician alone determines whether a person will be admitted to a hospital and when he or she is to be discharged.'

He says:[19] 'Stress is placed on the necessity of faith or trust in the practitioner in short, on *imputed* rather than demonstrated competence'. And later,[20] 'Insistence on faith constitutes insistence that the client give up his role as an independent adult and, by so neutralizing him, protects the esoteric foundation of the profession's institutionalized authority'. He says:[21] '*Belief* in the extraordinary character of the work ... sustains the ... claim that ... he must be independent and autonomous' and[22] it leads to professional pride.

He says:[23] '[The physician] does maintain the right to diagnose and prescribe according to criteria evaluated by colleagues, not by laymen. This is certainly the very heart of professional autonomy.' And he states:[24] 'autonomy of technique is at the core of what is unique about the profession': out of it comes control of the occupational environment. He goes on to argue:[25]

Emphasizing the position of an occupation in a political economy ... the Ethic called professionalism does not distinguish professions from other occupations and is not useful for explaining the character of ... self-regulation ... the Ethic I did find useful and necessary ... was one that was derived from the 'situated actions' of consultative, practical work.... The general Ethic seems to reflect primarily the occupation's task of attempting to persuade society to grant and sustain its professional status.

But, he adds[26] that since the weaknesses of professions 'stem from professionalism itself, professions cannot be expected to be able to rectify them'. This is so because[27] 'the critical flaw in professional autonomy' is:

by allowing and encouraging the development of self-sufficient institutions, it develops and maintains in the profession a self-deceiving view of objectivity and reliability of its knowledge and of the virtues of its members.... Consulting professions are not baldly self-interested unions struggling for their resources at the expense of others and of the public interest. Rather, they are well-meaning groups which are protected from the public by their organized autonomy and at the same time protected from their own honest self-scrutiny by their sanctimonious myths of the inherently superior qualities of themselves as professionals – of their knowledge and of their work.

Freidson argues[28] that critical elements of professional behaviour, including ethicality, vary not so much with training as with the working environment, because practitioners are part of the environment. Despite this they are predominantly from the bourgeoisie and[29] there is a 'curious ideological ambivalence in the premedical student, certainly composed in part of an inclination to assume a service orientation in the form of wishing to help people, but countered by an inclination to desire prestige and money as well'. He offers two possible reasons:[30] 'Sponsorship ... facilitates the careers of those selected and relegates those not so selected to a position where they compete under decidedly disadvantageous terms'. And more recently:[31] 'the class theories [of professional] specialization may be divisive and fragmenting.... Rather, at bottom is the fact of higher education, which ... can be seen as a common cultural experience.' And[32] 'a critical criterion lies in some degree of exposure to higher education and the formal knowledge it transmits'.

From a different perspective Rueschemeyer[33] suggests a number of other burdens my thesis has to bear. He summarizes the 'functionalist model' of professional work:[34]

> [T]he model begins with a knowledge-based competence held by experts, a competence accepted as pragmatically relevant for problems which are important for those directly beset by them.... Individually and, in association, collectively, the professions 'strike a bargain with society' in which they exchange competence and integrity against the trust of client and community, relative freedom from lay supervision and interference, protection against unqualified competition as well as substantial remuneration and higher social status. As guarantees of this self-control they point to careful recruitment and training, formal organization and informal relations among colleagues, codes of ethics, and professional courts or committees enforcing these codes.

He goes on:[35] 'A crucial question is whether the quality of an expert intervention can be judged by evaluating the result'. He argues[36] that 'there are many other bases of professional privilege and especially of professional autonomy than the bargaining chips identified by the functionalist model'. The privileges of the professions generally are similar to those held by any group that ranks high in social status.

> This suggests ... that we should expect 'survivals' of uncertain duration, which have their original basis in past patterns of culture ... though part of their power resources may be used to acquire new functions in a changed political economy.... Other factors, not included in the model, buttress professional privilege and autonomy – even in the face of a considerable gap between reality and claims to effective self-control. This gives credence to a view ... which sees the machinery of professional organization as a tool for acquiring and maintaining a privileged and autonomous position and only secondarily, if at all, as an instrument of professional self-control.

He adopts Freidson's conception of a profession as[37] 'distinct from other occupations in that it has been given the right to control its own work', and Larson's view[38] of professional self-control arising out of 'expanding potential demand in the course of urbanization, increasing market exchange and capitalist industrialization'.[39] Having considered the role of scientific knowledge, he says[40]

> Being learned in major cultural traditions, consensually accepted as valid and pragmatically relevant – at least in basic outline and on the part of dominant social groups – confers quasi-charismatic prestige and constitutes a powerful source of expert authority and legitimation of privilege.

In short, Berlant and to an extent Freidson on the one hand have conceived medical practice as an economic activity and, on the other, Rueschemeyer has blended the functionalist approach with structuralism. I have had a different emphasis. I called it 'idealism'. My approach leads me to review much of the evidence upon which particularly Berlant and Rueschemeyer rely.

I do not agree that high status in society or high incomes have much to do with the essence of professionalism. I have said, and will return to argue, that implicit in the idea of the professional medical man is the concept of the Pythagorean gentleman. Such a gentleman does not turn his mind to the connection between work and wealth. He is not concerned with his own labour and thus not with his role in the 'division of labour'. In so far as he does, he is less than the ideal. It follows that once income – or rather the capacity to have spending power – is taken for granted, there are greater opportunities to reach toward the ideal. Despite this many have associated the rise in income with a rise in professionalism. To do so however is to forget that for large periods of history most professional men were relatively poor,[41] indeed even today, on a not unduly wide understanding of 'professional', many (particularly women in nursing for example) still are. It is also to fail to recognize the essential ambiguity in the idea of the wealthy professional man.[42] The morality of service is a part of professionalism: to reap the rewards of this world is almost to contradict its own values.

I doubt also that patients have ever gone to doctors because of an empirical assessment that they are in fact successful. It appears more likely that for a variety of reasons they went (and still go) because patients have believed that doctors can help. As the earlier discussion of 'cure' shows, it is not necessary to rely on a placebo effect. In the Middle Ages, as Finucane suggests, the doctor's failure was excluded by reference to divine intervention. Some of the reasons for consulting doctors have been suggested by Horobin.[43] To describe them, he uses words such as 'commitment',[44] 'comportment',[45] and 'probity'. He argues that service is 'a moral imperative'.[46] These are, of course, modern expressions of the Hippocratic ideal.

I go further than Horobin for I see in these imperatives not a mere morality but fundamentals of the relationship. It seems real to say that professional practice (including its altruism) is not just a means to live, it is also 'the first necessity of living' – it is a vocation. Indeed, a divorce between service and reward is essential to professional practice. The doctor wields his authority within the doctor–patient relationship by means of the trust he creates. This creation of dependence is central to the activity and not as in Berlant's reconstruction a mere strategy for monopolization. The trust, as in effect Ladd argues,[47] is placed under strain precisely where the supposed expertise can be judged by results. Thus it is the successes of modern medicine which are challenging the essential base of Hippocratic medicine – the peer group may not be any longer the only forum in which competence is evaluated.

The ideal–typical gentleman

It is for these reasons that it is necessary to turn to the link between the practice of medicine and the concept of the gentleman. In this it is important not to confuse the ideal with everyday practice. Of course, within the 'political economy' – I prefer the term 'body politic' – ideals are not realized but their existence still directs much behaviour. We have seen the links between Hippocrates and Pythagoras. The highest of the Pythagorean ideals has close links with what Hirschman called *vita contemplativa*. It presupposes a way of life which does not depend upon the earning of income to support it. One of the earliest, and probably still the most perceptive, descriptions of the attributes of the ideal–typical gentleman is Baldesar Castiglione's *The Book of the Courtier*[48] written in the early Renaissance. Later I shall seek to show the relation of this ideal to the modern medical profession. I shall argue that this description is applicable to the personal attributes of the ideal physician and that we expect doctors to aspire to it.

It is helpful first to summarize his model and assess its effect without direct reference to medicine. *The Courtier* was influential throughout Europe including Tudor England. Della Casa's *Galateo*, 1558,[49] was clearly influenced by it. That was however written for a less scholastic and less lordly audience. The first English translation of *The Courtier* was by Sir Thomas Hoby in 1561. Elias[50] says that the decisive work was Erasmus's *On Civility in Children* published in 1530. Since Castiglione was apparently writing between 1508 and 1516[51] it would appear that he was the first. The point, however, matters little: the date of the change – the early Renaissance – is clear.[52]

The work sets out to describe the characteristics of the perfect courtier (*cortegiano*) – the term gentleman (*gentilomo*) is used as a synonym. It is important in understanding it, that it offers not only a description but also a possibility. Just as Machiavelli brought science and cynicism to state craft, so Castiglione brought them to manners.[53] *The Courtier* shocked[54] precisely because in rejecting the basis of stability of medieval society it joined the older ideas of the chivalry of the nobility to the Renaissance cult of the individual. The Renaissance, Castiglione, and Machiavelli provided the challenge to the privileges of the nobility of the later Middle Ages.

In large part, the attributes Castiglione describes are capable of cultivation[55] and produce a discernable, but not necessarily economic, reward. Indeed, because attributes are not always recognized the perfect courtier should 'bolster up his inherent worth with skill and cunning'.[56] Castiglione's perfect courtier is well-bred[57] but this is not because blood was an inherent guide to attributes but rather because good family links indicate that the desired qualities are more likely to be present. Coleman[58] makes the same point for the nineteenth century: 'it was normally not the first generation of sons who were ... dispatched [to the Public Schools] to learn the gentlemanly arts, but the second, ie the grandsons or grand-nephews, as the whole family moved up the scale of wealth and status'.

In physical accomplishments, to Castiglione, it is important[59] that the gentleman should be good at the kind of sports lords enjoy (and particularly that he should avoid losing at other sports, for example, wrestling, to common people); his physique[60] should be graceful, beautiful, but manly and not effeminate. His clothing[61] should adopt the style of the majority but be 'sober and restrained rather than foppish'.[62] He should be enterprising, bold and loyal in small things or great.[63] He has 'liberality, munificence, the desire for honour, gentleness, charm, affability'.[64] He should be able to 'laugh, jest, banter, romp and dance'.[65] He should not 'profess to be a great eater or drinker'.[66] Taking a point whose importance will appear later in my argument, 'Laughter' in particular 'is seen only in men'.[67]

Proportionate modesty[68] is esteemed because it implies self-confidence and the self-praise is implicit and not expressed: that is to say modesty is essential but it can be both overdone or underdone. He argues[69] that the right amount of modesty does give personal advancement. The 'universal rule' is:[70]

> to steer away from affectation at all costs ... and to practise in all things a certain nonchalance which conceals all artistry and makes whatever one says or does seem uncontrived and effortless ... true art is what does not seem to be art; and the most important thing is to conceal it, because if it is revealed this discredits a man completely and ruins his reputation ... to reveal intense application and skill robs everything of grace.

The emphasis is on nonchalance not incompetence. The perfect courtier thus does not do things in which he is not accomplished. He is, however, capable not merely of physical prowess but he can also paint, make music, enjoy poetry, and is a scholar.[71]

> You know that in war what really spurs men to bold deeds is the desire for glory, whereas anyone who acts for gain or from any other motive not only fails to accomplish anything worth while but deserves to be called a miserable merchant rather than a gentleman. And it is true glory that is entrusted to the sacred treasury of letters, as everyone knows except those who are so unfortunate as not to have made their acquaintance .... The kind of glory of which they have experience is nothing in comparison with the almost everlasting glory about which, unfortunately, they know nothing; and since, therefore, glory means so little to them, we may reasonably believe that, unlike those who understand its nature, they will run few risks in pursuing it.

This search for glory is to be accompanied by a rejection of flattery and even with some protest against justified praise. The gentleman is to be cautious[72] since all men like to find fault with others. He participates[73] 'as an amateur, making it clear that he neither seeks nor expects any applause. Nor, even though his performance is outstanding, should he let it be thought that he has spent on it much time or trouble'. And always[74]

> he can do everything possible and ... everyone marvels at him and he at no one ... [he] praises the achievements of others with great kindness and goodwill; and although he may think himself a man to be admired and by a long chalk superior to everyone else, he should not reveal this.

Since perfection is not possible, he should avoid seeming ignorant[75] by implying a greater understanding than he has, and if need be, but only where necessary, he should be prepared to admit total ignorance.

In Britain, the medical profession did not begin to achieve the accoutrements of the gentleman's status until the Industrial Revolution was well advanced, until, that is, the second half of the nineteenth century. For example, navy and army surgeons were not given an equal place to that of full combatant officers until the very end of the century. There was for example an early grievance (in 1831) of members of the Royal College of Surgeons that its Council did not object to the exclusion of Navy surgeons from the King's Levées. In the army the matter is somewhat confused because different regiments did different things and what was said was not always done.[76] Medical men generally were underrepresented in the Sovereign's honours lists.[77]

It seems there are at least two possible causes for the transformation. First, as Coleman argues:[78]

> The social structure of pre-industrial England had only one really important division: between those who were Gentlemen and those who were players. For all the elaboration of status and hierarchy distinguished in the seventeenth and eighteenth centuries, the line of greatest consequence was that older division which distinguished gentility from the common people.

And:[79] 'Training was for Players; Gentlemen were educated'. It followed that the medical profession generally could not lay claim to the status of the gentry until at least the emphasis of their total learning experience had shifted from the apprenticeship types of training, as with the former styles of apothecaries and surgeons, to an immersion in one of the University medical schools.

A second reason for the transformation in the social status of the profession generally might have been personified in the cricketing career of Dr W.G. Grace. If, *per contra*, the career (or its retrospective appreciation) was only a symptom of rising status then what follows does not make my point.[80] Wakley, founder of *The Lancet*, considered that chess was important to doctors.[81] That however relates to a view of intellectual accomplishment rather than social status. James says[82] that the Victorian middle class

> wanted a culture, a way of life of their own. They found it symbolized for them in the work of three men ... Thomas Arnold ... Thomas Hughes ... and W.G. Grace. These three men, more than all the others, created Victorianism, and to leave out Grace is to misconceive the other two.

James is right. Sport, like art and culture, can not only be a part of a way of life but can also symbolize it. Like them also, it can do more: it can provide the training for the readiness for action.[83] And it is sport, in particular cricket (pre-eminently the gentleman's sport) as an instrument of training, as well as Grace as an example, that make his sport and his achievements important to his profession.

Of course physical accomplishment and grace and courage are important elements in all competitive sport. But nonchalance, together with these other qualities, pays its highest rewards in cricket. Further, the cricket ethic and morality are more highly developed than their counterparts in other sports. That is to say, in cricket there are more unwritten rules of behaviour than elsewhere. Indeed the phrase 'It isn't cricket' means unethical behaviour. It is also significant that most games and sports are governed by 'rules' but cricket has its 'laws'. The difference is that 'rules' are sufficient within a framework of more general activities but the existence of 'laws' implies a special correlative morality.

The origins of the game were as sport for rural artisans and noblemen: the urban bourgeoisie were excluded.[84] By the middle of the nineteenth century all social classes indulged in it. In this it enabled aspiring gentlemen, under the influence of Arnold and Hughes, to 'play the sport that lords played'.[85] It enabled them to play a sport which was both nostalgic and contemporary and moreover one in which there was a sharp divide, even amongst almost full-time participants, between 'gentlemen' (who played as amateurs) and 'players' (who were paid to play).

Graves argued:[86] 'The public desire is that the best man, the best team, the best performance shall be definitively hall-marked as such. Hence a proliferation of championships, of athletic leagues, and the evolution of an endless series of records'. Once more cricket is, or was, structurally best suited to appeal. This is so because the pace at which it is played enables the results (at least) of each player's actions to be seen unmistakably: the game focuses on each one at a time and there is a large element of objectivity in the measurement of each player's achievement (runs scored, wickets taken, catches held, and the rest). Nevertheless cricket is a team game; the individual performer rarely shines entirely alone. To the player and spectator, cricket is a game that best reconciles the 'social' with the 'individual'. The Victorian roots of the game and its penchant for nostalgia are shown by the fact that *Wisden's Cricketers Almanac* was first published in 1864 and is still published annually.

If, as Hirschman argues, western society is on an oscillation toward the private (that is, the individual) this would explain the decline in the popularity of social (collective or team) sports, particularly cricket, where an essential part of the game is its social ethic and morality. C.L.R. James suggests that roots of the 1929–30 'bodyline' controversy lay in the First World War. He says:[87] 'Modern society took a turn downwards in 1929 and "It isn't cricket" is one of the casualties.... Much, much more than cricket is at stake, in fact everything is at stake.'

Cricket, along with other sports, is, or was until recently, given a high priority at English medical schools. But these others have neither a general public appeal nor, inherently, a capacity to distinguish the best man. In rugby a try is almost invariably the result of a team effort. In rowing the individual is entirely absorbed into the group. In, for example, baseball (which has no significant following in British medical schools), although there is room for the individual to be seen to shine, the range (but not necessarily the depth) of the accomplishment is less. That game is played with a scoring ark of 90°; cricket has 360°. The bowler, unlike the pitcher, makes the ball bounce. Cricket, therefore, has literally as well as metaphorically an extra dimension.

It is against this background that Mandle argues[88] that W.G. Grace won fame for himself as a cricketer and as a doctor: 'W. G. sits all night at an accouchement, then scores a century the next day'. It is indeed arguable that the existence of his profession, his prowess at cricket, and his enduring health and courage all combined in the popular imagination to enhance each of these attributes. And, if cricket is pre-eminently the gentleman's game, it moulded well with the medical profession's aspiration to that status. The sporting success of this doctor did not hamper the expansion of iatrocratic power.[89]

Grace, however, despite his amateur status and considerable wealth,[90] never received a knighthood, that is, formal state recognition. Although he received much acclaim, it was from the masses who saw him and who read about him. The failure of the campaign for the knighthood speaks of the gap in society that had to be bridged. A knighthood would have been conferred not only on the best known, and possibly best admired, Englishman of his day, but also on a medical officer of a poor provincial parish. It is arguable that the campaign itself raised the possibility of such recognition. If this is so the status of general practitioners generally was necessarily advanced.

Professional morality

Thus far my discussion has largely assumed a uniformity of ideas among individual members of the profession. It is similar to Freidson's:[91] 'When men work together in the same place, on the same terms, and with common work problems, they will develop a set of standards and procedures by which to judge and manage those problems, and they will discourage deviance from those standards'. My assumption must be explained; and for this reason I touch on the work of the self-styled 'Guildsmen' of the early part of this century[92] and, in more detail, that of Emile Durkheim.[93]

First, however, I must digress briefly to explain my view of 'self' and 'society'. Hawthorn[94] quotes Kant: 'I am conscious of myself as myself. This thought contains a twofold "I", one as subject and one as object ... it is the foundation of an intellect. It marks the complete separation from all beasts.' On this basis there is no need to construct 'society'. But even if society does not exist, 'I' exist. And, so also 'we' exist, 'you' and 'they' exist. Groups, as I shall argue, exist because pluralities of individuals are different from each of their members. 'Society' is a construct to describe one or more groups. It is as artificial as 'rational economic man', but the fallacies of each can teach us both by their insights and their error. That is how I can use Durkheim's approach to groups but not other parts of his method: they assume the existence of the 'social fact' which in turn assumes the existence of 'society'. As Hawthorn says:[95] Durkheim's failure was 'in his central purposes, a characterization of morality, a defence of the compatibility of individual autonomy and social order, a causal account of structural and ideal features of societies' but 'subsequent sociologists have pointed to the immense fertility of his ideas' – and, as I shall suggest, it is in this that they are right.

Turning then to the guildsmen, it is not necessary for my argument that I offer an extended discussion of their position. As will be seen, having used a different route I accept considerable parts of it. I take just one of them, Penty. He ignores groups other than those in trade.[96] To him, the most important social form enabling individuals to realize their own creativity was the Guild, and central to the Guild and its regulations was the 'Just Price'.[97]

> The Just Price is necessarily a fixed price, and in order to maintain it, the Guilds had to be privileged bodies having an entire monopoly of their respective trades.... Only through the exercise of authority over its individual members could the Guild prevent profiteering, in its forms of forestalling, regrating, engrossing, and adulteration....
>
> But a Just and Fixed Price cannot be maintained by moral action alone. If prices are to be fixed throughout production, it can only be done on the assumption that a standard of quality can be upheld. As a standard of quality cannot finally be defined in terms of law, it is necessary, for the maintenance of a standard, to place authority in the hands of craftsmasters, a consensus whose opinion constitutes the final court of appeal.

According to Penty, we ought to return to the Medieval Guild and the structure of society which it reflected and of which it formed part. He regards as mistaken and undesirable social forms which gravitate to the materialistic – a term he tends to equate with individualistic. Accordingly, he applauds the community basis and the freedom of the Medieval Church (and in particular Gothic art).[98] He is critical among ideas, of the Renaissance and Protestantism, and among men, of Rousseau, Adam Smith, and Marx. His greatest condemnation is reserved for unregulated currency and the influence of the Roman law of Justinian (which was, he argues,[99] in all its essential forms, including its centralization, applied in England). The former, he argues, led to the downfall of the Greek and Roman civilizations and the latter represents a military, capitalistic system to enable rich men to live among poor.

The question is therefore what is there so important about the guild. Is it only as Freidson suggests[100] that the autonomy is

organized and does not arise not by default as with a plumber? I
think not. Durkheim, and this is where I rely on his insights, sees
in the ancient past and persistent survival of the guilds[101] 'a proof
that they do not depend upon some merely contingent or hapha-
zard circumstance peculiar to a given political regime, but on wide
and fundamental causes'. He argues that this decisive institution
existed from the days of prehistory;[102] as an institution the guild
has had several forms with similar functions. It is necessary to
understand the causes of their survival in order to understand
professional codes of ethics. Durkheim argues:[103] moral and juri-
dical facts ... consist of rules of conduct that have sanction....
Sanction is ... a consequence which results not from the act taken
in isolation but from the conforming or not conforming to a rule
of conduct already laid down. Clearly relying on Rousseau –
morality is formed by society and only society can eliminate
inequality, dependence, and oppression – Durkheim argues, as
regards rules to which sanctions apply, that these are of two kinds.
These are:[104]

> divided into two groups: those concerning the relation of each
> one of us to his own self, that is, those that make up the moral
> code called 'individual'; and those concerning the relations we
> maintain with other people, with the exception of any particular
> grouping. The obligations laid upon us ... arise solely from ...
> intrinsic human nature.... The function of the rules of the
> individual moral code is in fact to fix in the individual con-
> sciousness the seat of all morals ... on these foundations all else
> rests.

Between these two extremes[105] 'lie duties of a different kind. They
depend not on our intrinsic human nature in general but on
particular qualities not exhibited by all men'. They vary because
people are in different circumstances:[106]

> But there are rules of one kind where the diversity is ...
> marked; they are those which taken together constitute profes-
> sional ethics.... We might say in this connection that there are
> as many forms of morals as there are different callings....
> These differences may even go so far as to present a clear
> contrast.... Here, then, we find within every society a plural-
> ity of morals.

Durkheim goes on:[107]

The distinctive feature of this kind of morals and what differentiates it from other branches of ethics, is the sort of unconcern with which public consciousness regards it.... The transgressions which have only to do with the practice of the profession, come in merely for a rather vague censure outside the strictly professional field.

He says, and the point is central to my argument:[108]

This feature of professional ethics can moreover easily be explained. They cannot be of deep concern to the common consciousness precisely because they are not common to all members of the society ... it is exactly because they govern functions not performed by everyone, that not everyone is able to have a sense of what these functions are, of what they ought to be, or of what special relations should exist between the individuals concerned with applying them.

Some who today take either a superficial or programmatic view of medical care may doubt the accuracy of this. After all, is there not widespread media and political interest in discussing the machinery for health care? Are not all the professions, including medicine, increasingly being called to public account? It is not easy, on their own terms, to rebut these views. Hawthorn cites Weber:[109]

What distinguished western capitalism was the remorseless intrusion of money-making into all social relations ... the western bourgeoisie was not merely one more group dedicated to material accumulation but the one group for whom this end had at once religious and thus moral significance.

If the professions are no more than the bourgeoisie then it would follow that the morality of money is the dictionary for translating moral codes. But I have argued that this is to mistake their other objectives and values, they are not to be judged solely by the criteria of what Freidson calls the 'political economy'.

We have seen that Pellegrino and Thomasma[110] talk of the 'insights obtained at the bedside'. But unless we have been there how can we know what they are, or indeed, if they are? Nor is it sufficient that we have been there, we must have been there in that role. Can we deny or assert the existence of things we do not know? One is reminded of the old-time school master's cliché – 'This is going to hurt me more than it hurts you'. There is indeed a special sense in which the knowledge of the professional act by the professional actor is at once unique and objective.[111] The knowledge of the professional act is understandable, if at all, only by those who have shared similar experiences. We know, do we not, that there is a point where explanation stops and understanding begins. It is similar to the collective consciousness of the Société Royale de Medicine which Foucault described.[112]

The argument leads Durkheim to the core of his teaching in the field. Moral power is always collective power:[113]

> Since ... society as a whole feels no concern in professional ethics, it is imperative that there be special groups in the society, within which [professional] morals may be evolved, and whose business it is to see they be observed ... we see in it a real decentralization of the moral life. Whilst public opinion, which lies at the base of common morality, is diffused throughout society ... the ethics of each profession are localized within a limited region.... [It follows] the greater the strength of the group structure, the more numerous are the moral rules appropriate to it and the greater the authority they have over their members.... Accordingly, it can be said that professional ethics will be the more developed, and the more advanced in their operation, the greater the stability and the better the organization of the professional groups themselves.

He argues that the converse is also true. Where individuals come together not as a cohesive group but merely by the fact of sharing a like occupation and by chance and furthermore where 'there is no corporate body set above all the members of a profession to maintain some sort of unity, to serve as the repository of traditions and common practices and see they are observed at need',[114] there is no common ethic.

In an earlier chapter, we saw how Hirschman attacked economic theory largely in its own terms. Its ideal was based in infra-human wantons. Durkheim provides new arguments to support this assault. In both classical and socialist economic theory, it is supposed that[115] 'economic life is equipped to organize itself and to function in an orderly way and in harmony, without any moral authority intervening'. He argues[116] that: 'this amoral character of economic life amounts to a public danger' for 'if we live amorally for a good part of the day, how can we keep the spring of morality from going slack in us?'. He says:[117]

> Clearly, if there has been self-delusion ... amongst the classical economists it is because the economic functions were studied as

if they were an end in themselves, without considering what further reaction they might have on the whole social order.

He argues:[118] 'in order that ... a group may persist, each part must operate, not as if it stood alone, that is, as if it were itself the whole; on the contrary, each part must behave in a way that enables the whole to survive'. Because, however, they are different, it is important that the conditions of existence of the whole should not be taken as the same for the parts. Popper, for example, regards[119] such statements as 'trivial' and 'vague'. However, the vagueness reflects its level of abstraction and the triviality the consequence derived from it. If, as here, the statement leads on to important insights both Popper's terms are misplaced. Because they are exterior to himself and because they are the interests of something that is not himself, these social interests that the individual has to take into account are only dimly perceived by him.

The force which obliges the individual to respect these external interests is a moral discipline. Individuals come together[120] not just to safeguard interests but also 'for the pleasure of mixing with their fellows and of no longer feeling lost in the midst of adversaries, as well as for the pleasure of communing together'. Durkheim compares the moral ethos created by the group to maintain its cohesiveness with the mechanism for cohesion in the family. Consanguinity[121] is not seen as important to the latter. What are important include shared ritual and the pleasure of enjoying life together. Indeed he argues[122] that 'the guild was formed on the very model of the domestic society, with banquets, festivals, worship, burial all in common'.

To Durkheim, a distinction must be drawn between the rules obtaining in such groups and 'workshop regulations'.[123] The latter are imposed externally to the individual; the former is a part of 'collective discipline'. To be sure, the former might use 'rules' of similar form to those of the workshop but that does no more than translate[124]

> into precepts ideas and sentiments felt by all, that is, a common adherence to the same objective ... beneath the letter lies the spirit that animates it.... As to the rules, although necessary and inevitable, they are but the outward expression of ... fundamental principles. It is not a matter of co-ordinating any changes outwardly and mechanically, but of bringing men's minds into mutual understanding.

And, it might be added, where the group expands its territorial cognisance so that individuals cannot meet, they are kept together by loyalties to places where they studied (in the field of medicine, the teaching hospitals) and by discrete specialist journals, particularly where they are run by the organizing authorities of the guild (again in the field of medicine, for example, the *British Medical Journal*).

Largely descriptively, I have already noted the development of the medical profession. It can now be seen how closely, at least in Britain, this history corresponds to Durkheim's theory and prescriptions. The medieval guilds have continued all the way through to today. But Durkheim says that in order to prevent the guilds being static, it is necessary for them to have national jurisdiction and responsibilities. In England they acquired it with the passage of the Apothecaries Act 1815, the Medical Act 1858, the expansion of the Provincial Medical and Surgical Association into the British Medical Association, and ultimately the 1946 National Health Act.

In great measure professional morality consists in the duties owed to these modern 'guilds' and their members. And what of those practitioners not in membership? Here, I argue that they too are infused with the same morality because these guilds are sufficiently large in number and in influence and sufficiently vague and overlapping in their 'fundamental principles' to provide a collective or common professional morality in which, as Durkheim argued, the duties are owed to the other members of the profession. Further, as he also argued, this morality arises out of functions not performed by everybody in society; its meaning is therefore not to be generally understood.

These rules, as Hughes said,[125] deal with mistake handling, they classify people, and they set up 'criteria for recognizing a true fellow-worker, for determining who it is safe and maybe even necessary to initiate into the in-group of, close equals, and who must be kept at some distance'. But as we have seen these rules are based in tradition, one which we can now recognize is shared by the initiates. This is why professional ethics as such are so inept at handling the moral consequences of novel technologies. But so also the tradition is largely exclusive to the insiders. It is the largely failed attempt by externals to be part of that tradition which has led to the exaggerated importance placed by many on medical values.

There are four further general points I should make. The nineteenth- and twentieth-century expansion in the numbers of doctors, the increase in specialization (and, with a considerable time-lag, in the increase in the numbers of guilds) have led to a broadening of this collective morality. The changes in the composition of the General Medical Council have followed. Whereas in origin it was a confederation of the interests of clearly identifiable guilds, now under recent legislation, there it is more real to say that it, and the people it registers, are now a unitary collective guild. One might say that in origin the State acted not as a party to a bargain but as arbitrator between those several interests but that now those concerns have been merged.

Secondly, no doubt connected with reasons concerning esteem and success and financial rewards, the specific organization and morality of the doctor's profession is the model to which other occupations aspire and under whose patronage they seek to function. This shows itself both in the typical composition of the governing councils (where the occupation is dominant with doctors providing additional membership) and in that the terms of reference of the disciplinary committees tend to adopt similar forms of words as the Medical Acts have applied to doctors. Thirdly, the existence and size of the health care bureaucracies, particularly the National Health Service, have in some ways complicated, and in others sharpened, the contrast between the professions and trade.

Fourthly, there is apparently a growing body of opinion among academic lawyers that a new Permanent Standing Advisory Committee should be established to review ethics and law in medicine.[126] The idea stems partly from concerns beyond the scope of this work, for example how to cope with the choices made possible by advances in medical technologies. Even here it is somewhat difficult to see what good could come of it. What is more clear, is that in so far as it would seek to intervene in areas that this book has discussed the suggestion is based on a number of fallacies. It assumes that medical practice is explicable to a world beyond its practitioners. It could provide an alternative focus other than the group for the maintenance of that particular brand of morality which Durkheim called 'professional ethics' and in so doing would, as he says, undermine them. It would be a centre for removing the art from medicine and for reducing doctors to mere experts. If successful, it would prevent the practice of medicine *qua* medicine.

Durkheim says that social groups, in order to preserve their cohesion, will naturally develop rules. Seen in this light the criticism of Percival's Code of Ethics and its successors that it is not concerned with ethics but with the prevention of unseemly competition is misplaced.[127] So also is that of Pellegrino and Thomasma[128] and of Kennedy[129] that they are drawn up by the profession. On Durkheim's view they are drawn up by the profession because only physicians are able to have a sense in depth of what the functions of the profession are.

So also Durkheim's insistence that values other than economic need to be recognized finds a more than ready acceptance by the medical profession than in some other places precisely because it is about the clinical act and healing rather than earning. Since historically this aspect applied to the profession, it was more capable of resisting the siren calls of classical economists and when its old guilds became outmoded, instead of abolishing them, it transformed them into their modern form. If I am right about the influence of loyalty to the places where doctors studied, we should expect to see a weakening of the guild within a generation or so of the expansion in the numbers and geographical dispersion of medical schools, more particularly where even the centres of excellence, of aspiration, are themselves dispersed.

The fact that doctors receive comfortable incomes should not delude us into concluding that this is the reason why they have adopted this occupation. As individuals, of course, it is a factor. There have been complaints, of course, throughout history concerning the very large incomes of some doctors.[130] But this is besides the point. I have argued that the very act of Hippocratic medicine requires that doctors practise on the basis of the manners of the Pythagorean gentleman. Implicit in that idea is not so much income or earnings as the capacities to spend, to consume, to have. Such considerations are moreover relevant to the individual; but the group is not the same as its separate members. Professionals certainly prefer comfort but, I am arguing, professionalism requires at least a substantial divorce between services and their monetary rewards. Where the link is direct, the occupation is a trade. When we consider professional ethics we are not considering the individual's ethics but those of the group. Collectively and institutionally it was, and is, the group which places its emphasis on other values than earnings. The individual may be seen therefore to modify his behaviour not in accord with some private ethic but in accord with the demands of the group. In so far as the modification is effective, so are professional ethics. Such an argument, it will be noted, judges effectiveness by the internal standards of the profession. The fact that this might, indeed does, make it more difficult for outsiders, who include lawyers, to make judgements about professional ethics is no reason for disputing the validity of the conclusion.

The growth of other groups with esoteric knowledge in the field of health care has challenged not only the integrity of the physicians as a group but also their claim to paramountcy. The extension of the ideas of 'profession' and 'gentleman' more generally has challenged the unique character of the few who once held the status. The concept of the 'brotherhood' has become more difficult to sustain. By being generalized, it has become debased. Further, it has taken place at the same time as the growth of the cults of the individual and moral pluralism, which in their degenerate forms are consumerism. No doubt they are the consequences of the 'morality' of the classical economists. Few individuals and no group have entirely escaped the impact of these ideas. With the sharing of values by health workers and the fact that they alone are 4 per cent of the working population, we are a long way from the close-knit professional guild that Durkheim saw as the originator of organized morality.

The fact that our society (but less than the United States) measures status by earnings and the fact that to gain, or even retain, a place in the 'earnings leagues' it is necessary to use the central device of classical economics (that is, sell labour and skill at the market price) has meant, even for those groups concerned with other values, a degeneration of the organizational purpose. There is therefore no surprise that there are greater calls for accountability since the professions are no longer unique, and at the same time, having less confidence in their codes of ethics (because they are more spread out, diffused) they are less able to resist these pressures.

It can be said, with much justice, that I am guilty of adopting a similar position to that of Parsons criticized by Berlant:[131]

> Even Parsons has noted that certain practices in the medical profession are illogical from the point of view of professionalism. What he does not seem to appreciate is that arguments in defense of these practices are more than deviations from a pure ideology of professionalism: they are intended to preserve central institutions of the profession, not peripheral phenomena.

In similar vein, Berlant also objects to Parsons' acceptance of the norms of the professional élite as general norms of the mass of practitioners. Again the criticism is true of my analysis. However, leaving aside any defence of Parsons, I do not think I have depended on an equation of interests of the élite and their masses. On the contrary, I talked of perceptions not realities, of aspirations not interests.

Briefly my reply to Berlant's critique is threefold. First, he has not paid sufficient regard to the differences of the British and American cultures. They relate to such matters as the organization (the depersonalization) of primary care, the existence of a fee for service, the far greater numbers of practitioners, a greater emphasis not only on scientific medicine but on scientism in medicine, and on a general culture which, because it is imbued with the emigrant philosophy of the New Frontier, more strongly emphasizes what it sees as the public and private dichotomy and consequently places less emphasis on group cohesion.

Secondly, as already anticipated, if it is right that medical men are motivated by the maximization of yield, why do they become doctors at all? To generalize, the difficulty of the criticism is similar to that of explaining why rational economic man consumes anything. Certainly, the emphasis on financial reward is difficult to reconcile with the long history of dangers faced by medical men. To take an example from the past, why should physicians have stayed in London to deal with patients, poor as well as rich, who had the plague?[132] Or to take a contemporary example which also distinguishes American from British practice, why do British general practitioners conduct so much of their practice by means of home visits rather than requiring the sick to attend on them?

Thirdly, Berlant does not sufficiently appreciate that, far from turning service into a commodity and disallowing every means of exchange except money, professionalism insists on activities without exchange: that is, it requires a separation of service and reward. When major changes in the system of health care are proposed both sets of protagonists have tended to react in economic terms to their opponents but not to the other values of medical and health care – pity, scientism, and the fight against nature and the rest. This ought to warn, as regards the profession, not against the views of self-interest involved, but rather the wisdom of accepting such understandings as to its role. It confuses what May[133] refers to as the internal and external catholicity of the professions. The former looks to the professional person and his relationship with the whole of a particular client; the latter to the relation of the profession to the whole of society.

Professional privilege and the bargain with the State

The view of occupational morality described in the last section stands in contrast to a frequent view among commentators that professional privilege is a bargain struck between the profession and society. As the Merrison Report put it:[134]

> An instructive way of looking at regulation is to see it as a contract between public and profession, by which the public go to the profession for medical treatment because the profession has made sure it will provide satisfactory treatment.

Freidson puts it in constitutional terms: 'The state has ultimate sovereignty over all and grants conditional autonomy to some'. He says:[135] 'The most strategic and treasured characteristic of the profession – its autonomy – is ... owed to its relationship to the sovereign state from which it is not ultimately autonomous'. This view of the state or the group or their relationship is not, however, self-evident. If, for example, Durkheim is right to utilize the idea of group-will manifesting itself in something like a guild, then the 'bargain' fails, as lawyers might say, because there are not two sides giving and taking by way of mutually agreed undertakings; the group does no more under the agreement than it would have done without it. Further, even if there is to be a bargain its existence is determined by the group; and Durkheim's simpler explanation of professional cohesion seems preferable.

Besides, if there is such a bargain, one would suppose that if it is shown to be breached, then either side may be entitled, again to use the language of lawyers, to treat it as repudiated. The consequence is that if the breach is demonstrated, direct state intervention to take over the regulation of medicine, as Merrison ostensibly anticipates, would become more acceptable. Aside from this narrow lawyer's point, this bargain theory gives no room for the professional organization, in its ideal form, like that of the professional practitioner, to separate service and reward. Further, when was this bargain struck? It cannot have been with the passage of the Medical Acts because the Royal Colleges existed before. It cannot have been with the grant of their Charters because, although these documents grant privileges, they are not their core. It is not irrelevant that the courts have been prepared, through the doctrine of passing-off, to use the civil remedy of the injunction to protect titles of occupations otherwise unrecognized by the state.[136] The truth is that state recognition has come and gone and come again; but it is not essential to it. My view denies any meaning to the question why has the state entrusted the professions with so much. It was on this basis that we saw in the previous section that in the 1858 Act the state did not grant powers to the estates of medicine: it arbitrated between them and used the results of its award for its own purposes.

The Merrison Report said:[137] that 'we recommend a predominately professional GMC. The ultimate safeguard of the public interest is the power of Parliament ... Parliament will be able to intervene if the contract to which we have referred is not operating in the general public interest.' This is either a statement of the obvious or (less likely) a forecast of the abdication of professional power. In its modern form the profession is governed by a balanced federation of group and state interests. For example, it is clear that the British Medical Association's origins were guild-like. Its current power is an amalgam of this autonomous power, of a public affairs pressure group, and an instrument of the state.

These are structural considerations. Functionally, too, it stretches interpretation to think of the 'privileges' of the profession as being in some way dependent on the state. Of course, such matters as the monopolies of appointments and the use of titles are protected by the state's criminal law. Other matters such as the enforcement of group ethics are indirectly linked to these but the content of the group's standards of competence does not concern the state.

In truth, there is no bargain and the profession has not 'been given the right to control its own work': unless the meaning of 'medicine' is to be wholly reconstructed, the phenomenon commonly associated with the bargain is the inevitable consequence of any mode of its operation and any form of its organization. It follows that all the state can do, if 'medicine' is to be carried out at all, is to seek to influence the modes or forms of regulation. It is at this point where specific bargains are struck.

I am arguing that elements within both the radical critique and contemporary sociology go against the evidence in conflating a number of specific agreements with each other and with the essential form of professionalism into one omnibus contract. If general state intervention over the practice of medicine were to occur, it would require extensive changes not only in the mode of practice but also in our ways of thinking about ideas of the doctor–patient relationship, of disease, of cure, of health, and of the rest. This is why I suggest that where there are differences in the mode of operation and form of organization of the medical profession we should expect to find differences in the central concepts of medicine. This is why comparisons between the United States and the United Kingdom are so difficult.

The external regulation

Freidson says:[138] 'Knowledge of the characteristics of the informal organization can explain what the formal organization does not concede and cannot explain – namely, how a diversity of technical and ethical practices can persist without strain'. He says also[139] that the 'attributes of organizational institutions ... can be determined empirically by the examination of' formal written documents. But this enterprise invites the skills of the lawyer. Accordingly, in addition to the insights of sociology and the other social sciences, in order to understand regulation it is necessary to use a legal viewpoint. Let us be clear about this utility. The law does not define these sorts of relationships, but it is a social phenomenon of which sociology and the rest ought to take account.

Freidson's early contrast between the formal and the informal is not one the law recognizes because the law lets the informal world of custom move into the formal world it will enforce. More recently, in his *Professional Powers*[140] he has recognized this: 'In essence, privately established standards are routinely adopted and given the force of law by public agencies'. He says that they are 'merely ratified' by them. As necessity arises the law requires the informal, the inarticulate, to define the formal. We might say that formal documents must mislead unless read in the same way as those who interpret them.

There is another reason for recognizing the importance of the inarticulate. As a University teacher, I have found some occasions when it appears impossible to make myself understood to those who, to adopt the saying of Hippocrates,[141] 'have not been initiated into the mysteries of the science'. There is no reason to suppose that my profession is qualitatively more introspective than medicine. There is a possibility then that medical men have the same problem in dealing with the uninitiated. Further, I have yet to see an account by one of the school of the 'true-view' that is both (a) intelligible to outsiders, and (b) acceptable to insiders. Once more I am led to the conviction that because the experiences of one individual or one group are never fully available to others, the search for an understanding of those experiences by externals is unlikely to be fulfilled.

In the face of these difficulties why should the outsider seek to gain any comprehension of what goes on inside, and how can he do it? As to the why, although the discourse is closed, its effects are not. As to the how, a variety of answers is possible. As we have seen, history and sociology provide some of the means. So also an ethical understanding may be sought. Such an analysis may not seek to penetrate any inner mystery (although on occasion it may deny its existence). It may merely seek an assessment of the practical or moral effects of a discourse upon the outside world. Its virtue is that it is necessary; its vice is that all too easily it degenerates into statements that the world should be different from the way it is. This analysis is necessary because it can give life to an assertion of interdependency of people, and thus provide a measure of external accountability. Its danger is that by confusing the 'ought' and the 'is' it can lead to the creation of false expectations or to reforms built upon sand.

But also, the outsider may seek to establish the existence and scope of internal regulation by describing the limits to the external regulations. This is a part of my method. Manifestly it is narrower (and in some eyes more tedious) than the other approaches. It does not answer the questions of how, nor why, nor even, to a considerable extent, of what they are. But one does not establish the existence of the molten plasma in the Earth's core by digging; one establishes it by measurement and inferential comparison *inter alia* of seismic waves. The regulation whose external limits I look at is to be found in the general (public) law of statutes and law reports. The inferences I draw are what are presupposed by it. If some characteristics, properties, of internal regulation remain unexposed by this method, so be it. It is, I think, preferable to making them up.

The most striking feature to note is that in England, as in effect anticipated by Durkheim, in no significant respect is the external regulation of the professions dependent on the existence of the National Health Service. Those practitioners who work within the Service, and they are by far the largest section, are therefore subjected to both professional and bureaucratic regulatory machinery. The two mechanisms are almost entirely severed. In the remaining part of this chapter, I discuss the former and in the next the latter.

As appears in the Introduction to the *Encyclopedia of Health Services and Medical Law*[142] the basic function of the statutory regulation of the profession is the maintenance of registers of practitioners deemed competent. The structure used to achieve this is the establishment of a council with duties (for example, to register those who satisfy the 'statutory' criteria) and powers (for example, to determine them). The efficacy of the registers is supported by the creation of certain monopolies (which might be shared with specified other groups) and which are protected by provisions preventing the recovery of fees (or limitations on the unregistered on the right to take appointments which might yield an income), and by the use of the criminal law to protect professional titles.

The conclusion drawn from the examination of the statutes – the external regulation – may be put shortly: at almost every point they assume an internal normative order intelligible only to and operable only by the initiates. Further, where the group has ambitions to achieve upward social mobility it may seek to utilize those which are functionally similar but which have already been successful. This applies to the constitutions and functioning of each of the professional councils, to the training and examination, to the establishment of criteria for the gaining of clinical experience, to the operation of machinery for the maintenance of standards of fitness to practice, and to the reluctance of the courts to intervene in such professional judgements. It is to be observed that because each of these depends upon the understanding by initiates, external challenge, say against the shortcomings of an individual, is commonly regarded as a challenge to the whole group. In brief, both the outward manifestation of internal forms and the relevant external law give regulatory support to the classical theory of medicine and are opposed to a discourse based on science or participation.

Some explanation needs to be given for this conclusion.[143] First, however, to take a point of general law, the courts say that it is not possible for an English statute wholly to exclude their jurisdiction: they will not accept even in plain words that this is what is meant. They assert the right to intervene to compel the performance of a duty or to correct an error 'on the face of the record'. The basis of this jurisdiction is the application of the rules of what lawyers in their jargon call 'natural justice' – that everybody shall have the right to a hearing and that everybody shall have the right to an unbiased tribunal. This general rule, however, stands in contrast to their treatment of disciplinary cases. Here, repeatedly the courts have said they cannot review professional decisions merely where they disagree with them. In *Leeson* v. *General Medical Council,* Brown L.J. put it bluntly:[144] 'the jurisdiction of the domestic tribunal which has been clothed by the legislature with the duty of discipline in respect of a great profession must be left untouched by Courts of Law'.

Under their original forms, the professional councils were given powers to strike off practitioners from their registers for 'unprofessional conduct',[145] and pursuant to this disciplinary committees were established. Because the register was the basis of the monopoly power, which itself was to be enforced by the general criminal law, it was necessary to provide for the composition and powers of these committees in the relevant statutes. In these circumstances, it is no surprise that much of the reported litigation has indeed concerned the transitional provisions under which individuals could continue to work on an older basis. Thus most of the early cases on the Apothecaries Act 1815 were about the issue of whether an individual had been in practice prior to its commencement. There was not dissimilar litigation concerning the use of titles after the 1858 Medical Act. Where they had been in practice before it, they were exempt from its licensure provisions.[146] However, and the point is more important, because the statutes were concerned to lend the state's power to the internal professional forms, they neither spelt out what conduct might be unprofessional nor made any provision for an appeal.

In 1950 the basis of the jurisdiction of the court in one regard was changed; a doctor (but still not, for example, a complaining patient) was given a right of appeal to the Judicial Committee of the Privy Council. The change however has not meant that the courts are substantially more willing to interfere with decisions of the professions' own committees. In one of the strongest examples showing the reluctance of the courts to interfere with the decision of a professional body,[147] the Judicial Committee took the view that no damage had been done to the public and that the complaint to the General Medical Council had been made on grounds extraneous to the charge – the reason for the complaint was that the defendant doctor was no longer willing to commit adultery. Nevertheless they held:

The Medical Acts have always entrusted the supervision of the medical advisers' conduct to a committee of the profession, for they know and appreciate better than anyone else the standards which responsible medical opinion demands of its own profession.

Generally, then, the courts adopt a hands-off approach to professional regulation. Most commonly the cases indicate that the courts are not prepared to comment on the specific internal rule alleged to have been breached, and where they do they normally support it. They do not attempt to argue against it. Although he supported the professional view, Lord Denning was characteristically unusual in disregarding the technicalities of the law when he observed:[148] 'No distinction can be permitted as to what can be done in the drawing-room or the surgery . . . . The doctor must resist temptation, not succumb to it.' Normally the content and nature of professional regulation is a discourse closed to nonprofessionals, to uninitiated laymen.

Take for example the changing basis of the jurisdiction of the General Medical Council. Until 1969 the Medical Acts used the expression 'infamous or disgraceful conduct in a professional respect'. In that year this was altered to 'serious professional misconduct'. The question which arises is whether these mean different things. The most commonly adopted formula at least used to be:[149]

> If it is shewn that a medical man, in the pursuit of his profession, has done something with regard to it which would be reasonably regarded as disgraceful or dishonourable by his professional brethren of good repute and competency it is open to the General Medical Council to say it is 'infamous conduct in a professional respect'.

In another case[150] Lord Parker C.J. said that the form of words in a professional statute does not matter. Misconduct could be variously described as infamous, disgraceful, unbecoming, serious. It amounted to the same thing if it reflected on the profession. On this view the change effected in 1969 is cosmetic. It is merely a modern expression of the same meaning. In the coarse view of the law there is no change in meaning. I argue, however, that the change of words reflects an alteration in the professional form. Put shortly the older set of words carried a meaning more closely associated with gentlemanly morality; and neither the breadth nor the definition was particularly affected by the limitation[151] that the conduct must concern either the patients or the professional brethren. 'Serious professional misconduct' is narrower. The change in the statutory language reflects the shift that the impact of amoral scientism has had on medical practice.

Anticipating events, in 1930 Scrutton L.J. put it:[152]

> It is a great pity that the word 'infamous' is used to describe the conduct of a medical practitioner who advertises. As in the case of the Bar so in the medical profession advertising is serious misconduct in a professional respect and that is all that is meant by the phrase 'infamous conduct'; it means no more than serious misconduct judged according to the rules written or unwritten governing the profession.

It is important to my argument that there is a qualitative difference between a profession and a trade, and in particular that the practice of medicine, at least as a collective phenomenon, is sharply distinguished from the process of being paid for it. Of course all practitioners, as we have seen, seek an income (which they may define as reasonable) from their occupation. A distinguishing feature between a profession and a trade is not the strength with which they press their claims but more prosaically the way in which they do or are supposed to do so. On this basis it is possible to classify occcupations into professions and trading professions; that is, into those within the Hippocratic tradition and those significantly infused with classical or neo-classical economics.

The distinction is not one of organizational structure but specifically of the attitude taken by their regulations to selling. Something of this shows itself in the old rule which distinguished physicians from other medical men. In the absence of an express contract Fellows of the College could not sue for fees; their income was obtained by the receipt of honoraria from patients, whether grateful or not.[153] The presumption against physicians' fees was reversed by the Medical Act 1858, except in respect of a member of a College which had a by-law preventing fees.[154] Not surprisingly, in my argument, the Royal College of Physicians maintains such a rule in respect of its Fellows. As regards licentiates of the College, surgeons, and apothecaries, until at least the early part of the nineteenth century, although they could sue their patients even on an implied undertaking to pay, the amount they could recover was that which the court (in those days, the jury) regarded as fair rather than any customary or usual charge.[155] Of some note was the distinction made between surgeons and apothecaries – only the latter were in 'trade' for the purposes of, for example, the Bankruptcy Acts.[156]

To generalize, the one thing the history of the medical profession, if no other group, suggests is that there has been a demand for upward mobility and it is symbolized in the erection of two 'ethical' barriers: the first enforces this withdrawal from trade and the second increases the formal – 'academic' – as opposed to the practical training. As Hughes says: 'Delegation of dirty work is ... a part of the process of occupational mobility'.[157] Lloyd's translation has Hippocrates condemning quacks. There may be some doubt as to what is meant by this but in any event we can be sure that at least since the foundation of their College, physicians have been concerned with two sets of rivals: these quacks and empirics.

It is not simply, as Freidson says[158] that from 1860 the 'distinction between the physician and the so-called quack needed no longer to rest on the academic certification of the superiority of one superstition over another'. Still less was it mere preference for the intellectual over the practical. Freidson explains part of the objection:[159] quacks are client-dependent and have 'no obligations to or identity with an organized set of colleagues'. Even as regards the apothecary, by the early nineteenth century at the latest, practising on the basis of 'no cure, no fee' was quackery and not part of his practice.[160] The rivals to medicine were objected to, and I argue still are, not on the simple but 'vulgar' basis that they damage the economic interests of the profession, but rather because their existence impedes the achievement or maintenance of the corporate morality which itself is needed to enhance its general social status. Competition induces behaviour contrary to what I have described as the idealized gentleman Pythagorean Hippocratic physician.

6

Administration and medicine

Still more history: the growth of
public health institutions

My concern is not so much with the workings of public health
institutions as with their relation to medical practice. In part
associated with industrialization but also in part with other events,
threats of mass illness became an issue which was perceived as
requiring State or community action. As we shall see, the schemes
which were set up gave the medical profession institutional state
power. This involvement was crucial. The effect was that the professional establishment became a part of the foundation of the
general bureaucratic apparatus of the State. Atiyah suggests that
this growth, and its associated legislation, ran counter to the otherwise prevailing ideas of economic liberalism and freedom of contract. It may readily be conceded that this contrast is clouded
by the attitudes of specific actors, for example, Chadwick. The
point, however, is of philosophy, not history. Full freedom of
contract and government intervention stand in contrast to each
other only to be reconciled by the complexities and compromises
of pragmatism.

Accordingly, I approach the institutions through practice and
through something of awareness of disease. In particular, I take as
examples occasions where the state used the prestige of the Royal
College of Physicians, despite its competence. My first example is
of 'exotic' diseases (those introduced from abroad). It had long
been recognized that some diseases were liable to importation by
ships which had visited far-off ports. It was believed that diseases
which were epidemic (localized in time) and even pandemic (localized in space), in so far as they were not caused directly by Divine
intervention, were contagious. Such beliefs, at least, had the effect

of reinforcing the idea that disease was preventable. As early as 1374, Venice ordered the inspection and exclusion of infected ships. In 1383, Marseilles imposed a forty-day detention for persons suspected of suffering from disease. In 1403, Venice, still concerned, applied a general detention of *quaranta giorni* (from which the word 'quarantine' is derived) for travellers from the Levant.[1] A limited form of quarantine was first applied in Britain by Henry VIII in 1518. Clark suggests[2] that it was done on the advice of physicians and might have caused or eased the foundation of the College in the same year.

The idea of seeking the advice and co-operation of the College remained a feature of its power. Thus for example the City of London had sought its guidance at the outbreak of plague in 1583 and the Privy Council did so at the further outbreaks of 1629–30 and 1665. By the 1620s it was also consulting the College on a range of other matters including the health aspects of fumes from an alum-works and the advantages of colonial over home produced tobacco. By the early nineteenth century the pace of this consultation increased. In 1828, following difficulties in applying a series of Acts which gave the College powers over private madhouses, it connived at a new Board appointed by the Home Secretary to supervise those institutions.

A more significant way in which the early nineteenth century saw the establishment of a state health bureaucracy concerned smallpox. As a major killer in Britain, it lasted for less than a century. One distinction between it and other earlier fearsome diseases is that leprosy and plague were generally fatal. With smallpox on the other hand, although death was common, so was recovery. By the end of the century and into the nineteenth, techniques of vaccination were tried out and they quickly became common. In 1807, Parliament turned to the Royal College of Physicians to supervise the newly established National Vaccine Establishment and in the 1840s[3] the Poor Law authorities were required to contract with qualified medical practitioners to provide smallpox vaccination for all persons resident in their localities. To anticipate events, the National Vaccine Establishment lasted until 1861 when it was taken over by the Privy Council. In 1871, it was transferred to the Local Government Board and, in 1919, to the Ministry of Health.

My third example concerns yellow fever. It became severe in Gibraltar and it was feared it might be brought to Britain. In December 1804, the Privy Council asked the Royal College of

Physicians to help. The College perhaps not unexpectedly advised strict quarantine but also, with greater novelty, the establishment of a Board of Health to make regulations. The Board began as a committee of the Privy Council. It set up a Centre of Epidemic Intelligence. The yellow fever threat receded and the Board was dissolved in 1806. In retrospect, what was important for the development of bureaucracy was that a central Board of Health dominated by doctors with power to make regulations could control disease.

My last example, cholera and the response to it, exploited this idea.[4] The disease was virtually unknown in Europe until the nineteenth century. According to Cartwright,[5] Britain was able to anticipate its arrival. Certainly in June 1831 the Privy Council established the Central Board of Health expressly on the model of the 1805–6 body with the President of the Royal College of Physicians at its head.[6] It is to be noted however that in December of that year an exchange in the House of Commons indicated that the cause of the first outbreak in England was unknown.[7] The *Annual Register* for 1832 remarked:[8]

> The cholera left medical men as it found them – confirmed in most opposite opinions, or in total ignorance as to its nature, its cure, and the cause of its origin, if endemic – or the mode of transmission, if it were infectious.

A few local Boards of Health had already been established – for Manchester in 1794, and for Newcastle in June 1831 – but later in 1831 the Central Board recommended one for each town and village. It also recommended the maintenance of the quarantine regulations and, later still in 1831, the Cholera Regulations. The local boards were to consist of the 'Chief Magistrate, Clergymen, one or more Professional Gentlemen and Principal Inhabitants'. These boards were to allocate special places (or, in the case of those who could afford better, approve other places) for those suffering from the disease. In November, the membership of the Central Board was reconstituted on a full-time basis. Its members then travelled urging and advising the institution of the local Boards and isolation hospitals etc. In February 1832, the Cholera Prevention Act gave powers to abate nuisances and to provide nurses and medicines for the sick poor. When the first epidemic of cholera receded later in 1832, the Central Board was dissolved.

It was in the same year that Edwin Chadwick came to some prominence. It was the year of Bentham's death and in some respects Chadwick was his intellectual and perhaps political heir. For a short while (1831–2), Chadwick had acted as his secretary. In considering Chadwick's influence, it is important to note that he demonstrated a considerable antipathy to what he called 'mere medicine'. In any event Chadwick was invited to assist the Royal Commission which led to the reform of the Poor Laws and the establishment of the Poor Law Commission. Chadwick was later to claim that Bentham had approved the outline of the Poor Law proposals.[9] Advised by Doctors Southwood-Smith,[10] Arnott, and Kay, his *Sanitary Report* was produced in 1842. It argued that illness had a quantifiable economic cost and much of it, by less expenditure, was preventable. It appears[11] that the germ of this idea was derived from the French medical statistician, Villerme – 'the gradations of wealth, or the means of providing comforts, may almost be taken as the scale of mortality'. The Report led directly to a number of towns conducting further investigation and securing private Acts for better sanitation. They not merely allowed the abatement of nuisances, but also the appointment of Medical Officers of Health, Borough Engineers, and Inspectors of Nuisances.

Although a connection is not commonly made, in 1848 a second wave of cholera struck and the Public Health Act was passed. The Act provided for an appointed but otherwise autonomous General Board of Health and for local Boards where the ratepayers petitioned for one or where there was a high death rate. The Act also extended the powers of local authorities. They became responsible for paving the streets, constructing drains and sewers, refuse collection, and the provision of water.[12] They could appoint Medical Officers of Health but at that stage few took the opportunity. The MOH. was given a variety of powers and duties including a right to search for infectious disease, removal of the sick from places of overcrowding, and vaccination of smallpox contacts. The General Board, upon which Chadwick sat, had no executive power and operated mainly by giving advice. Chadwick's personality and the continuance of cholera led, in 1854, to his fall.[13] As *The Times* said:[14] 'we prefer to take our chance of cholera and the rest than to be bullied into health'.

After the departure of Chadwick the General Board continued. It was then largely guided by Sir John Simon. He continued the work of showing the link between cholera and contaminated water and proposing action accordingly. He began investigation into infant mortality and into industrial injury and disease. A series of *ad hoc* institutions and inspectorates were created. These were rationalized in the 1872 and 1875 Public Health Acts. The Local Government Board was established in 1871 with powers over both the Poor Laws and public health. In due course, government became more concerned to apply, or to re-emphasize, the principle of less eligibility: within the Department an emphasis on the poor law administration gained the ascendancy. Significantly, but in retrospect not unexpectedly, the political importance of public health was diminished.

More important than these twists and turns of fortune were the underlying facts that the growth in concern for public health itself laid the foundation for the modern state bureaucracies and medical practice was seen to be opposed to classical economics. In a rather different way, I have noted Foucault's suggestion that the clinic reflected economic liberalism but that the Pythagorean Hippocratic physician also had other, and more mystical, objectives. Both these, taken with the strengthening of the internal regulation within the profession, laid the foundation for the distinction I shall come to that the law has made between professional practice and other forms of 'economic' activity.

The trends were applicable in countries other than England. Ideas of economic liberalism were generally applied in revolutionary France. Closed centres of power were opposed and the old guild and university systems abolished. However, these goals were not universally accepted or applied. For example, Cabanis[15] distinguished occupations where consensus could judge the utility and therefore value from those where either the object of the occupation was itself a market criterion (as gold is for goldsmiths) or it concerned the activities of an individual who would otherwise be a party to determining value (as health and life are for medical practice). In these cases, the state must not determine the value of the occupation but it must judge the capacity and moral worth of those who pursue it. This reason too served to distinguish medicine from the normal bounds of classical economics. It is important that doctors were involved with the foundation of the bureaucracy two decades at least before the profession had any specifically scientific basis for action.

Public regulation – bureaucracy and law

In much legal writing there is a separation of consideration of bureaucracy (the necessary result of large scale administration) and law. That cannot be sufficient for my purposes. Freidson correctly points to two structures:[16] 'It is common' he says 'to note an administrative hierarchy that is parallel to the professional hierarchy but that is insulated from influencing the conduct of what are defined as professional or technical affairs.' It is necessary however to go further and describe the administrative and its link to the internal norms. Further, as I shall argue, out of its collective engagement, the administration provides the means, including litigation itself, for the resolution of problems precipitated by the untoward.

This book does not offer any practical account of the law and administrative machinery. Works such as *Encyclopedia of Health Services and Medical Law* describe the strictly legal arrangements. However, they provide no basis for a theoretical understanding since their definition of 'law' is entirely formal, that is, they assume that statements which are pronounced in legal form are 'law' and those which are pronounced in extra-legal form are not. What the definition fails to do is to indicate the scope of the norms governing medical practice, or even offer a method of ascertaining them. This dogmatic or atheoretical approach is by no means rare. The bulk of legal writing does the same. At the level of practice there is no harm in it; it provides the methodology required to satisfy litigation and prospective litigation. *En passant*, at the level of teaching, it is dubious if this is satisfactory; the methodology, although it is detailed and specialized, does not contain the essence of that esoteric knowledge and understanding of inherited traditions which are necessary for either truly 'professional' practice or its critique. What it also fails to do is to offer a method of isolating extra-legal normative statements from those which are non-normative because it ignores them both; or, perhaps more seriously, it fails to isolate those statements in legal form which are normative from those which are not, because it tends to equate them both.

Specifically, legal theory endeavours to meet this last problem by speaking of mandatory or directory as against permissive statements. The terms are useful for courts in distinguishing 'shall' from 'may'. But there are occasions when statutory language cannot be refined enough either to isolate its normative elements or to define them. Thus the courts have held[17] that the allocation of resources within the health service is legislative and their distribution, discretionary; that is, the distribution of resources is usually for bureaucratic and not legal regulation. In *ex parte Hincks et al.* the court said that the duties on the Secretary of State in sections 1 and 3 of the Health Service Act of 1977 are limited by the exercise of discretion within the resources available. In that case the applicants were four patients on a waiting list for orthopaedic surgery. They complained that a planned expansion of a particular hospital had not taken place. The need for the hospital was admitted, but the court held that the Secretary of State and the subordinate health authorities were limited by the resources available in their fulfilment of their duties, both as regards present provision and future planning. In this case, the court therefore held in effect that, despite the legal form of the duty, it was a duty understandable by the bureaucratic system and not the law. Such a view ignores any normative element internal to the administration.

It can be agreed that both the bureaucracy and the law seek in their own ways to influence the methods of practice of an occupation whose history pre-dates them both; whose area of discourse is at the same moment, in one sense unique and individual and, in another, global and international; and, whose ends, the attainment of health, are (to adopt the means of measurement used by the others) more obviously subjected to popular approval than either the bureaucracy or the law. For example, note the question put by three doctors seeking further resources from the government:[18] 'Should a doctor ever allow a patient to die of a treatable disorder because he is ordered to do so by a representative of the state?'.

I start by asking whether there can be any help in distinguishing the 'public' and the 'private'. In at least two ways the law has distinguished between them. Thus, there used to be special periods of limitation in litigation against public authorities.[19] They may be said to have restricted not only the pursuit of rights but also the development of the English malpractice action. They were progressively abolished from the mid-1950s. More recently the law has sought to apply the same words (with apparently different meanings)[20] to determine the correct mode of procedure in the courts.[21] In both these ways the words take technical meanings; there is no necessary correspondence with their ordinary use. Accordingly an alternative route must be attempted. I do so with the thoughts that: these public and private law distinctions are at best misleading;[22] that the search for the boundaries of the two is unsatisfactory for the simple reason it seeks a difference of essence where there is none; that all law in the state courts is public, irrespective of who the parties are; and that the truly private 'law' in biomedicine consists in the rules of the professional guilds. On this basis, no private law is the concern of practising lawyers until recognition is sought for it in the courts. What appears to have happened is that lawyers have myopically confused their formal working categories for reality. For example, the courts are concerned, not with contract law, but with the law of breach of contract. On this basis the norms of contract law are rarely the concern of lawyers. They are for practical application and for economic or other investigation. They are the private law. When there is a breach, the matter may become public and of concern to lawyers. Seen in this light both the bureaucracy and law are in the realm of the public and its contrast with the private does not take us far.

Turning to bureaucracy, we may follow Weber's postulate that 'domination' is the probability that a command with a given specific content will be obeyed by a given group of persons, and his distinction between three ideal types of 'legitimate domination': the charismatic, the traditional, and the legal. For the current purpose and as far as medicine is concerned it is sufficient that these three types of domination are thought of as chronological and that today it is regulated by a competition between the traditional and legal ideal types. Thus far, the analysis enables us to understand from a different angle the nature of regulation internal and external to medicine. The previous chapter discussed the current extent of traditional domination – internal regulation – in part as defined by state machinery. In effect it showed that the extent of this last definition is the extent to which legal domination has accommodated rather than replaced the traditional, in this the law follows the understandings of the initiates.

Here I am concerned with other aspects of the legal domination of medicine. To Weber, 'traditional legitimate domination' was derived from the routinization of the charismatic, and itself led to formal rationalization. As it did so, there was a tendency formally to maximize rationality and efficiency and reach stability. This last not only increases the scope of legal rules but also the range of bureaucratic regulation. I have noted the ideological consequences of the contrasting theories of medicine. I have also noted the rise both of the scientific imperative and of coercive medicine and a similar rise in bureaucratic health care systems. Mommsen says:[23] 'The "disenchantment of the world" closely associated with the progress of modern science as well as the irresistible advance of bureaucratization left less and less room for value-oriented forms of domination'.

As an ideal, the elements of Weber's concept of bureaucracy that directly concern its regulation[24] are that: it has a specified function, or functions; its operation is bound by rules; the organization of personnel is on the basis of hierarchy; the scope of authority within the hierarchy, and the rights and duties of the officials at each level are defined. Other elements of the ideal typical bureaucracy are: records are used; the staff are 'subject to authority only with respect to impersonal official obligations'; staff are appointed and promoted on the basis of impersonal qualifications and merit; and they are paid fixed salaries, have fixed terms of employment, and the employment is permanent.

This ideal type contains a number of difficulties.[25] One example is the fact that within every bureaucracy there is an informal sub-system operating alongside the formal.[26] Staff at every level have discretions in which they will make use of formal and informal organizational patterns. Or again, as contrasted with the power to err (which is maladministration) the functions of the bureaucracy may be several and be in conflict. Or further, within the hierarchy necessary expertise is likely to be exercised by subordinate rather than superior staff. As Thompson puts it[27]: 'the most symptomatic characteristic of modern bureaucracy is the growing imbalance between ability and authority'. Nevertheless the importance of Weber's model for the current purpose is precisely that it serves to identify those aspects of organizational behaviour susceptible to regulation, whether formally by law or otherwise.

Rarely are legal rules and principles expressed in a form descriptive of an individual. More commonly they are general statements about categories. It is not unrealistic to regard these statements as operating on ideal types. It is inevitable that rules in statutes and decisions by judges are made on the basis of the relation of the ideal to reality – facts found or supposed by Parliament or the court. Where however the analysis is reversed and the reality is used to describe the ideal and hence the rule, the perception of the reality and the ideal becomes confused. In practice, the precedent system of the common law always does this; but the wider the rule that is stated, the greater the scope of the possible confusion. In large part, the appeal procedures of the common law systems are concerned with the resolution of conflicts of values. Since, as I have already noted, all such litigation is a part of public law, such appeal processes necessarily involve public interests or public policy. The particular problem for the court is that the wider the interests it takes into account, the larger the probability of its departing from reality. One of the reasons why so much legal theory in this field is unsatisfactory is because, in the main, it is espoused by academic lawyers who tend to be impatient with the detail (reality) of the dispute between parties to litigation.[28] It follows that we must search elsewhere for such a description.

Presthus has suggested:[29]

Authority can be defined as the capacity to evoke compliance in others on the basis of formal position and of any psychological inducements, rewards, or sanctions that may accompany formal position. The capacity to evoke compliance without relying upon formal role or the sanctions at its disposal may be called *influence*. When formal position is not necessarily involved, but when extensive sanctions are available, we are concerned with *power.* . . . Authority, power and influence are usually interlaced in operating situations.

Thompson has argued[30] that those in positions of formal authority make use of two types of device, which he calls 'ideological' and 'dramaturgical', to translate authority into influence. The former set are concerned with the importance of leadership; the latter are 'stage' effects (size of office, protection by secretaries etc.) used to create impressions of managerial importance.

Considering the literature, Hill notes three approaches to the problem of leadership:[31] the functional;[32] the cultural;[33] and the orientational.[34] He himself adds a further type of orientation, the 'political' – the relation of the group to the rest of society.[35] The orientational approach requires some explanation. In Etzioni's theory organizations are either 'utilitarian' or 'normative', that is, the major means of control is either by remuneration or by internally determined goals. In a 'normative' system where the control is internal, use is made *inter alia*[36] of 'rituals and manipulation of social and prestige symbols' – there are more likely to be shared values. The orientation analysis of leadership distinguishes the leader from the led. To the leader what matters is whether he is 'expressive' or 'instrumental', that is, whether he is concerned with maintaining the group or with achieving a specific goal. To the led what matters, even more than the perception of the leader, is the means of control. If these means are 'utilitarian' then the leadership can be instrumental with cash. If the means of control is 'normative', then instrumental leadership becomes more difficult because the leader may have to change the values of the led.

An example may help. In *Royal College of Nursing* v. *DHSS*[37] the issue was whether a particular way of carrying out abortions was 'performed' by the doctor or by the nurse. If by the doctor it was lawful; if by the nurse, unlawful. By a majority the House of Lords held that, having regard to the degree of supervision by doctors over nurses, it was done by the doctor. The importance of the decision in terms of Etzioni's analysis is that it cast doubt on the 'normative' – shared value – means of control implicit in the idea of nursing as a profession. The nurse was seen to be controlled by 'utilitarian' methods. The conflict in question was between the emerging aspirations of a group (the nurses) to have their values reckoned against not only another group (the doctors), the expression of whose values might accordingly be more difficult but also between them and the tendency of the bureaucracy to diminish the role of the values of both them and the doctors.

Arguments of this type can be seen either to be based on the psychology of the actors or on the idea that authority is institutionalized power. Either way they do to some degree explain the operation of bureaucracy. A somewhat complicating feature in medical care is that although there is a bureaucratic (administrative) structure roughly corresponding to Weber's model there is, as we have seen, at the functional end a second system, that of the medical profession (itself collegiate but now also partly bureaucratic). Weber's ideas go some way to aiding the understanding of the bureaucracy; Etzioni's that of the professional hierarchy, and, perhaps also, the doctor's role in his relationship with patients. These are points to which I shall return.

The British National Health Service

This is not the place to describe the policies and events leading to the wholesale reforms effected by the National Health Act (1946). It is however convenient to cite the assessment offered by Abel-Smith:[38]

> For a century or more medical care in hospital had been regarded, as the education of children was always regarded in the United States, as a responsibility for which the community should in some form provide. It was this heritage of shared opinion which was responsible for the widespread acceptance in Britain of what others chose to call 'socialized medicine'.

.... While the nationalization of hospitals represented a large increase in government ownership, it also involved a substantial transfer of power to the medical profession.... Regional boards, boards of governors and hospital management committees were all given a generous proportion of medical representatives.

The Act represented a major rationalization but it was not a wholly new structure. The associated National Assistance Act of 1948 abolished the Poor Laws but kept, for example, the idea of coercive medicine in the provision that people could be confined to hospital where they were found to be incapable of looking after themselves.[39] Under the health service general practitioners receive their incomes by way of a complex formula but which in essence has regard to the numbers of patients on their lists. Except in a few areas they are not paid in respect of specific services which they have rendered. Although in practice it is not exercised to any great extent, in formal terms both doctor and patient have a choice, in the primary sector, as to whether they will enter the relationship. In this way the service and the reward are severed – practice can continue without regard to its economic consequences for the Service, the practitioner or (apart from payments for prescribed pharmaceutical items) the patient. In secondary health care, the undertaking to provide the service is given by the health authorities and they merely employ staff, including medical staff, to discharge it. Broadly, practitioners in both sectors, having discharged the obligations of their contracts with the Health Service,[40] are free to undertake other work. Many do, but only to a small extent.

The theoretical implications are not to be missed. Parsons had in his model described the way in which patients perceiving themselves as ill present themselves to the physician. McKeown had added that the physician's role included not only treating the sick but also reassuring the well. A system where the patient can meet the doctor without charge most closely approximates to the reciprocal Parsons–McKeown model. Earlier doubts that the removal of the contract nexus would mean that doctors would be taken for granted and thus interfere with 'trust' seem to have evaporated. As the British Medical Association argued:[41] 'The ideal personal doctor service ... can exist only when the limits to it set by the state are so wide that in day-to-day practice there are no practical constraints'. Any other system must introduce control devices, be they economic or bureaucratic, and which are extraneous to the reciprocity of the doctor–patient relationship.

Whereas the Secretary of State's duty is generally 'to provide' health services (including of course the hospital service), his duty as regards primary health care is more circumscribed. He is bound 'to secure' it by 'making arrangements'. These arrangements endeavour to provide that those who supply them shall remain in legal form independent contractors. As I shall argue, the issue does not affect clinical freedom. The effect is to give to the providers of primary health care a feeling of clinical autonomy. It is, however, not an insular autonomy. They are not divorced from the bureaucratic structure which has the Secretary of State at its head.

What is more important than the specifically legal question of the independent contractor status of the professions is their incorporation in the structure. Despite the House of Lords decision in the *Royal College of Nursing* v. *DHSS*, bureaucratic control is largely, in Etzioni's sense of the term, 'normative' (value-orientated) and increasingly so. Throughout the nineteenth century, the medical profession consolidated its power as a bourgeois profession. In the middle of the century the nurses,[42] the dentists, the pharmacists deliberately began to organize in the same way. In this century other health care professions, in part reflecting the advance of the new technologies and therapeutic measures, have emerged. They include the suppliers of ophthalmic services and, in the main, those centred round the Council on Professions Supplementary to Medicine.

These groups, particularly the older ones, sit on a host of committees. Specifically, for example, each Regional Health Authority and each District Health Authority is provided with separate advisory committees for medicine, dentistry, nursing and midwifery, pharmacy, and ophthalmic and dispensing opticians. These are in addition to the executive committee structure of the authorities (where government has in recent years attempted a policy of de-professionalization) and also to the negotiating machinery between professional bodies and their employers. But their position is more complex because in addition to these structures they also provide a second, and different hierarchy at its functional end, that is, the gradations of medical ranks in the hospitals – consultants, and the grades of junior doctors. This second structure is not subordinate to the National Health Service administration if that relation is to be measured by performance indicators set for the bureaucracy or by the status its members have in the organization, or, except in the resources made available, the control that the administrators have over them. It is a professional and not a manager who determines what should be done and to whom. As Freidson says,[43] '[professional] autonomy is sustained by barriers to supervisory information.... Even without legal support, concern for the privacy of the client has insulated the work of many professionals.... And it is the professional worker who creates [case] records.' He adds[44] that the professional view varies according to whether it is expressed by an ordinary practitioner, by a member of the professional structure, in England for example in the British Medical Association or the General Medical Council, or in one of the directly executive bodies. On this basis, it may be remarked the introduction of lay management serves to sharpen professional positions.

It is this second hierarchy that provides the links with associated organizations, that is, the Universities. And it is to be noted that particularly since 1974 when Regional Hospital Boards gave way to Regional Health Authorities, the demands of education within the system have been increased. The whole country is now within the jurisdiction of the teaching hospitals. And, although much of general practice continues as before, its tendencies to group practice have facilitated the expansion of the learning process there as well. Supervision and the opportunity for Etzioni's 'normative' control are both greater.

The untoward

People do something we do not like, and we say there ought to be a law against it. Something untoward happens, and we say there ought to be an inquiry. People are injured, and we say they ought to be compensated. Can any meaning be given to these sayings, these reactions? So also, with the best will in the world (and it is not always present) things continue to go wrong. Mistakes happen. Accidents occur. Ethical codes are breached. Professional interests are trespassed upon. Forecasts go awry, probabilities are not realized, and the unsought happens. Sometimes too, individuals are injured in their hopes or in their persons.

It is not surprising that each of the social structures involved in medical care, including the administration and the law, make provision for responding to these occasions. What perhaps is less expected is the spectrum of procedures that has been created. The quantity of the literature relating to empirical or theoretical investigation in some of the fields set out below varies, so far as I can tell, from whole libraries to nothing. Clearly, the issues and questions dealt with in these mechanisms are not always (or, indeed, often) similar. But what they share is a concern for malfunction and for disturbance, not so much of order, as of aspiration.

There is one other opening point. In particular cases, these types may often be used concurrently or seriatim. If a general point can be perceived, it is that an administration will conduct some form of its own inquiry before launching or participating in some mechanism controlled by other hands. For example, in an allegation (which itself might have originated in a wider investigation of the untoward begun without suspicion of blame) that an employee of a health authority has acted negligently or unprofessionally, there could be an internal investigation, and also a separate professional investigation. If either or both of these lead to penalties, not infrequently we can expect resort to the more ordinary law. There are occasions when this might offend ideas relating to 'double-jeopardy' (that is, an individual may be punished twice out of the same set facts) but this is not a common risk.

The *Encyclopedia of Health Services and Medical Law* identifies, within its field, administrative, professional, and legal mechanisms for responding to the untoward. The administrative includes: (1) inquiries (which themselves may have varying levels of formality and types of intent); (2) the Health Service Commissioners; (3) Community Health Councils; (4) the Service Committees and the Health Service Tribunal; (5) investigations under the Department of Health's circular HC81/5 (and the Health Service Complaints Act 1985); and (6) the Health Advisory Service. The professional includes: (7) the General Medical Council and the other professional registration bodies; (8) the power of the defence societies to refuse to represent a member; and (9) the powers of the Royal Colleges and the British Medical Association to investigate unprofessional behaviour. The legal includes the potentiality of (10) civil and (11) criminal liability.

The task here is to isolate the theories which explain these mechanisms for responding to untoward occurrences. Beyond the clusters suggested above and a relatively fuller discussion of litigation, I have not sought a classification. This task would be necessary if I were to attempt to describe their procedures.[45] I do not make the attempt for two reasons: first, in so far as I am describing medical practice, these procedures are responses to exceptions;

and, secondly, as I have said, the emphasis of the literature is unbalanced. The theories, then, are five. I term them historico-anthropological; economic (loss adjustment); economic (class control); administrative; and psychological. It is probable that none of them alone tries to explain all the devices, still less their variety. The overview, however, presents points of comparison, and of joinder, which make it useful.

The historico-anthropological approach looks towards individualized threats to social order, most often disputes. I might have called it 'traditional' were it not for the fact that I have already appropriated the word twice, once on my own account to describe some aspects of Hippocratic medicine and once, following Weber, to describe what can be called pre-bureaucratic societies. Undoubtedly it is the most common way, in our culture, of thinking about the untoward. It has informed most previous descriptions of systems. Birkinshaw says:[46] '[his] examination will tell us something of value about ... the *loci* of official power'. And:[47] '[The method of the law] is to transmute conflicts of political, economic and social moment into disputes between *individuals* based upon individual entitlement and duty'.

This first approach almost naturally leads to, if it does not start with, ideas of wrongdoing, blame, and sanction. Thus Stein[48] suggests that in a stateless society there is either conformity to the old ways or the likelihood of dispute for which 'the ultimate sanction ... is expulsion'. In a way which is reminiscent of evolutionary theory, he goes on to describe, still within such societies, methods of mediation and arbitration. And then, with the emergence of central social structures (which apparently he associates with statehood) he discusses adjudication. The possibility of organized investigation outside individual dispute is dismissed in half a paragraph.[49] The modern tribunal system, as contrasted with the courts, and arbitration are described but in terms which imply they are some later stage of evolution. Conciliation is not mentioned but it would fit the same pattern.

Roberts[50] is less cultural-centric. Focusing on social order, he argues that the control mechanisms we associate with centralized government can be absent in a society which is nevertheless ordered. Thus there need be no articulated rules, or means beyond talk for resolving disputes, or any authority to enforce decisions:[51]

At the root of everyday life in any society there must necessarily be some patterns of habitual conduct followed by the members, providing a basis upon which one member will be able to predict how another is likely to behave under given circumstances and how his own actions will be received. But in some small-scale societies a normative base for these regularities is not clearly conceptualized or articulated; people simply do not always think in terms of rules and obligations.

It is right, of course, to emphasize this aspect of small-scale societies, but the point, I argue, is wider. Our civilization is made up of dynamic, changing, and interlocking groups. The reason that obligations are not always articulated is that they are directed toward single human beings: where their selves are incorporated in greater wholes, the rules and obligations lose their capacity to describe. Rules there may be, but in order for them to be treated as obligations they have to be translated from the language of the group into that of the individual.

So also, in my argument, the groups in our societies have autonomy, have, that is, existence, divorced from the communities of which they are part. Roberts' point is applicable to the maintenance of order within them. At least in western culture it is another description of some of the attributes of the guild. One aspect can be brought out. The absence of articulated rules does not imply that the 'small-scale society' – a group or guild – does not have either the means to resolve disputes or to enforce decisions. At whatever its level of sophistication, a good reason in any society for not having an articulated rule is that the events to which it might be directed have not occurred before, and it is scarcely less good a reason that they are so unlikely as not to be worth thinking about. So long as there is a common understanding of what is acceptable, precise definitions of what is not are not live issues. In our interlocking groups and bureaucracies the point is recognized even by the central government. The legislature commonly uses a 'broad-term' whose meaning is intelligible only in its application. This explains why it can use phrases such as 'serious professional misconduct', why the courts have left the meaning to the professions, and why therefore the various formulations have each elicited the same hands-off approach by the courts: the term indicates an action threatening to the habits of the group and the group is its judge.

Although this sort of explanation is helpful in responding to man-made untoward occurrences, it is not sufficient. At bottom it says that communities are in general ordered. Occasionally disputes occur. The community can cope with these either by recognizing the result of a fight or, which may be the same thing, institutionalizing dispute resolution techniques and their sanctions. The explanation does not touch on a crucial element of dispute, namely in many (in our culture, most) cases the party who has cause to feel himself aggrieved does nothing and commonly forgets about it. This may be, I might suggest, a symptom of the maturity or stability of the culture. It might explain differences in the *per capita* rates of litigation in seemingly similar economic and social systems. It does not explain why when litigation is precluded by cost, normally the dispute (but not always the social relationship) is ended. Nor, as I have indicated, does this approach (it can perhaps be called the idea of the safety-valve) touch untoward occurrences for which human intervention is not overtly responsible.

The second theory of the untoward (the economic – loss adjustment) again, most often, focuses on individual responsibility. At its crudest it says that where a loss has been suffered the person who can be held to have been responsible shall make amends and all is satisfied. The reason for this is that a potential injurer will know the costs of causing the injury and therefore will want to avoid it if he spends sufficiently on some other course of action. In this way, by way of deterrence, it is linked to blame.[52] A variant of this theory in the hands of Posner[53] is used to evaluate the wisdom (that is, economic efficiency) of many legal rules. Applying his analysis to the British context, it objects to the malpractice action against doctors[54] because the costs of determining the existence of malpractice (that is, medical 'negligence') are disproportionate to the gains in safer medical practice from imposing damage liability on careless doctors; and also because judicial fact finding is so prone to error as to remove any deterrent effect that the costs of wrongdoing may ordinarily be supposed to have caused.

The theory tries to show that in a more rational world, 'medical injury' (the term is inherently uncertain but some states, such as Sweden, have tried to give it formal meaning) would be dealt with in a different way. However the theory not only assumes rationality (which it is about) but also the possibility of medicine (whose social structures it ignores). I have sought to show the senses in which medicine is necessarily irrational. Following McKeown, medicine consumes resources which, in order to achieve its commonly stated goals (for example, the prevention of illness) could more efficiently be spent in other ways. Medicine presupposes inequality of knowledge between doctor and patient because their ways of knowing the disease must differ. It also presupposes an inequality of bargaining because the patient is under the duress of the distress of illness, and because the moral agency of each in relation to the patient possibly differs between doctor and patient, and in my argument necessarily does.

The second difficulty of this loss adjustment approach, as with the previous method discussed, is that there is no room for nature, that is, where loss is suffered without anyone else gaining or being at fault. The work which has come nearest to bringing economic theory to these issues is Calabresi and Bobbitt's *Tragic Choices*.[55] The task they set themselves is however not how to cope with choice in the face of tragedy *per se* but with how much of a scarce good should be produced and how it should be allocated. They say that there are four approaches: pure market; accountable political; lottery; and custom. The first three are the stock in trade of economics. Custom, on the other hand, they say, avoids choosing but only at the cost of openness and honesty. In the United States, for example they argue (in terms reminiscent of Parsons) it has close affinities with a pure market but becomes a haven for the powerful in the face of changing technology. Although they admit that openness and honesty are not fundamental, there are difficulties with this critique. Although for example their analysis helps understanding of the distribution of kidney dialysis machines, by definition since it is concerned with choice after tragedy, it says nothing about the incidence of kidney failure. So also, by placing custom in contrast to openness and honesty, they tend to imply a possibility of proceeding without it. Thus they deny the necessary inequalities between doctor and patient that I have described.

The third approach to the untoward (economic – class control) says, for example of a legal system, that it is a part of a superstructure of a society whose foundations are described by the relations between the material conditions of its social classes. Accordingly, all that the legal system does is determined by those relations. It is sufficient with two exceptions here merely to mention the theory: any further description would, by its definitions, include not only the means of coping with the untoward (man-made or otherwise), but its discussion of the material conditions of social classes. It is a task too far beyond my present concerns.[56]

It is however worth noting a complexity inherent in the approach. On their face, the general rules contained in the legal system are applied regardless of the social class of the parties. Social class does not bring people to doctors nor does it bring them to the courts. Whilst it is probably true that health and ill-health are influenced by class or at least by material circumstances, this is less clear of the chance mismanagement in care. Further, in so far as there is a reality in the critique, it is as true of medical practice as it is of law. If there is a greater likelihood that upper classes will receive better medical care, it is likely also to be technically more advanced and so increase the possibility of injury being serious.

The approach does however have a near relation which it is worth pausing on. It is now quite common. Davis has had a marked influence.[57] He argued that official discretion relating to individuals can and ought to be cut down by the use of rules. If Weber described an imperative in the growth of rationality, Davis responded to it. The approach says that since everybody is subject to events beyond his control, all misfortune is the result of the unintended. It rejects responsibility and blame. (Because it has much in common with sociology, that discipline is often, either wrongly or mischievously, held to adopt this view.) It directs attention towards the rectification of ill luck. At the same time it moves discussion from authoritative solutions (as for example the ordinary legal system) to devices designed to expose the merits. In other words, with blame and other concepts of the adversary process in particular gone, there can be the creation and investigation of other, and more wide ranging forms of procedure. It is worthy of note that although the English legal academic tradition refuses to look at procedural law in the formal legal system, it is quite happy to do so in this informal arena.

Because 'merits' (as the lawyers describe the issues legal technicalities disguise) are exposed and because merits are values, the approach is available to all shades of the political spectrum. It enables formalism to be disowned. A criticism of this style is offered by Abel. He says:[58]

> Within the substantive civil law we find reforms in divorce, probate, residential land transfer, and tort that are ostensibly intended to decrease the magnitude and complexity of state intervention in those transactions.

Biomedicine continues the process with the medicalization of conduct previously criminal and trends to no-fault compensation for medical injury. Abel argues:[59]

[The] erosion of formal rights is a necessary concomitant of the progressive penetration of state and capital into areas of personal autonomy: The individual must be given the illusion that his dissatisfactions will be heard and redressed as he surrenders more and more actual control over life.

In fact he suggests, in line with the Pearson Commission[60] for example, that although there are no fault compensation schemes for various specific types of accident, claimant plaintiffs, prefer to use the formal law. Beyond this, but importantly for that discourse, suggesting a political dichotomy, he does not seek to penetrate that preference.

The fourth of the approaches to the untoward is the administrative. Under this scheme, the purpose of *ex post facto* inquiries is to rectify not the past but the future. It is conceivable (although in Britain, rare) that a common law court can be directly involved in the application of this theory.[61] Indirectly, and most often partially, it underlies a considerable part of the rationale of the contemporary method of handling disputes involving governmental agencies. More directly the approach is an important element in the inquiries which lead, for example, to the Department of Health issuing hazard notices to health authorities.

The explanation is much wider. In litigation, for example, damages are awarded in order to make the future as much as possible like it would have been if the injury-causing action had not taken place. The administrative approach – we might call it rationality – is happier with no fault systems of compensation, because the payments can be met out of an anonymous fund; but it is quite content to award damages in the next best set of circumstances, that is, where the defendant is insured. The interest of reason is only partly in these conceptualizations of matters which the other approaches have already described. What is novel is its capacity to include forms and issues beyond them. Because of its concern with the future rather than individuals, it can encompass the investigation of events without looking for attributable fault. It can look instead for ways of reorganizing systems, whether they be social,[62] or mechanical.[63]

Commonly, however, at the outset at least, there is a possibility that someone may be blameworthy. Because rational inquiry normally and most happily exists outside and alongside formal systems, it can manifest a variety of forms. It includes the permanent system of coroners' courts, and the use of powers of formal inquiry under the National Health Service Act 1977.[64] It can take the form of the Health Service Commissioner, inquiries under HC81/5 and the Health Service Complaints Act 1985, and by the Community Health Councils. Because, although it is not particularly interested in faults, it can investigate them.

So also if the occasion warrants it can utilize the prestige of judges and lawyers, not only in courts, but in a host of *ad hoc* investigations.[65] In these inquiries, it is intended that specific action will be recommended. Two points should be observed. First, the action is recommended not implemented. Secondly, although some commentators would wish to make a distinction between administration and policy, what is notable is that commonly the action that is eventually recommended combines the two. The expectation is that the inquiry will approach its task in an unprincipled commonsensical fashion. However there are clearly occasions when other methods would be more efficient. It is clear that despite the prestige of lawyers, their skills are not always the most relevant. So also even where their skills are relevant, their method of investigation, for example of questioning witnesses, is not best designed to look to the future. These are no doubt among the reasons why the Health Advisory Committee includes no lawyers.

Indeed one suspects that in the use of these inquiries, as with the preference for formal law identified by Abel and the Pearson Commission, another factor is at work. There are occasions, when although there is concern for the future, the past lies heavy. The need here is for a cathartic cleansing, a purification of the emotions by formally reliving the past by personal or vicarious experience.[66] This then is the fifth of the approaches to the untoward. Clearly, it reaches beyond mere rationality. Clearly too, it is an ingredient in the ritual of the court-room and why to complain about its lack of reason is often beside the point. But it is more. It represents a fundamental need formally to re-create, and so exorcise, catastrophe either on the grand or on the individual scale. Unfortunately, the literature does not reflect investigation of this form and my remarks do not do it justice. What we need to know is when such a cleansing is appropriate and when, by contrast, the fear of the creation of a scapegoat or a martyr prevents it. Clearly this device allows the investigation of the breach of non-legal norms but we need to be able to describe the perception of the relation between them and the law. What I have indicated are the beginnings of reasons why a formal inquiry, particularly involving lawyers (because of the sense of stability and continuity that the law generally conveys) is sometimes used even where such recommendations as it might make are predicable and predicted in advance. It begins to explain why inquiries are used where the costs clearly absorb resources which could have been directed to cure the problem, or where the grand inquiry is powerless because the law (with its emphasis on obligation) insists that individualized investigation is alone capable of making decisions, as where there must be a formal determination of some civil or criminal liability.[67] Of course any civil liability can be compromised or settled, but only between the parties: this device, technique, by-passes that chance.

Litigation

The most formal approach to the untoward is litigation. It is a method of constructing a workable but partial reality. As a description of the whole it must fail. First, there must be a winner and a loser: a proposition in contrast to so much other activity, including medicine. Secondly, because it is general, law is, in my argument, always crude and even within that limit is not always effective or predictable. Thirdly, we shall see that Burt describes oscillations which preclude the consistent application of rules (that is, general articulated commands). Fourthly, the law must deal in retrospect. The deepest wish in a case of malpractice is to return to the *status quo ante*, and with that impossible the law is left to pick up what pieces it can.

Fifthly, despite this, it fails to notice that it looks through the distorting glass of money which turns that part into the whole. For example, the legal system (and lawyers) are satisfied by enforcing money payments for loss of arms, legs, eyes, life. Within its terms of reference there may be no other way, but it is only a cause of satisfaction in the moral sense Weber attributes to the western bourgeoisie – it is the one group for whom material accumulation had at once religious and thus moral significance. Risk is part of life and the more so with higher technologies, but the risks are not always financial. Awards of damages (and insurance, cash in any event for greater cash if the risk materializes) are a poor translation. To continue the metaphor, without that pervasive refracting medium, the incommensurables are almost too obvious to be mentioned: the most irrational form of rationalism is economics: a whole science devoted to the proposition that money can join units of value which are not compatible.

Kennedy says:[68]

> [There are] two propositions [which are] both wholly untenable.
> The first is that anything to do with medicine, by virtue of its
> being 'medical' is best left to the medical profession since they
> are the experts. The same argument has been used as regards
> medical ethics, though I doubt if it would be as strongly held if
> business ethics were being discussed and the view put forward
> that the adjective 'business' entailed that it was a matter only for
> businessmen.... The second proposition is that the law really
> has no place in regulating medicine, that it is too clumsy a tool,
> too blunt an instrument for the subleties and complexities of
> medicine and the doctor–patient relationship. [But] ... Law
> is not necessarily clumsy ... Furthermore, law cannot be kept
> out of the consulting room or surgery. It is there already.
> Whenever someone lays hands on another ... society takes it
> sufficiently seriously that it looks to its most formal method of
> social ordering, the law, to make sure the line is held between
> the tolerable and the intolerable.

Both these propositions are worth some examination because I
have argued for precisely that which Kennedy regards as 'unten-
able'. The view that the law has no place in regulating medicine is
based on positive and negative considerations. On the positive
side, medicine, as I have sought to say, is an art and a vocation.
Quite simply, it mistakes its fundamentals to equate it with business: we each have a greater (and prior) interest in our bodies than
in our bank accounts. Indeed one of the difficulties contained in
the notion that medicine is only an applied science is that it
compels us and doctors to think of the link between service and
reward. When we go to our medical advisors, we need to know that
the advice we receive is unbiased, that is, not motivated by the
advantage to them. In crude terms, we need to know whose side
they are on. And, if medicine is a business, if doctors have a
financial interest in what they do, whatever the other competencies
they may have, the one thing we cannot know is whether the
advice they offer is on the whole for us or for them. On the
negative side, the law has no substantial place in regulating medicine because although some rules establish structures, the law's
prime concern is with the untoward.

Kennedy's second proposition that the law need not be clumsy
is also questionable. Law's clumsiness arises out of its generality. If
it is not general, it scarcely deserves the name of law. Of course,

when it is applied, it can be as finely tuned as the wit of man can devise: but, as far as only those with the authoritative right to define it (the judges) it can only be applied in retrospect. Since the idea of regulation of an activity presupposes that the actor may know what he can and cannot do before he acts, the law is bound to be crude or coarse.

So also the suggestion that the law is already in the surgery deserves rebuttal. I have observed that God has been put in a pigeon hole. Now in Kennedy's hands, in place of an omnipresent all-seeing God, we have an omnipresent all-seeing law. He is wrong. Although it is true that the law is potentially capable of being applied to all activity, it does not follow in any meaningful sense that it is. Most of the time, most people proceed without regard to it. Nor is it true that the law is the 'most formal method of ordering society'. The word 'formal' is a statement of procedure. The law becomes formal when it is invoked in the courts. By then, of course, what happened in the surgery or anywhere else is a matter of the past.

The traditional conception of the basis of the liability of the doctors is placed in express agreement in contract or in the more general torts of 'trespass' and 'negligence'. The *Encyclopedia of Health Services and Medical Law* challenges this. It suggests the idea of *situation liability*. Briefly, the *Encyclopedia*'s idea separates clinical freedom from patients' legal rights. It suggests that the existence of duties to provide medical care, the standards to be adopted, and whether there has been breach are each dependent upon the situation of the doctor's occupation; it suggests that its relation to the patient is established by reference to the normal expectations for the time being created by, and accepted within, the medical profession. A consequence of using the idea is, as that work shows, that many obligations can be, and are, determined by the customs of the profession. The idea allows the courts to decide issues that are brought to them without making themselves alternative interpreters of what professional standards should be. It explains why they are disengaged from these controversies, and yet it renders evidence and discussion of professional morality, etiquette, and practice relevant to litigation. If the duty for which there may be liability arises by operation of law, then the content, the standard, can be defined and imposed by the same means.

If the duty arises out of an undertaking given by the defendant, out of what Pellegrino and Thomasma call the 'act of profession', the extent of the undertaking is defined by his intention. His intention is not necessarily a specific subjectivity; it can as well be an 'ideal-type' of intention. Thus, where a man is possessed of skills and has undertaken to use them his intention is crucial to the determination of the standard of care. Hence, the situation of the defendant and the consent of the plaintiff are the necessary preconditions of liability, and the standard of care to be applied by the defendant is that determined by his intentions. A further consequence of situation liability is that it supports both the classical theory of medical practice and the necessary creation of internal professional standards. That is, the practice of the Hippocratic Pythagorean physician is supported by this approach. It is also not dependent on medical practice having a 'scientific theory'.

The *Encyclopedia* argues the basis of the liability of the medical attendant was fixed at an earlier time than either what we now recognize as the development of the action for breach of contract or the action for the tort of negligence. The medical profession was largely insulated from the forces and events which led to the flowering of those actions. The *Encyclopedia* also argues that the theoretical basis of the liability – the legal incidents of the situation of the potential defendant – has remained unaltered. The content of the liability itself has been altered by forces and events contemporaneous with those affecting contract and negligence but they are not otherwise connected with them. (Perhaps only a lawyer of a particular sort could think they could, or should, or must be.) The practice of medicine has been altered by changes in its science and in society. The direct influence of the courts has been insignificant.

The patient's place: situation liability, consent, and self-determination

Thus far, my analysis of the doctor–patient relationship has been one-sided. It has concentrated on the doctor and his relationship to the patient, to his profession, and to society. I have not considered these issues from the position of the patient. I do so now because litigation requires the conflict and resolution of interests (albeit translated, as I say, into those of individuals). Among the issues which arise are how far it is possible to be consensual where need on one side and expertise on the other is presupposed? What is the effect of the doctor's authority, or influence, or power, or prestige on the patient's willingness to enter the relationship? What is the scope of the mandate given by the entry into the relationship? How far do the patient's needs for cure and relief of pain and suffering prevent a meeting of minds? How far, as Canguilheim suggests,[69] do variations in understandings of the biological normal (which he argues is a value, not a statistical reality) stop even this being a meaningful question? Is a meeting of minds also prevented by the over-optimism of the patient described by Parsons or by the Hippocratic tradition that 'life is short and the Art long': that is, by the different knowledge of illness held by doctor and patient. In other words, do the motivational factors on both sides of the doctor–patient relationship – the desires to exert authority and to practise the calling on the one side and the need to seek help on the other – create incommensurable objectives for its parties?

Disregarding all this and even assuming that there is a possibility of full agreement, how can it exist with an inequality of information and understanding? Both codes of professional ethics and the law speak of 'consent'.[70] Do they intend the same meaning or in practice are they given it? What role is there for the externals, particularly relatives of the patient, close by habit as well as by blood? Ramsey argued:[71] 'Patient and physician can say and ideally should both say "I cure"'. In this he has assumed that they are 'joint adventurers in a common cause' and, I would argue, takes for granted a common view of medicine, disease, and cure. To take Ramsey's road is to take the road to self-determination. It is also to reject Hippocratic medicine. It is to treat medicine as scientific.

As I mention below, Beauchamp and Childress seek to provide a theory of medical ethics in what is in effect a unity of the ideas of Mill and Kant. Giesen[72] argues that there is a common view of the patient's role in both Anglo-American (where utilitarianism prevails) and European jurisprudence (where Kant is highly influential). J.S. Mill's view, expressing the former, was that:[73]

> As soon as any part of a person's conduct affects prejudicially the interests of others, society has jurisdiction over it.... But there is no room for entertaining any such question when the person's conduct affects the interests of no persons besides himself, or need not affect them unless they like.... In all such cases, there should be perfect freedom, legal and social, to do the action and stand the consequences.

Mill also wanted to achieve a 'general unanimity of sentiment' by way of similar educational experiences[74] but it is this dictum that has proved more influential. The difficulty with it is that it places its emphasis on the idea that individuals are controlled by law and is in this way opposed to control by sentiment. Further, it is, as we would now say, the bottom line of his approach that the 'sentiment' comes before the 'but'. By a further extension, the dictum is in many ways applied not only to the adults to whom Mill would have confined it but also to those being educated; the opportunity to acquire the 'general unanimity' is being undermined.

It is worth pausing on the *Encyclopedia*'s idea of situation liability. In any particular case disclosure of certain facts or possibilities may be seen to help or hinder that co-operation. As it was put in *Slater* v. *Baker*,[75] 'A patient should be told *what* is about to be done to him, that he may take courage and put himself in such a situation as to enable him to undergo the operation'. The amount was not conditioned by giving enough information to bring the patient into the tactical considerations of the decision to operate or not. I would argue, in this as in other fields, that the idea of giving orders requiring somebody else to take unreasoned courage is less applicable than once it was. Tennyson put it[76]

> Not tho' the soldier knew
>   Some one had blunder'd.
> Theirs not to make reply,
> Theirs not to reason why,
> Theirs but to do and die:

It is perhaps true that, as with so many other social forms, subservience of this degree was destroyed by the Great War. What does seem clear is that the amount of information now required to enable people generally to take courage is greater and that submission is no longer unreasoned: there is now an insistence on making reply and on reasoning why. I would argue that the medical profession has responded to this change. This is not to say that true self-determination has become common: rather it is to say those in authority, in particular, doctors, have recognized that greater degrees of explanation are required in order to secure the patient's compliance. The philosophical divide between compliance and liberty remains.

It seems likely that compliance in this sense is itself based in the religions of the western world, particularly in the various Christian sects. For most of them information is not required for the sake of participation in decision-making; it is required in order that the patient 'may put himself in a situation' to enable him to undergo the operation. The purpose of this is that he may make self-determined arrangements with his priest and others (concerned with his spiritual and social existence) rather than with his doctor (concerned with his body). Possibly the change in the quantity of information to be given reflects a secularization of this religious view.

What appears to have happened is that the advocates of informed consent theory have attempted to apply the ideas of the protection of the individual developed in one tradition, that is, the religious (where the future of the soul was at issue) to the other, the scientific mode of medicine (where the body was concerned). This religious tradition corresponds to what I have termed classical or Hippocratic medicine. The grafting of part of concepts on to separate traditions has caused the legal and policy confusion regarding 'informed consent'. The scientific theory of medicine is itself, as I have argued, open to serious doubt. Its effective emphasis on the objective nature of medicine (that is, the subject-matter of the malpractice action) lends itself to negligence theory. It is not unreasonable to suspect that the limitations on the one are applicable to the other. (At times, it has also led its advocates to consider that consent is itself therapeutic.)[77]

One of the elements of a critique offered by Kennedy and by Lord Scarman and Donaldson M.R. relates to whether a doctor's competence is limited to therapy or whether it extends to the giving of 'advice' – the preferred word is 'information' with the indication of the possibility of choice. Kennedy says:[78] 'Advice-giving is to a solicitor what diagnosis and treatment are to the doctor, namely what their skill consists in'. And, to an extent Kennedy is right. Because to Kennedy, as to Lord Scarman and Donaldson M.R. medicine is a science, the advice (information, warning) is outside. On the contrary, I have argued that medicine is not scientific and also (in effect) that because it is authority based, communication is essential to it. It is to be noted that the Health Service Commissioner (who is precluded from inquiring into 'clinical matters') does not investigate complaints relating to alleged failure of doctors to inform patients. If Kennedy, Lord Scarman, and Donaldson M.R were correct it would be difficult to explain this. To re-emphasize the point, patients conceivably could determine the rules for the exercise of biotechnology. They cannot determine them for Hippocratic medicine since doctors have not only skill but art.

It is not a part of my argument that members of the profession can do what they like. Kennedy says:[79]

> In the context of the disclosure of information, the very notion of a professional standard is something of a nonsense. *There simply is no such standard*, if only because the profession has not got together to establish which risks should be disclosed, to which patients, in which circumstances.

Of course any standard adopted by a formal mechanism is more likely to be an aspiration than a representation of a state of mind. But I have sought to show that the guild creates its customs by practices, not by resolutions or externally imposed rules, although each may influence the other. Its practices are conditioned by the culture in which it operates. The particular practices are those which relate to conduct at the bedside. Therefore I argue that as subservience has declined so the requirements of disclosure imposed both by the guild and by the law have increased. But crucially, as I shall argue in the next chapter, subservience within a static relationship may rightly be condemned as outmoded; but it may be the cement of a dynamic one. And since, as we shall see, static social forms are not descriptive of human relationships, externally imposed strategies designed to eliminate obedience may, to the extent that they are successful, dissolve society.

The matter may be put another way. It may be agreed that 'we' have to agree on common standards. In the face of the impossibility of finding the means to do so, we adopt an agreed procedure to define them. In the field of disputes we ask lawyers to tell us how to resolve them. In the field of medicine, we ask doctors to tell us what we should know of sickness and health. It is procedure, not reason, which makes us accept their verdicts. They give us the 'right' answers because we give them the job of defining answers: they define them for the simple reason that our needs require a definition and our procedure gives that task to them. What we cannot do is to change the procedure and merely assume that either the lawyers or the doctors will be able to carry out the same job as before.

7

Conclusion

Selves: singulars and plurals

The questions concerning the patient posed towards the end of the last chapter are framed largely within the same philosophical framework as the law. Central to them is the hypothesis of an 'autonomous self'. If, instead of postulating society as comprising a finite grouping of biological individuals, an alternative is adopted, the 'coarseness'[1] of the law may be avoided. Take then two postulates: that human beings are in more than biological, instinctual, relation with each other, that a distinction can be made between human society and a colony of ants; and that their relations vary over space and time. Robert Burt[2] has sought to explore the consequences of these ideas for the doctor–patient relationship including the modern doctrine of informed consent. Put briefly he argues that co-existent with the biological entities to a two party relationship there is another to which each of them has a relation. It is the relationship itself. In the static world of autonomous beings, A and B = A + B; in the dynamic world of social beings, A and B = A + B + AB; that is, in any two person relationship there are three 'selves' to be considered.

The conclusion that in the social world of A and B there are three not two selves transforms the problematics involved in issues of consent. It is accordingly necessary to explain how Burt arrives at it and to consider its implications for the question as I approached the patient's place. He describes four sets of relationships where the psychology of the actors demonstrated both omnipotence and impotence. His attention is thus directed to an empirical rather than metaphysical examination of the effect of power, and powerlessness, on individual. In each case the questions that Burt poses centre on who it was who was choiceless.

The first example is of a man who suffered intense burns causing profound pain, severe and permanent disability, and disfigurement. Crucial to the discussion is the fact that the injuries prevented him from caring for himself in any way at all, even to the point of his not being able to take positive steps to kill himself, and yet despite this he was able to object to receiving treatment and to express a desire to die. The issue arose on a psychiatrist's investigation as to whether the court should make a civil commitment order which under the State law would empower the doctors to override this expression of volition.[3] He said he wanted to die. To Burt, the individual could be seen either as seeking to implement his own choice or that of others; that is, was the perception of his isolation and the pain his existence caused to others responsible for his expressed desire to die? To Burt, the medical staff and potentially the lawyers were personally involved because they could not avoid interpreting that wish but at the same time as seeking to apply impersonal solutions or, which amounts to the same, to shift the responsibility for decision to others.

In Burt's second example[4] standards of etiquette expected in public street behaviour were violated[5] and neither acceptable evidence of competence was offered (in this case, giving an address) nor a need for help accepted. In effect, Burt argues that the adoption of impersonal, responsibility shifting postures (particularly in categorizing somebody else as choiceless) is unsettling to those in authority: the rejection of the help of the authorities could be regarded either as failing to acknowledge 'that they have any cohesive self-determination' or as an inability[6] 'to hold in their minds an image of some "other" ... who, in turn, would view them as a coherent self, worthy of recognition as such'.

He concludes:[7]

> When we understand the idea of 'self' as a product of mutual interactions among people rather than as fixed presentations of a priori separate self-delineations, we then see that neither the patients in the first two examples nor anyone who saw either of them could coherently ask themselves whether to enter social relations. The coherent question rather was how the various actors could disentangle themselves into separately conceived integers.

Thirdly, Burt discusses Milgram's experiments.[8] These had sought to establish how people would willingly inflict pain on others. Subject-teachers administered what they supposed was an increasing intensity of electric shock to actor-learners. The former were told that he was testing the effect of punishment on learning. In fact what he was testing was how far they would impose punishment. *Ex facie*, the results seem incredible. The subject-teachers were paid a small fee whether or not the actor-learner responded. They were told that although pain might be inflicted no permanent tissue damage would be occasioned. What they saw and heard and had every sensual reason to believe was that the 'punishment' which they were inflicting was causing not only great pain but also injury and in some cases death. Nevertheless most of the subject-teachers were prepared to impose any amount of pain and danger in response to commands to do so by the experimenter.

Burt suggests that the subject-teachers were disoriented. The actor-learners could be regarded as fools or liars, or the experimenter as malevolent or insane. But because the original source of the volunteers was a public advertisement and because the experimenter clothed himself with all the trappings of science, it was his authority that prevailed. On occasion indeed the subject-teacher would only inflict more pain if the experimenter re-undertook 'responsibility' for anything that might happen. In other words, as in Burt's first two cases, pain inflicting actions were imposed where responsibility could be allocated elsewhere and also where one side of a relationship could be conceptually obliterated.

Burt expands his analysis of irrationality by describing what he calls 'the rule of opposites'. He explores[9] 'the way that all infants learn the self-other distinction' because 'no adult ever abandons his earliest infantile beliefs that he and the universe are indistinguishable ... the adult's rational belief in the self-other distinction remains juxtaposed in his mind against its opposite'. But how and why do these distinctions remain? Because[10] 'the very progression by which his caretakers lead him to believe ... in the self-other distinction is perceived by the infant to contain an implicit promise that his espousal will permit him to achieve the abolition of the distinction'.[11] There is thus, to Burt,[12] 'a coexistence between diametrically opposed ideologies, each of which is an internally consistent world view that excludes the other'.

Accordingly, this is a psychological paradox which must influence relationships between all adults. The more dependent the one becomes upon the other, the more polarities (the distinction, or compounding, of self and other) are brought into focus. He argues:[13] 'the pessimism that peculiarly afflicts the abusing parents in their perceptions of their children, and that triggers their abusive conduct, is everyone's common perception of' those in pain and close to death or those whose personal oddities appear alien. Further, the power polarities assumed by abusing parents in respect of their children and by medical staff in respect of such people is very similar. The only difference is that because in the latter case the power is exercised through the medium of a bureaucratic structure all the actors except the patient can[14] 'avoid confronting the question of the power of irrational thinking in his own mind'.

This irrational mode is therefore likely to be accentuated where the physician faces extremes in his patient. Moreover, and centrally,[15] 'medical care always addresses, in some guise, the issue of mortality'. Leaving aside extremes, Burt explains the common phenomenon of patients not taking prescribed medication[16] as at least suggesting 'the paradoxical conclusion that the patients sought out physicians precisely in order to disobey them'. In these non-extreme cases such postures do no harm.

In extreme cases, the struggle concerning the patient's identity remains an issue throughout the relationship. Those who, through the medium of the informed consent theory, would defer to the patient's expressed views most commonly apply J.S. Mill's view of self-determination even to the point of self-destruction. But, Burt argues, that is based on a static view of the freely consenting adult. If, however, there is anything in the above discussion, Mill's paradigm hardly exists. Every individual, including every adult, is in a state of oscillation between polarities; between perceiving himself[17] as choice-making or choiceless, as adult or infant regarding others. Even if statistically most of the population most of the time is oriented to the adult, choiceful polarities, the view is static and it obscures the dynamic reality. Therefore, the psychology of Mill and his followers[18]

> misconstrues both the way in which equality is reliably experienced in relations and the roots of the equality norm itself in the structure of human thought. Equality is learned and repeatedly experienced as alternating inequalities among people, of alternating relations of dominance and submission, and not as a static equivalence among all or even some people. This is because every individual inevitably oscillates between the poles in his social relations and, more fundamentally, in his thought processes.

Support for Burt's view comes from Santarcangeli's discussion of the role of the jester.[19] This suggests that this figure is historically enduring and that he is 'by turns creator and destroyer, a strange being who grants and refuses, duper and duped'. Santarcangeli quotes Schlegel:[20] 'Society is a chaos to which only humour can give form and harmony. Unless we joke and make fun of passion, it condenses itself into thick masses and darkens everything.'

Burt goes on to argue that the change in the self-depiction of the doctor as the practitioner of objective science, separate from his patient, attempts to break the psychological link between them. Its result inevitably has led to the patient's self-depiction increasingly emphasizing self-determination cumulating in recent years in the legal doctrine of informed consent.[21] The traditional characterization of the express psychological interdependence of doctor and patient still shows in, for example, the use and efficacy of placebos. He notes that a century ago their mechanism was as well understood as any other healing mechanism. The twentieth-century success of curative techniques has transformed most physicians' conceptions of themselves as practitioners. Rational objectivity is the organizing ambition. Its cornerstone is the physician's effort to draw sharp distinctions between self and other. This change, he argues, was marked in the United States' courts by the expansion of the role of consent[22] 'to follow [the] parties step by step throughout all of their dealings ... contemporary courts no longer assume that the relationship of doctor–patient is necessarily characterized as a psychological fusion of identities'.

Burt calls this conception a 'fantasy'. He sees in the search (for example to find the biological villain in cancer) an endeavour to find a cause that enables the physician to manipulate the disease. Whether the research is justified or not, its motivation is an expression of the same fantasy. So also, he argues, is the claim for public interest control over medical science both at the level of society's institutions over medical technology and at the level of the individual's claim to control what happens to his body. On both sides there is a claim that the other side has an unnecessarily narrow view but both rest[23] 'in the unattainable premise that posits the pursuit of objectivity, of clear-cut fixed separation between self and other'.

This pursuit[24] contains constructive and destructive aspects. In the first aspect, it suggests manipulable constructs on the otherwise 'senseless' flux of intrapsychic impressions; in the second, the extension of the reach of rational control becomes transformed into the desire to ignore everything that seems beyond control. It is the adult refraction of the confusion between self and other on which all infants rest their faith in the nutrient character of the universe. He says:[25] 'the special intensity of their confusions regarding self-boundaries and their motives to fix those boundaries inspire[s] a reciprocal intensity from all those who [see] them'. One such response is, in face of the patient's sense of helplessness, from the authoritarian physician who assumes total control of the joint self. In such cases and where the patient places himself wholly in the physician's hands there is a soothing effect. But the effect is equally pronounced where the patient claims full or almost full self-determination, and the physician can and does respond by withdrawing into bureaucracy and specialization. The imprimatur of 'responsible medical practice' – scientific medicine – is that[26] 'any treatment modality should be equally effective in the hands of any physician'.

In recent years the courts have sought to readjust a balance against physicians locking 'themselves and their patients with a progressively univalent choicemaking–choiceless role allocation'. But the judges have done so at the cost of placing themselves in the same authoritarian role. Burt argues:[27]

> They fail to see themselves as participants in a dialogue between physicians and patients, as instruments to unsettle the rigidity of role allocation that the stress of illness provokes in both patient and physician. They see themselves as authoritative dispute resolvers rather than as *agents provocateurs* of disputes between physician and patient on the question whether either one is univalently in command of the other.

Burt maintains that at their best the law and the courts do not (particularly prematurely) settle disputes; they coerce each of the parties separately and jointly into reconciling the oscillations between their psychic polarities. The plea is therefore for a legal strategy designed to induce conversation rather than an exchange of monologues (as where the physician in order to discharge his legal obligations considers his task is done when he merely recites the statistics concerning risks), or a premature decision giving omnipotence to one side or the other. So also this strategy should include coercion toward the provision of full evidence of this conversation in form of extensive record-keeping.

There are moreover special dangers in the use of law. The idea of 'government of laws, not men' expresses the same authoritarian, impersonal psychological view as does bureaucratic, specialized medicine. Burt argues:[28] 'The judge's mind is no more free from the alternating ideas of separateness and self-dissolution, rationality and madness, than anyone's'. At least so far as the doctor-patient relationship is concerned, it is better that the law is not invoked until the conversation has ended and that during the conversation what it will say should remain uncertain.

Such are Burt's analysis and the implications he sees for the law. The two questions that arise are does he go far enough, or too far? He has recognized the practical reality of every individual's intrapsychic fantasy in the sense that it provides functional understanding of an oscillation, in particular, of feelings toward others. He has not examined who are 'others' in this fantasy world. Burt is convincing as regards the motivation and capacity for the mind 'to conceptually eliminate' the humanity of those it perceives as threatening. But more fundamentally, does the mind make a distinction between sight, vision, or imagination? If, in the intrapsychic world no distinctions are made even for some of the time, it would follow that Burt's analysis can be applied as much to figments of the imagination as to real other human beings. For example, as an author I can understand my friends and colleagues who have seen this book. I cannot relate to its readers except through the image-making capacity of my mind, my imagination.[29] So also whilst they can relate to the physical reality of my words, they cannot relate to me except through the same process. We all not only understand but also feel for the hero of a novel and against the villain. We can 'get lost in a good book'. In the pursuit of our lives we measure our own success, or failure, and those of others, by the extent to which the mental image and the seen reality (either of which may be of our construction) coincide. Intrapsychic images have emotional and physiological realities.

Burt almost casually observes that the retrospective adjudication of a dispute between two parties by a judge may have a precedential effect. He fails to observe that the judge in creating a precedent is likely to be influenced by the present intrapsychic fantasy that the future represents. So also in considering in retrospect both the actions of these parties and the meaning of the case law cited to him, the judge is not concerned with the past but his present intrapsychic fantasy relating to the actors in those events. It follows that in so far as Burt is right in his description of the impossibility of objective judgement about individuals with whom we have a relation, he ought to have applied it to every aspect of judging. It may be that the law (that is, sanctions external to ourselves) ought to maintain a strategy of encouraging conversations between participants to relationships but this cannot be achieved by the simple expedient of curtailing the declaratory judgment nor even, at least for the reasons he gives, by maintaining uncertainty as to its meaning.

At the core of the argument is that the strategy is only likely to be successful and then only to a limited extent by broadening the involvement. A strategy that is centred on the patient, the doctor, and the judge must fail because it has assumed in social relationships A and B = A + B. A strategy based on the relations of the doctor to the wider community and hence the patient is more likely to maintain conversations between individual relationships. Doctors live in a community and each member of the community contributes to its values and expectations. Accordingly doctors absorb those contributions. Doctors also work within a group – I have called it a guild. The guild, although it has a life and function of its own, is also affected by the wider community. In a malpractice action the patient, who has made some (even if small) contribution to society and hence the medical guild, is alleging a violation of the values of the guild.

On such a view individual patients are not ignored. There are more, and sometimes more effective, ways of contributing to society than by the use of formal powers. 'Informed consent' theory, by seeking to impose rigid and external structures on the doctor-patient combination, hinders the relationship of both with the wider society in which it and they participate. In seeking 'justice' for the individual it is compelled (by its own forms) to do so at one point in time and place. My argument, but not informed consent theory, recognizes the collectivism which lies at the heart of Foucault's analysis of the clinic[30] and the mutual (although in my argument, separate) responsibility recognized by Pellegrino and Thomasma.[31] Where, on the other hand, the law insists that the participants to a medical relationship are 'rational economic men', particularly where the relationship is governed not only by consent but also by contract, as I have suggested, medicine *qua* medicine is impossible. The patient becomes the object of biotechnology. A simple strategy is a siren call.

Incommensurables and social cohesion

The solution of the previous section does not solve all the problems. I have suggested that two features of the Renaissance and the Enlightenment created a dilemma from which medicine has not recovered. It encouraged medicine to think it was scientific and it brought men's minds to think of themselves as individuals. Because the basic unit of science is the individual (whether it be atom, planet, organism, or whatever) medicine was compelled to depart from holism. Because individuals then and now, in their desire to be rational, to be able to express a reason, wish to conceive of themselves as separate and choiceful, they too are inclined to reject a social system where they are 'a simple aliquot fraction of the whole'.[32] It is not easy for adults to recognize either their own dependency or that of others on them. It is not easy to recognize, still less to rationalize about, the immersion of the self into a greater whole.

Both medicine and law, each classically conceived and currently applied, ignore the problem. If medicine were to do otherwise, it would transform itself. And there are many who say it should, even if they concede that it has not done so already. But, even if it did, what then? The dynamics of Hirschman and the oscillations of Burt will not go away by wishing. But even apart from these, the existence of human beings rather than organisms is defined by social relations. Indeed, perhaps the core of my concern regarding medicine is that the radical critique, malpractice actions, an a priori universalization of a right to self-determination and an ill-informed application of consumer ideology are most likely to alter medical practice; its mode could be propelled from one which is, by and large, tolerable to one which is not and which moreover would require very different forms of regulation. At its extreme, nothing will remain except a private capacity to enrich its practitioners at the cost of those who are, by definition, most in need and capable of help.

If we have to accept the group's own assessment of its non-economic standards and hold back our sharpest, that is most reasoned, criticism of the group's failures[33] – for most surely it, like all other groups, can be self-serving – we do so not for the sake of the group or its power or its values but for the concepts which we value, because they are part of what it means to be civilized. Besides, most often our reasoned criticism is based on information from a professional from which we conclude his fellows fail to achieve the standards the group as a whole sets itself. As Freidson points out[34] expert testimony 'is an intrinsic necessity in those cases in which experts are themselves the object of suit'. Castiglione was perhaps cynical in the expression of the idea that it was possible to teach oneself the arts of gentlemanly behaviour. He did it in a culture which valued these things. His successors have so extended individual self-fulfilment as to exclude those arts from the litany.

The important question that remains is what has motivated this transformation. Castiglione's achievement went beyond making possible entry to the rank to gentleman. It was itself part of the triumph of the aristocracy. It enabled tradesmen to aspire to those ranks. However, in that aspiration not all could forget the values of their trade and in particular the moral importance of material accumulation. There is some truth in the idea that this conflict within the new rich of seventeenth-century England led to the Civil War, the Restoration, and the Protestant Revolution of 1688. In any event, those events laid the basis for political debate through the eighteenth and nineteenth centuries. It is commonly described in terms of competition between 'Whigs' and 'Tories'. Although the terms are somewhat ambiguous and changeable, some themes can be discerned.

Whiggery was, or is, more concerned with temporal than with humanly interpreted spiritual authority. It demands that the individual be responsible for himself. It calls for an atomized social structure. It fosters what Oakeshott[35] calls 'rationalism'. It recasts obedience from being merely acceptance of an unchallenged order of things to the conscious desire to see some benefit to those who might obey. It welcomes theories of social contract to explain social cohesion. Because of this, it compels the successful members of such a structure to take a particular view of the relationship between change and progress: out of their success, change is progress. Whiggery's political commitment to material rationality compels social relations to be interpreted in terms of classical or neo-classical economics. Structures become described as strategies and their material advantages opened to analysis. Whiggery's commitment to an atomized society, at times based in a social contract, does the same for the moral agency of the parties to any relationship, including that of doctor and patient.

Toryism on the other hand holds a different view of the world. At every one of these points, it opposes Whiggery. It postulates a hierarchy with superiors and subordinates which is dependent on the members of the social order knowing their place and recognizing mutual sets of responsibilities and privileges. Authority and obedience are part of the natural order of things and they, not some rationalized creation in the form of a social contract, explain social cohesion.[36] Change is, if anything, undesirable rather than morally advantageous.

Although no one put it in these terms, the history of medical practice I have set out reflects these themes. It is the residue of the conflict between Whiggery and Toryism which goes a long way to explaining the criticisms of the ways doctors go about their occupation. The foundation and style of the College of Physicians reflected a need for a medical hierarchy headed by that body. Politically, in the seventeenth century, it was aligned with the Royalist cause, and afterwards with the Court. For much of the period it reflected a Tory view, of change in knowledge as much as of change in general: it was not to be welcomed. The rise of the apothecaries can be seen not merely as a series of challenges to the established ways of doing things, but also, and perhaps more simply, as medicine's Whiggery.

Of course there has been confusion. On the one hand, as much of my account has argued, the apothecaries and after them the general practitioners have aspired to the Pythagorean Hippocratic ideal – to the virtues of the aristocracy. On the other, each time they opposed the College they were concerned with change, with rationalism, and with material and measurable benefit. From the negotiations leading to the grant of the charter of the Society, through the quarrels regarding the policing of the apothecaries and the establishment of the Dispensaries, to the compromises of the 1858 Act and the reforms of the General Medical Council in 1886, the challenge has been accommodated by the physicians in Toryism's way: the aftermath of even forced change becomes part of the new natural order of things.

By the time of the establishment of the National Health Service in 1946–8, rational Whiggery was almost, but not quite, triumphant. The scheme itself may be seen as an achievement of an alliance between two philosophies which have much in common – aristocratic Toryism in the form of the consultants in the voluntary hospitals and egalitarianism socialism in the form of the government of the day. Not only was there the consultants' acceptance of the Service, but also, and more important for my thesis, there was the maintenance of the historic relationship between doctor and patient, the incorporation (or rather re-incorporation) of the consultants into the management, and the continuation of hierarchies within medical practice. The socialist government got a service available to the whole population but, so long as the server (the doctor), could choose at least when to reject a patient the Tory, aristocratic, paternalistic basis of practice could continue.

If this view is so, it was the high point of the alliance of the socialists and the Tories. Rationalism was on the march. In the hospitals, the visible success of surgery was raising the status of the 'cutters'. In primary care and the associated public health, the rationalism of Whiggery was undermining the prestige of the old centres of power and the old ways of doing things. In all sectors of medical care, as elsewhere, scientism was establishing itself not only as a (measurable) success but also as a moral force.

We should expect to find that the common law's approach to medical practice shows something of these changes. The point is often made that the common law is highly influenced by ideas of *laissez faire* economics; and it is that theory in its turn that underpins the prospectus of Whiggery. I would argue that in its modern form this philosophy has close affinities to consumerism – they differ only, and only at times, in the latter's view of progress. It follows out of this that we should expect to see an alliance formed between the common lawyers and consumerists (of whatever ostensible political party). This has indeed happened by way of the common lawyer's reaction to informed consent theory.

True it is that the English courts, as contrasted with some of the judges, have not yet adopted the full rigours of this idea. What is significant is that the minority of judges and the majority of academic lawyers and others who favour it are also those most willing to accept other aspects of the prospectus of what I have just described as the modern form of Whiggery, consumerism. It may be a convenience for my argument, and the evidence is scanty, but the majority of judges, in rejecting the theory, appear to be influenced by the other side of the dilemma facing the general practitioners, the aspiration to Hippocratic medicine. Quite possibly, as that aspiration weakens, and is weakened, so the judges' support for it will decline, and informed consent theory will be adopted. Just as possibly, however, the contradictions within Whiggery, some of which are specific to medical practice (such as the different view of disease of doctor and patient) and some of which are general (such as the impossibility of an atomized view of human relations being a social philosophy) will prevent both the abandonment of the Hippocratic ideal and the general adoption of informed consent theory by the courts.

I have dealt with medicine and law because they are devoted to the management of bodies. My interest is in something else – opposite or antithesis are not the right words – the management of minds (souls) by rules. That is why empiricism would be so useless. So far even the best of modern techniques of social survey can describe only inclinations, not motives. At stake are non-economic standards, non-measurable standards – those values which Horobin used to describe professionalism. Values described by words such as 'commitment', 'probity', 'comportment', and, I might add, 'propriety'. They are not confined to that range of occupations described by professionalism. In general, they are other regarding virtues; that is, they do not conceive of individuals as being alone – they have no meaning except in relation to others. Rational economic man by definition cannot have them except, perhaps, as an expression of cynicism. Reason may tell us they are unnecessary; history and experience and intuition deny reason. As James said of 'bodyline', much more than cricket was at stake, in fact everything was at stake. 'Bodyline' was cricket's expression of rational economic man. In its rationality, it debased everything else. By making an applaudable spectacle of rationality in an arena whose metaphors were synonymous with morality, and by rejecting an ethic which rational economic man (what Hirschman called an 'infra-human wanton') cannot know, the controversy was both a symbol and a beginning of our new amoral secularized society.

Hawthorn says the logic of the Enlightenment, although he concedes[37] that no one put it quite in these terms, was: if 'the good was the right, the right the true, and as scientific enquiry was demonstrating, the right was also natural (since nature manifestly conformed to reason), so the natural must be the good'. The absurdity of this view is forced upon us almost everywhere in the field of health care. Lifestyles are built out of the notion that the natural is the good and the good is the normal. 'Natural' environments, 'natural' foods, even 'natural' birth and 'natural' death are better than man-made or man-controlled ones. The idea forgets that misery, pain, disease, and death are also natural and normal.

Hawthorn says[38]

The Enlightenment is ordinarily thought of as a French affair ... France ... still was ... a primarily Catholic country; England, a Protestant one. To the French the model of intellectual and institutional authority was the hierarchical and absolute Catholic Church; to the English (as to a man of Calvinist inspiration like Locke), it was the individual . . . . To the English, there was no longer a collective authority which demanded submission . . . . His contact with nature was as direct and unmediated as was his contact with God.

Despite this there was an English Enlightenment of which the prime exponents were Locke and Bentham. Both were influenced by those best known for their contributions to what had become theory-driven experimental natural science: Locke by Boyle[39] and Bentham by Priestley. Of this last Bentham, for example, said:[40] 'Priestley was the first (unless it was Beccaria) who taught my lips to pronounce this sacred truth – that the greatest happiness of the greatest number is the foundation of morals and legislation'. It was Locke's individualism which taught us the fundamental right in property. It was Bentham's which taught us that legislation could solve problems. Their Enlightenment contains two contradictions. Both lie in the wonder in man's achievement. Because the good is natural, it leaves no room for that wonder. Secondly, the achievement, being of all of us and over time, is a social statement made against the background of an individualist philosophy.

In this connection, I argue, our times are heavily influenced by Whiggery's view of change, of reason, and of the individual moral agent. There is, is there not, a deep acceptance of the notion that all change is progress and all progress is for the better: that the present is always better than the past? Secondly, arising out of this we lack a sense of time. It is easy to forget that whereas between the Renaissance (say 1500) and the Enlightenment (say 1800) there were 300 years, between the Enlightenment and today there are less than 200. Change may be of many sorts. It is helpful to distinguish three of them: change in technology, change in social relations, and change in social ideas. Although each will influence the others, there is no reason why they should all proceed at the same rate. Part of our present problem lies precisely in the fact that these changes are moving at different speeds. It is obvious that technology is moving at an accelerating pace. It is scarcely less obvious that many types of social relation are undergoing rapid alterations. What is less obvious, and indeed may be doubted, is that the ideas by which we organize our relationships to the world are moving as fast.

One of the ideas of the Enlightenment is, as we saw Hume saying, that only that which is measurable is worthy of our attention. It is an idea confirmed by the advances in the natural sciences and technology. This emphasis on the measurable means that these other changes have difficulty in being accommodated. Out of this has come a valorization of the results of technology. Quite simply, one of the most important social ideas of man is morality. Because we cannot get rid of it, we give a moral value to technology and to the things which it produces. If we could recognize their amorality, we could become free to acknowledge morality in non-material things: it is common and ultimately pathetic to blame or praise the material world for what mankind does with it. This acknowledgement of morality in non-material things would be however to recognize that there is a valuable social idea not necessarily connected with the measurable (and therefore the knowable).

We are bewildered. There is the Renaissance and the Enlightenment and their aftermath, with the emphasis on reason and the unitary nature of experience. They rid us of old ways of thinking but not necessarily the old habits to which they gave rise. To us the glory of the Enlightenment is magnified by the technical wonders whose beginnings are associated with it. Because we have placed the heart of morals in the material world, by an irrational leap we have placed great store on the achievements of that period: at times we forget the cementing character of those habits. It is probably true that the contemporary interest in Foucault's work is because of his rejection of the universal rationalism of the Enlightenment. He had the vision to individualize knowledge over time. He picked up two themes of our age: the emphasis on the individual and on doubt. And both the individual and the doubt arise out of the contradictions of the Enlightenment.

There is however another theme. It is, as we saw Hirschman suggesting above, that there is the shift from the public to the private. We now abstain from public action. The choice, however, is not to be responsible for history or be resigned to it. Abstention is not condonation. Hirschman's shift is the expression of a complexity but one which is largely independent of the things about which we used to act. Even in our private world, we are still capable of caring. Difficulty, complexity, frustration may be reinforcing our posture of individualism, of retreat from expressions of public concern. It is a shallowness born out of ahistoricism which says that the retreat is permanent. And there are profound intellectual, moral, and even physical dangers in rejecting a social dimension to our world.

Freidson argues:[41] 'Our civilization emphasizes choice over constraint, the individual over group, and the actor over the environment. In reflecting that emphasis, our legal, religious, and educational institutions, even our scientific institutions, reflect a moral value.' One may say it is a moral value which if need be insists on the manufacturing of choice for where there is no option, the possibility of choice does not occur; it is reason which is used to create these possibilities.

In this creation of choice there is a demand to find goals which are obtainable. And in doing so, people in our age and in our culture are becoming specialized and fragmented. It follows that actions are looked upon for their effects on the individual and not society. To the extent that they are social acts, they have no meaning when judged by the criteria of individualism. Increasingly, the reality of whole ranges of human experience – all those feelings which are other related (love, sorrow, compassion, pity) – are rejected or reconstructed. To take one example, where individuals face each other within a joint relationship, the calibration of individualism uses the language of exploitation (and its subset of paternalism) to describe its effects on one or other (and quite commonly both) of them.

Individualism has appropriated morality and the judgement of what is good for society. Because they are other-regarding virtues (which it condemns as mistaken), among the standards it rejects are honesty and truth telling. Machiavelli did this for relations between states. This modern doctrine does it for relations between people. Lies are blameworthy only if they are found out,[42] but not always even then, for individualism is more concerned with purposes and results than with means. Thus, by a perversion, trust itself has become anti-social. Simmel argued that trust was foundational to relations between men. It is now little wonder that people are confused and inward-looking when outside ourselves the foundations of human intercourse have become anti-social. Reason may tell us that there is no alternative, no other way; our intuition (perhaps, our spirit) tells us that this is no way at all.

To reject individualism is not to reject human dignity. On the contrary I see it difficult for the individualist to object to the degradation of another. It is only with a social perspective that we can become concerned for others. An important distinction must be made: individualism (and the law) wants peace but always on terms; humanity, I suggest, at least in some of its moods, yearns for an unqualified peace. The former reserves a place for the single human being in social relationships; it compels that being to be on guard against breaches of the conditions. The unqualified, or unconditional, peace which I say humanity can desire does neither of these things: although it may exist either temporarily or even for a specified time, whilst it exists (and to that extent) single beings merge their individualism within the greater whole described by the relationship. And yet, unless this is done, tranquillity will be a matter of the peace being on terms rather than being unconditional.

Jaques remarked:[43] 'one man in his time plays many parts'. To him, the parts were played chronologically. And to be sure, man exists as a biological entity whose changes are of course in part chronological; there is change from birth, childhood, adulthood, old age, and death. In some ways the human condition can be described in these terms, and also in terms of the ranges of health and illness that occur throughout these stages. In these ways it can therefore be defined by the biological sciences. But individuals exist also as social beings.[44] In this sense, rather than the biological, existence varies not only in time but also in space.[45] As a social being we are concerned with self, with near-others, and with far-others. We are concerned with our own being, that of our family, of our neighbours, of our workmates and playmates, of our near-community and of our far-community. But only some of the time. We find a commonality with other individuals of our sex, our race, our faith or lack of it, and our nation. But again not all of us all of the time. Moreover, as a social being, we exist not only at that place and time where our physical persons are located but also everywhere that others discuss us, use information about us, or otherwise respond to our existence.[46]

For simplicity we may say that as a biological entity we are governed and limited by the laws of the biological sciences. However, our existence as social beings is not. The hypothetical construct of individuals alone in the state of nature does not and never could exist. Our existence is dependent upon our relations with our fellows. The poets express it best. Thus Shelley in 'Love's Philosophy':

Nothing in the world is single;
All things by a law divine
In one spirit meet and mingle.

And John Donne, in *Devotions, Meditation XVII*:

> No man is an Island, entire of itself; every man is a piece of the Continent, a part of the main.

Indeed the existence of each may be, perhaps has to be, defined in terms of other individuals, and, just as relations change, so does the definition of existence. As Tawney said[47]

> The conventional statement that human nature does not change is plausible only so long as attention is focused on those aspects of it which are least distinctively human.... Man steps into a social inheritance, to which each generation adds its own contribution of good and evil, before it bequeathes it to its successors.

Change within each of us indeed may be influenced by a biological state (that is, there may be a correlation between mood and physiology and psychology) but it is conditioned by its relation to our perceived past and prospective relation to others. The change may be an oscillation or a progression. It may occur in short or long chronological periods. There is no reason why the temporal existence of the social being should be coterminous with the biological. In our culture it is not. As Horace said, 'Non omnis moriar' (I shall not altogether die): for example, we maintain a law of succession based upon the 'will' of the dead. Thus the dead live.

I have argued that medicine is not possible in an individualized, atomized society. That may not matter. Just as there can be more important things than health, so, and more clearly, there can be more important things than medicine. What does matter is that in accepting atomization we have also to reject the arguments for the collectivization of medicine. That too may not matter. But, if we reject that, and apply the rejection generally, what remains of civilization – what is there left that is particularly human for which we may care? This century, if no other, has taught: that not all change is for the better; that much arises out of exaggerated reaction to error.

It is my argument that the conceptions of the individual 'self' inherent in common law legal theory are defective. The necessary contradiction of the individualist position is that it seeks to address the external world as if man were at once separate and yet a part of it. If he were completely separate, there could be no relevant external world. Liberty which allows the single being to have perfect choice cannot allow that being to enter any social relation for the simple reason that any such relation limits choice. Thus liberty of the individual is not to be confused with freedom. Liberty in this sense is in contrast to free humanity. Humanity's freedom requires the incorporation of the self within the varying complex of social relationships. Collective action is not, of course, the only necessary condition for free humanity but it is essential to it. So also, I have argued that man has to live his life under many normative regimes. Among others I have mentioned: law, morality, ethics, aesthetics, instinct, emotion, habit, economics, science, biology, and medicine. His freedom comes of his choosing and judging between competing rules. When one of these systems is raised to a primacy, freedom is imperilled. There are indeed words to describe regimes where some of these exclude the others, words such as tyranny, anarchy, bestiality. It is no surprise that each of these can be used in opposition to civilization.

At the opening of this book, I said I would try to be like Russell's drugged balloonist in rejecting ideas merely because they are 'useful in ordinary life or seem like necessities of thought'. In the end, what I have done is to reject the necessities of reason in order to preserve necessities of life. Reason's truth may or may not be; all that we can know of it is by way of a mirror. And then all we know is that it keeps changing. The mirror is like the patterns in a kaleidoscope. The image (of truth) is certain and fleeting and never quite repeated.

Dahrendorf says, if we are to avoid the 'Road to Anomia', we must build institutions.[48] The ideas discussed in this book, from disease and illness via medicine and health to liberty and freedom, present incommensurable values. They cannot be weighed against or with each other. They are part of us, but they are in different worlds. We deceive ourselves if we do not recognize that there is no right answer to the proper balance between them. What is even more difficult to reconcile ourselves to is that we necessarily lack the means to determine which are the wrong ones. I, at least, am left with a feeling that the process of which Dahrendorf spoke is best done (indeed can only be done) not be seeking to build afresh but rather by more or less extensive refurbishment and restoration. Perhaps the lesson to be taken is that neither courts nor legislatures or indeed rationality can do that job; but each is very capable of demolishing the institutions which make our world a social world, a human world.

Appendix: The *Hippocratic Oath*[1]

I swear by Apollo the physician, by Aesculapius, Hygeia and Panacea, and I take to witness all the gods, all the goddesses, to keep according to my ability and my judgement the following Oath:

'To consider dear to me as my parents him who taught me this art; to live in common with him and if necessary to share my goods with him; to look upon his children as my own brothers, to teach them this art if they so desire without fee or written promise; to impart to my sons and the sons of the master who taught me and the disciples who have enrolled themselves and have agreed to the rules of the profession, but to these alone, the precepts and the instruction. I will prescribe regimen for the good of my patients according to my ability and my judgement and never do harm to anyone. To please no one will I prescribe a deadly drug, nor give advice which may cause his death. Nor will I give a woman a pessary to procure abortion. But I will preserve the purity of my life and my art. I will not cut for stone, even for patients in whom the disease is manifest; I will leave this operation to be performed by practitioners (specialists in this art). In every house where I come I will enter only for the good of my patients, keeping myself far from all intentional ill-doing and all seduction, and especially from the pleasures of love with women or with men, be they free or slaves. All that may come to my knowledge in the exercise of my profession or outside of my profession or in daily commerce with men, which ought not to be spread abroad, I will keep secret and will never reveal. If I keep this oath faithfully, may I enjoy my life and practise my art, respected by all men and in all times; but if I swerve from it or violate it, may the reverse be my lot.'

Afterword to the Transaction Edition

My adolescent dream was always modest. It was to make a better world—in those days people actually did think like that. Although I had not read them when this book was first published, instinct attracted me to the emancipation of the human spirit in the kind of social philosophy found in P.B. Shelley, John Ruskin, and William Morris. Chance, as I explain in the Introduction to this edition, led me to look at medicine. This Afterword does four things. First, again, it explains the purpose and method. Importantly it now makes explicit the different ways we know our world. Secondly, it disentangles its different subjects, its several themes: What is medicine? What is professional practice and how far is it understandable from the outside? What are the origins and force of the internal and external rules governing practice? What do the rules governing practice teach about social cohesion in general? Thirdly, partly because the professions always borrow from each other and partly for reasons that will become apparent, this Afterword compares the values in the medical profession with those of other professions, particularly of lawyers. Finally, it reflects on how far values and mores have changed and must change in response to the events and changes of the last ten years. The 1987 publication of this book came at a time when optimism was permissible. Given the most likely prognosis, that day may be gone. Accordingly, with more ambition than sense, I now try to find what needs to be done in order to get away from the ideas that we can only be motivated by the knowable, that the knowable is always both objective and measurable, that altruism and trust are impossible and that we are irretrievably selfish.

There is, however, a difference between this chapter and the others. When I first wrote this book, I tried merely to make sense of things as they are. I still try to do that but now, because this book led me to conclusions, this Afterword has an express commitment that is lacking in much of the original. Certainly, there is rejection of the neo-liberalist tradition, what this book calls whiggery. There is not a commitment to the old left or right, nor to new this or new that. Nor is it an inclination to any third way. Rather, although this is not a history book, it recognizes a need to learn from our history. In particular, it wants to know how to apply the good things, the socially cohesive things, that our traditions can teach us.

In a way, I set myself a task impossible for the modern age. In a way, I tried to be like Ruskin of whom Hobson said:[1]

> He never addresses the intellect alone; in his writing there always lurks a double appeal: he ever seeks to touch the heart as well as to convince the understanding. The system which underlies this process is thus one of . . . the blending of passion with argument . . . is apt to cause confusion and distrust in those who like to have their reasoning dry. Moreover, this . . . mode of exposition, proper though it was for Mr Ruskin, often beguiled him into the opposed errors of discursiveness and excessive condensation.

A number of reviewers criticized this book for its digressions into too many disparate fields. They misread me. The asides are part of the plot. This is not a work of the narrow academy: its reasoning is not intended to be dry. Any search for the complexity and vitality of social cohesion should not be that. If there is fault in these digressions, it is that there is too little, not too much, of life's experience. In particular, the force of the arts, including literature and architecture, scarcely show themselves. I like to flatter myself that this book is intellectual in Said's sense:[2] 'it is a lonely condition, yes, but it is always a better one than a gregarious tolerance for the way things are';'Least of all should the intellectual be there to make his/her audiences feel good: the whole point is to be embarrassing, contrary, even unpleasant'; and,'At bottom, the intellectual . . . is neither a pacifier nor a consensus builder, but someone whose whole being is staked on a critical sense, a sense of being unwilling to accept easy formulas, already made clichés, or the smooth, ever-so-accommodating confirmations of what the powerful or conventional have to say, and what they do.'

Other societies and other ages have found their own harsh ways of dealing with these contrary, unpleasant opponents of the powerful and the conventional. In our times, with some exceptions, the main device is to ostracize or to ignore. It is a spiritual exile. The intellectual is lonely not because he or she wants to be, but because this is the way our society copes with this form of disturbance. And this is a great cruelty but it is the price of being concerned for the state of society.

Prelude

On its face, this book is about the regulation of the practice of medicine. It is more. Directly it is about power within groups in society of which the medical profession is but one. Indirectly it is about liberty. There are three odd things about the method. It is odd because it is concerned not so much with the realities that have informed the élite and the rule makers as with the images in their minds. It is odd because there is an emphasis on groups and guilds, which, more so than when it was written, seems strangely, alas, outmoded. Finally, it is odd because, for a lawyer's book there is a great deal about medicine and its practice and very little about legal doctrine.

It is helpful here to explain what is going on. The book is founded on a sense of a mismatch between what doctors were saying and what others said about them. During the 1980s, as I wrote, this book's ambit spread and spread. It is about rule making but not in the sense of the procedures by which rules are made. It is not about legislative processes even within sub-units of society. Rather, it is about the aspirations of rule makers: not with their agenda, but with why their agenda takes the form it does. We are all familiar with meetings where debate is coded. This book is about the code, not the debate. In the course of doing that, mischievously, it talks variously of irrational idealism, mysticism and the limits of reason. These expressions are not intended to alienate my readers, but to gain their engagement with the problems I was facing. They are designed to provoke my readers to step outside the ordinary bounds of thought and even to question their own premises. This is not done out of any sense of arrogance or superiority. It is done because I, too, have tried those assumptions and found them lacking. Indeed, one of the things that the reading for this book taught me is how different the world is when the same phenomena are viewed from different perspectives. For example, Ruskin's view of the Renaissance (a 'foul torrent')[3] and Penty's of the Roman Empire ('a military . . . system to enable rich men to live among poor')[4] stand in contrast to the usual view of these things. This technique underpins so much of my argument which accepts a sociological and rejects an economic imagination. I have no doubt that one of the reasons why some have found this book difficult is because it insists on a sharp divide between these views. But in this, I am unrepentant.

More specifically, one of the main assumptions I find wanting is that rules, norms of behaviour, are made so to speak from the bottom up. It is one of the basic tenets of democratic belief. It is the omnipresence of that creed that is in question. It may satisfy egalitarian ambition but it belies experience to deny that leadership exists. In order to describe it, I have tried not to see the world as I, too, want it to be. I take leadership to be a social fact, whether it is social (verging toward what Weber called charismatic) or structural (based in hierarchy). Moreover, this is not all. Historically, and I argue still, leadership is provided by élites (whether defined by merit or structure) and it is these who provide the aspirations of the led. Commonly, what they provide is not based on conscious resolution, but for the most part is the result of historic and traditional experience. It is of course true that the reality is, as it probably always has been, that these élites have feet of clay. Our age, however, takes an unusual delight in looking only at these toes and ankles rather than anything higher.

Like it or not groups are led by these élites and groups thus have collective ambition. Once, the possibility of their aspirations was recognized by leaving them to achieve their own goals. Now, and it is one of the characteristics of public service in our times, this recognition is given in the attempts to define these goals by imposing performance targets. And, most often, these targets are set by the outside or under outside pressure. Where this is not done, the other technique, again normally from the outside, is to impose competitive practices. I shall return to the point when I discuss *new public management* and the 1997 White Paper, *The New NHS*. I shall suggest that these economic devices ultimately destabilize social cohesion. This book thus follows Titmuss[5] and questions 'the philistine resurrection of economic man in social policy'.

One of the problems of performance target culture is that it looks at life in little boxes. It pretends that an occupation cannot be a vocation, and, by its pretense, makes reality. This book is not intended as a counterbalance—nothing can be that—but to provide some answer to 'little box' theories. Despite the almost universal application and apparent success of Taylorism's 'time and motion studies',[6] I doubt they have ever been true even of manufacturing industry. Job satisfaction is not only to be measured. It can also have an inner quality. All work is capable of being dull but it is also capable of having its dignity and arousing the passion and the pride of the worker. The stress and satisfaction of work, and relationships formed there, need not be carried beyond the workplace. But they always can be. It offends, even insults, common experience, as some economists have done, to interpret fraternalistic devices (the pleasure of communing with fellow workers, as Durkheim put it) merely as the means by which internal competition is eliminated.

As regards what used to be called the learned professions, they must be wholly re-conceived rather than merely re-organized for these 'little box' theories to be applied. This is de-professionalization. Much of this book is about the possibility of ending professionalism in this way, and a plea against it. The process, as the occupations move from dependence on experience to valuing expertise, is one of ceasing to be learned in the old sense. At the same time, as the values that previously distinguished them become derided, they stop being professional in any specific sense. And it is a process which, far from emancipating either the practitioners or their clients, imprisons them in measurement and numbers. It introduces what Ruskin termed[7] '*cold* cutting'. Thus, in worrying about rules, my concern is with liberty. Perhaps in the endeavor to be concise the point is not sufficiently emphasized in the original chapters. But it is a liberty more profound than what Matthew Arnold called[8] 'an Englishman's heaven-born privilege of doing what he likes'. This liberty cannot be confused with the licentiousness of any cult of the individual. It was liberty in Ruskin's sense:[9]

If by liberty you mean chastisement of the passions, discipline of the intellect, subjection of the will; if you mean the fear of inflicting, the shame of committing, a wrong; if you mean respect for all those who are in authority, and consideration for all who are in dependence; veneration for the good, mercy to the evil, sympathy with the weak; if you mean watchfulness over all thoughts, temperance of all pleasures, and perseverance in all toils; if you mean, in a word, that Service which is defined in the liturgy of the English church to be perfect Freedom, why you do name this by the same word by which the luxurious mean license, and the reckless mean change; by which the rogue means rapine, and the fool, equality; by which the proud mean anarchy, and the malignant mean violence? Call it by any name rather than this, but its best and truest, is Obedience. . . . The noblest word in the catalogue of social virtue is 'Loyalty', and the sweetest which men have learned in the pastures of the wilderness is 'Fold'.

By their different routes Penty and Durkheim (both of whom this book discusses) found this liberty of the spirit within autonomous groups called guilds. It is in this respect that in the last ten years, with greater emphasis than hitherto, that Britain has become *Americanized*.[10] The United States is not only the land of the free, it is also the land of choice. The emigrant (not immigrant) foundation of its culture requires individualism. Even its groups are held together by choice not chance. The last ten years in Britain have accentuated the movement to ensure that the only power in the State is the State. It has seen attacks on trade unions, on the sense of locality that used to be found in our towns, villages, and counties (that is, our local government) and on the professions. That is the stuff of politics and other than the last is not my current concern. All however represent a diminution in autonomous pockets of power beyond the reach of government. These attacks have been underpinned by the changing economy—labour must be mobile, jobs for life have gone—by patterns of home ownership and family life and by the expansion of concerns from national to continental and global matters. My *Republican Crown* talked of the hegemony of whiggery. The organizing categories of individualism have become so pervasive that it is well nigh impossible to see the world without them. Piece by piece the cement that was social cohesion has been removed. The process is not new but it is now almost complete. It is the final victory of the Enlightenment. Kiernan made the point this way:[11]

> What was overthrown with the Guilds was the principle of social authority. Economic individualism had fostered a growing irritation with regulative measures and this false sense of freedom undermined the communal arrangements which had promoted the contentment and stability of life as it had existed in England until the close of the seventeenth century and in France a half century later. The transition was made from a corporate arrangement of society to one in which the individual was dependent on his initiative to survive or perish.

The last way in which this book is odd is, as I say, despite being a lawyer's book, it has a heavy emphasis on medicine and its practice. Reason told me I could not use my lawyer's skills on a social institution without understanding its form, its modes of change, its strengths, and its weaknesses. I could no more do that than a sculptor can fashion marble without knowing his tools, the material in general and the piece in particular. It was all this that required me to know about the relation between law and the behavior of a tight-knit group. In order to do that I had to determine what the group was doing and by what means and by what values it held together. It was for this reason that I was led away from general social theory. My training in the common law method suggested that theory would come inductively, from the particular to the general: not deductively from *a priori* assumptions about society. It is not that I doubt the wisdom of social theory. Indeed, as the book shows I plagiarize bits. I call them 'insights'. My problem remains that social theory as it is commonly conducted is too abstract and too general to make it (easy) to apply to concrete social relations.

At one point in his Foreword Donald MacRae suggests that I have rediscovered the approach to sociology adopted by Vico in early eighteenth-century Naples.[12] I confess that until reading that Foreword I, too, had never heard of Giambattista Vico. Nevertheless, there is much in MacRae's remark. Indeed, had I been versed in Vico, the book would have taken more and better shape than it does. At one point (p. 26) I said that I was not attempting a theory of epistemology. I went on to say 'it seems clear that some things will always be beyond reason, that perfection is impossible, and some goals are worth having despite being manifestly unattainable'. This book talks of the need for inter-disciplinary and multi-disciplinary study. The sentiment would have been the same but the passage would be different if I had then read Vico. Such study is essential because as Vico told us:[13] 'language, art, polity and religion all interpenetrate one another'. More importantly, the haunting doubt of reason, which the book shows throughout, could have become more specific. Rather than talking generally of the Renaissance and Enlightenment, I might have focused more directly on Descartes, Voltaire, and their followers. I would certainly have agreed with Vico about their defects, which include:[14] 'disregard for everything except the absolute truth of which it is the criterion'. They neglect the wisdom of experience, eloquence, and all that depends on judgment. They have a universal application of geometric method. They use deductive logic and reject inductive methods and argument by analogy. They fail to use metaphor or rhetoric. It is a method that has achieved a great deal. Its problem is that it cannot achieve everything and it does not know that.

Certainly, the book would have been stronger if it had expressly used Vico's distinction in ways of knowing. The book says much about the limits of reason and science. It rests its argument on the importance of mystery and the unknowable. Unknown to me then, was the fact that Vico had faced the same problems. Science, to Vico, was knowledge by understanding the causes of things. This *knowledge by causes* is refined, reflective, and deductive. It is cold and austere. It precipitates specialization. For reasons the book explains, by its own definition, it can never be complete. This is because there are other ways in which we know our world. There is a distinction between this *knowledge by causes* and *knowledge by conviction*, what Adams translates as *certitude*. It is this second way in which, for example, we know our bodies. (This incidentally is why MacRae says I have regarded the body as a social construct). This form of knowledge comes from the imagination, from poetry in Vico's sense (metaphorical statements that describe a perceived reality) and from history. The third way of knowing is knowledge by (divine) revelation. I take it that in the worlds with which this book is concerned this now has little influence.[15] Three excerpts from Berlin might help explain the differences in *knowing by causes* and *by conviction*, the one so common in the academy and the other so usual in life:[16]

> This kind of knowledge is not knowledge of facts or logical truths, provided by observation or the sciences or deductive reasoning; nor is it knowledge of how to do things; nor is it knowledge provided by faith, based on divine revelation. . . . It is more like the knowledge we claim of a friend, of his character, of his ways of thought or action, the intuitive sense of the nuances of personality or feelings or ideas. . . . To do this, one must possess imaginative power of a high degree, such as artists and, in particular novelists require.
>
> One must possess a developed *fantasia*—Vico's term for imaginative insight. . . . This is the capacity for conceiving more than one way of categorising reality, like the ability to understand what it is to be an artist, a revolutionary, a traitor, to know what it is to be poor, to wield authority, to be a child, a prisoner, a barbarian. Without some ability to get into the skin of others, the human condition, history, which characterises one period or culture as against others, cannot be understood.
>
> The use of informed imagination about, and insight into systems of value, conceptions of life of entire societies, is not required in mathematics or physics, geology or zoology, or—though some deny this—in economic history or even sociology if it is conceived and practised as a strictly natural science.

Adams refers to this kind of understanding as *vulgar*, but it is not vulgar in the sense of being common. It is vulgar in the less usual sense of not being the product of reason. It is what I mean by mystery; and, Vico's discussion of the limits of *knowing by causes* explains what I mean by the unknowable. *Knowledge by conviction*, as I use the expression, requires a holistic approach. It is warmed by being human. We abandon it at the peril of our humanity. If we leave it, we can only return to a selfish, individualistic, primeval solitude. If we think of ourselves as without it, we think of ourselves as what Hirschman calls 'infrahuman wantons' (see p. 75). Titmuss puts the point clearly. He quotes Edgeworth as saying in another context:[17] 'We cannot *count* the golden sands of love; we cannot *number* the "innumerable smiles" of seas of love'. Titmuss goes on:[18]

> It is here that we can discern some of the fundamental distinguishing marks of social policy which differentiate it from economic policy. Because it has continually to ask the question 'Who is my stranger?', it must inevitably be concerned with the unquantifiable and unmethodical aspects of man as well as those aspects which can be identified and counted. Therefore, in terms of policies, what unites it with ethical considerations is its focus on integrative systems: on processes, transactions and institutions which promote an individual's sense of identity, participation and community and allow him more freedom of choice for the expression of altruism and which, simultaneously, discourage a sense of individual alienation.

This is why there are so many digressions in the book. It is why the book does not follow Plato or Rousseau in looking at the world as it should be but insists on facing it as it is. Specifically, it is why the book rejects a world based on numbers and the deductive logic of geometry; and why, instead, it bases itself on a view informed by as many sources as it can imagine. The book talks of mystery because it talks of the world beyond the manmade. *Knowledge by conviction* is what Hippocrates meant when he referred to the 'mysteries of the science' (above p. 1). *Knowledge by conviction* is acquired by the experience, imaginative or otherwise, of immersion in a situation. The fact that *knowledge by conviction* varies with time, place, and circumstance does not detract from its verity, or its force, at any moment. It is *knowledge by conviction* that helps us distinguish what our hearts and our heads tell us, and which sometimes enables us to listen to our hearts.

Most importantly, *knowledge by causes* insists on a single, so-called objective truth. Partly because of its tendency to specialization and partly in its desire always to find a cause, it is prone to confusing cause and effect. The successes of *knowledge by causes* eclipses *knowledge by conviction*. But this is the device that explains why the same phenomena mean different things to different people. In Vico's hands, it was the method to understand history. In this book, although there is some of that too, its main use is to understand the thoughts, hopes, and aspirations of those who have particular experiences. It is in this way that the book reflects on the world of those who have sat at the bedside of the sick. Today, it may be obvious that people who have lived in distant times had different experiences to our own. It is still not so easy to grasp that those who live in our times but who have had a different education and have had different occupational experiences may be as unlike ourselves as the subjects of history. The essential difference between these methods of knowing lies in the kind of things that may be known and whether the truth about them is single or multiple. It is important that each of us can uphold a single moral vision even where different people validly view truth as different. This is no more than saying I can understand someone else whilst disagreeing with them.

In chapter 7 (pp. 188ff), this book says that there is an 'important distinction: individualism (and the law) wants peace but always on terms; humanity . . . at least in some of its moods, yearns for an unqualified peace'. In one of the most celebrated legal decisions of the twentieth century, Lord Atkin said:[19] 'The rule that you are to love your neighbour becomes in law, you must not injure your neighbour; and the lawyer's question, Who is my neighbour? receives a restricted reply'. So, if our neighbours injure us, we can sue them. To the law, then, we are at peace unless we are wronged. It is a conditional peace. Titmuss, however, tells us that social policy is concerned with the other question, 'Who is my stranger?' He says that his book,[20]

> has . . . advanced three inter-related theses. First, that gift-exchange of a non-quantifiable nature has . . . important functions in complex, large-scale societies. . . . Second, the application of scientific and technological developments in such societies . . . has increased rather than diminished the scientific as well as the social need for gift relationships. Third . . . modern societies now require more, rather than less, freedom of choice for the expression of altruism in the daily life of all social groups.

Lord Atkin's neighbours are those who are connected by causal links, and they are links that are increasingly expressed in numerical terms. Unquantifiable and unmethodical aspects of man and ethical considerations connect Titmuss's strangers. We recognize Lord Atkin's neighbours with *knowledge by causes*, Titmuss's strangers with *knowledge by conviction*.

Theme 1—What is medicine?

This beginning required the book to explore what medicine and its practice are. When I started out, general discourse offered platitudes. The few doctors I had met did not match the stereotypes portrayed. The platitudes are still there, and they now inform debate and policy more so than before. At that time, as now, the general press was in thrall to the consumer movement, which I have always intuitively felt to be intellectually and spiritually inadequate.[21] More specifically, the law itself left gaps. It left important questions to others. For example, abstaining from any view of its own, the law left the issue of what incompetent practice was and is to witnesses from the profession.[22] Instead of following fashion by condemning the abstention, the book wonders why it does so. This is the first example of where the method of describing the world as I see it rather than how I want it to be leads the book from orthodoxy. It was thus that I turned to what some doctors said about themselves and about what they did. Often, there was engagement but not reason.[23] Accordingly, the book itself spends much time with writers who give substance to the passion. I have tried always to be informed by empathy with the concerns of those who understand a different world because of their insights gained at the bedsides of the fragile, the vulnerable and the sick. It is Vico's method.

Adopting a somewhat theoretical mode the book proposes three ways of conceiving medicine: the scientific; the participatory; and, because the first two are found to offer inadequate descriptions, the classical. It is not that the first two do not contain important elements of truth. It is that in major respects they are incomplete. The purpose of this excursion is not so much to explore what is meant by medicine. If that were the task, the omission of important factors such as primary and mental health care would be serious errors. These three conceptions are described only because they give rise to conflicting regulatory regimes, and I needed to know how far each was built on sand.

The central characteristics of the scientific mode of medicine are, or would be if it were valid, twofold. First, just as a scientific experiment ought to produce the same results if similar conditions are applied, medicine should not vary either in its application or in its result between one practitioner and another. Second, because science as knowledge is ethically neutral, medical ethics would be no more than a branch of general ethics. The first point is largely true as regards medical research. But then, such research, such deliberate acquisition of new knowledge, is carried out by scientists who commonly are, but equally commonly are not, doctors. As doctors move from knowledge to its application, necessarily they are concerned with particular settings and particular patients. They apply their knowledge, practice their art or skill on the basis of informed intuition born out of experience. Again to talk of Vico, they apply both the *knowledge by causes* and the *knowledge by conviction* their profession gives them. First and foremost, practice is not intended to acquire new knowledge, although it always does: it is intended as the right action for the particular patient. At bottom, the supposition that the scientific mode of medicine is a complete description confuses the means with the aims. That does not matter until regulatory structures are built on or resources allocated because of that idea and until management is made to depend on it.

There are three main structures affecting medicine that are in fact built on this only half-true doctrine. They are democratic theory using, for example, ideas of egalitarian citizens, informed consent (both in terms of practice and in terms of what the law might require), and the modern machinery for resource allocation between possible subjects of medical care. Each of these is made possible by translating the discourse of practice into conventional economic terms. The book insists that the classical mode of medicine (I describe it in a moment) is both the better description and creates the possibility of the most favorable conditions for its practice, that is, favorable for its practitioners as well as those they treat. This idea is anathema to democracy. Democracy cannot tolerate closed or even élite knowledge. This is no place to begin a critique of democratic theory. It suffices to say that it is in this that Western mass democracy is at its weakest. It is one thing to accord everybody equal dignity and equal civic rights. It is quite another to denigrate special skills and understandings. Besides, the argument that medicine must be scientific because otherwise it is incompatible with democracy has no persuasion: it raises a conclusion to an assumption. The same objection exists to the assumption that practice must be primarily an economic activity.

I shall come to the administration of health care in due course, but one remark is worth making now. At one time, scientism had appeared to herald a new democratic means of delivering health care. The reforms, which led to the 'internal market' within the NHS and the application of *new public management,* were founded on this idea. As it falls away, as it does with the new 'clinical governance' under the 1997 White Paper, democracy in medicine is transformed. It moves from emphasizing equal moral right and agency and to equal moral worth. Medical practitioners are left to their experience and expertise. But they are bound to use them for all patients equally and without discrimination on any social basis. Thus, they can withhold treatment from a smoker on the ground that it will not work because of the smoke. They cannot withhold treatment because smoking is morally repugnant.[24]

The assumption of the possibility of equal knowledge by practitioners and their patients (it suggests the former only have to explain and parity is achieved) also underlies the modern legal doctrine of informed consent. This book surmises that this doctrine has its base in religion.[25] It dates from times when surgery was extremely dangerous and patients needed to make their peace with God. The (autocratic) doctor was treating the body, but there was a soul over which medicine had no jurisdiction. With God now shoved into another little box, the modern mind is incapable of even imagining a process of secularization.[26] Leaving such issues aside, the possibility of equal knowledge asserts equal interest. This too is manifestly false. The engaged practitioner does not have either the patient's pain nor can he or she share the same hope of cure; the one wants restoration and the other, if no more, a job well done. In a nutshell, medicine deals with patients, sick people. It does not deal with citizens.

This book argues that the basic reason for the resources poured into medicine (particularly secondary and tertiary care) is not that it is a cost-effective method of reducing unease or *dis-ease.*[27] Rather, medicine gives us hope against brute nature, that is, hope against our own mortality. Once more, it follows Vico:[28] 'Man in the face of death is conscious of the desire that there should be power to overcome death on his behalf, a God superior to nature'. Increasingly, as this book notes, God has been marginalized. The need to have the power to overcome death remains. It is for this that we value medicine.

The force that society gives to medical practice is that it gives hope over experience. Nowadays we are not much motivated by the suffering of others: we might be by the potential of our own. It is medicine, and medicine alone, that opposes sickness, pain, (and with the demise of the God and the Church) those ills that we can call brute nature. We value medicine's dictates because it enables us to deny reality. At the governmental level both in Britain and within the European Union, we establish scientific committees not merely to advise us, but to tell us how to live. Whereas once people smoked and ate beef[29] for pleasure, they now do so in guilt and defiance. Forgetting we must die of something, we are led also to believe that if we do this, we will not die of that. Having thus focused our concern on one issue, we are led to forget that we will therefore die of something else. What was medical advice has shifted to an imperative. Here then is an apparently strange thing. Having devalued expertise in the name of democracy, we accord it legislative force over our very lives. It is the recognition of the difference between professional *knowledge by conviction* and scientific knowledge.

Both the other ways of conceiving medicine, the participatory and classical modes, insist that it is not possible to separate the question of what is medicine from what is its practice. Like the scientific, both also have elements of reality and both also inform policy. Within them medicine uses, but is not encompassed by, *knowledge by causes*. There is more to each than the mere application of technique. The relationship is asymmetric: the patient trusts and the doctor cares both for the disease as well as the patient as an individual. The knowledge of the 'pain' cannot be anything other than different. To the patient, although the pain may bewilder, there is the hope, the expectation, and the demand that the doctor will remove it. To the doctor, the pain creates the opportunity for medicine to be practiced. As Parsons argued,[30] typically the patient overestimates the seriousness of his illness and underestimates the time for recovery. So also, as Hughes put it:[31] 'The professional mind . . . appears as a perversion of the common sense of what is urgent and what less urgent'. The participatory and classical modes differ in the way they involve the recipient of care. In its participatory mode, the patient always retains a moral agency. However firm the trust and however sound the judgment, patients are always at liberty to reject the advice they receive. In its classical mode, medicine suspends the patient's moral agency. The physician gives orders, not advice. Plainly, then, the participatory mode is closer to notions of informed consent. The enterprise itself requires the willful participation of both parties. The problem for the law and the egalitarians is that although the consent is free it cannot be full. The asymmetry of the relationship prevents it.

Classical and participatory medicine have much in common. Indeed, I have been tempted to portray the latter as the modern development of the former. This book traces a history. This makes it sufficiently clear that for most of the period from the ancient Greeks to very recently the classical mode held sway, if not as a mode of practice at least as a mode of aspiration. It argues that this has been true for most but not all of the time, nor in all places and not among all classes or types of patient. Participatory medicine becomes possible when under the influence of egalitarian and democratic theory it becomes necessary to accord moral rights to everyone. This, however, still seems to be a proposition more of hope than of description.

The general truth, uncomfortable as it may be, is that classical medicine is still generally applied. This is, for example, why the curious word *patient* is used to describe the object of the profession. Other occupations have *clients* or *consumers* or *customers*. Clients define objectives but they are dependent on the supplier as to the means. Consumers define what they want and customers merely have to ask and pay. They are 'always right'. Only medicine has patients: passive recipients whose duty is to wait and who get what the practitioner thinks is right for them. The different meanings are clear but their consequence is that it becomes impossible to apply the organizing social categories of our age. The term *patient* is incompatible with conventional economics. It does not suit our egalitarian democracy. It renders medicine immune to being ordered by publicly accessible statistics.

Theme 2—What is professional practice?
How far is it understandable from the outside?

Medicine may then be taken to be the right healing action for the particular *patient*. The difficulty is finding the procedure to define what is right. Once we move away from the simplicities of medicine as a science, we move into a world of values, full of choice. The interesting questions are: How are those values made and expressed and who makes the choice and on what basis? The behavioural edifice we know as practice is built on the answers.

The foundation of this structure lies in these two concepts—the ideas of the patient and of the right healing action. It is on these that the rest is built. One of the key ideas underpinning the patient is the concept of, not so much illness (that is a matter for science and society), but of being exposed to unwelcome danger. Despite the fact that in Foucault's terms the patient is a carrier of discourse and despite the fact that the moral agency is suspended, medicine cannot be other than a social activity directed at the vulnerable. Inevitably, it involves the powerful and the weak, and the moral issues which that relationship throws up. True, at times, it is the discourse that becomes dominant. This does not mean that the carrier must be irrelevant to the relationship. The suspension of the moral agency does not mean that it is abrogated. It is the pretense of science to universality that makes the carrier irrelevant. So also, the ethical neutrality of science makes it unable to distinguish between the suspension and abrogation of moral agency. It is also true that science, now as was not once the case, is a *sine quo non* for defining the right healing action. But, crucially, it is not now, as it never was, sufficient. Mixed also into that definition are considerations of the patient, of culture, of circumstance, and sometimes too of resources. Because of these other factors, practitioners who merely apply science deny the possibility of professional responsibilities. At their crudest, when the emphasis is on the application rather than the science, they verge also on empiricism, denying the possibility of intellectual discipline. This is why, although modern medicine can learn from alternative therapies, it can never be happy with them.

The ideas of professional responsibilities and of intellectual discipline are themselves built on these two foundational concepts. They take their shape from them. It may be an accident but it is medical practice that has done most to teach the world the meaning of professional responsibility. It has a longer history than either the law or the Church. More importantly, because of the re-discovery of the Hippocratic corpus in the Renaissance, it was available for adoption in a more mature form at the outset of the modern age. I think now that this book places too much emphasis on the decisive character of that time. At any rate it does not notice enough that what was adopted was essentially pre-Renaissance. The Renaissance, and in particular its ideas of self and of the individual, has worked its way through the Enlightenment, into the modern and the postmodern ages. As it did so the contradictions of what was done in the early sixteenth century (for example the foundation of the College of Physicians) have become more apparent. It was medicine that taught the central ideas of professional responsibility, and it taught it in essentially pre-Renaissance terms. First, it said:[32] 'Life is short and the Art long; the occasion fleeting; experience fallacious and judgment difficult. The physician must not only be prepared to do what is right himself, but also to make the patient, the attendants and the externals co-operate.' Secondly, by regarding teachers as parents and other practitioners as brothers, it created not only the idea of a closed community, but one where property (particularly that, including intellectual property, related to the occupation) was held in common. Thirdly, the idea of professional confidence goes beyond the utility of the relationship: it extends to all information about the patient however acquired. Fourthly, practice is directed to the patient. Exploitation is forbidden. Finally, there is an amalgam of negative ideas. These revolve around not doing things beyond the practitioner's competence, not doing things unless they are for the benefit of the patient and not doing things for personal aggrandizement.

Perhaps each, but certainly in total, these are incompatible with the modern world. They all lift professional responsibility beyond the confines of a two-party relationship. They extend it to co-workers and make it timeless. These ideas place the professional worker within a group that is not delimited by his or her will. They make professional judgment that of the group not the individual. Professional acts always and must be in common. The professional is trusted by society but is isolated from it. The modern world can make no sense of any of this. They are all collective and not individual forms. They all reject the conditional time-bound, choiceful emphasis on self of the Renaissance and Enlightenment.

It is at this point that this book departs from any ideas founded on this besieged and isolated self. It therefore has to reject any worldview informed by only one discipline, for example, conventional economics. As with many others, discipline asserts universality. By its account all social activity can (or must) be viewed in economic terms. True to the idea that there can be more than one way of looking at the same thing, this book sets out (at p. 112) some of the phenomena that both the sociology of medicine (and more generally of the professions) and economics can bite upon. It mentions the economic justifications. Taken together these reasons describe medicine as a cynical, disingenuous, and almost dishonest occupation. This book asks: How then does the organizing discipline of our age arrive at this critique of what is surely almost the only occupation to maintain a generality of public esteem? The answer is that there is a confusion of cause and effect. For example, the vilification by the profession as 'quacks' of those who practice on the basis of 'no cure, no fee' is a strategy that, to be sure, makes external criticism difficult. For that reason it can be seen to protect the economic interests of the profession. It is however also a strategy based on—it may even be a consequence of—the different knowledge of the illness possessed by the doctor and patient. It is a device that underpins the trust that is essential to medicine. Why, one may ask, is it necessary to insist upon only one of a variety of possible explanations?

So also, there is the suggestion that the profession creates scarcity by licensing and by the monopolization of supply in the form of the control of education. In this way it maximizes the possibility of income. Again, we can see that the profession gains economically by persuading those with legislative power to grant these 'privileges'. This then is clearly an *effect* but to leap from that to say that is a *cause* seems unnecessary and dangerous. These devices (of licensing and of education) can at least additionally be viewed as consequences of the nature of professional knowledge and its associated intellectual discipline. At this point a digression is appropriate. This book demonstrates how the practices of law and medicine have learned from each other over time. On balance, one may conclude that medicine has been the senior partner, not in terms of social status where the upper strata of law have been on a par with any in the land. Medicine has been the senior partner because it provides a more coherent and comprehensive ethical system for practice. Law could once have adopted this role. The physical arrangements in the Inns of Court could have, but did not, provide an ethically based legal profession.[33] Perhaps what stopped it was that the leaders of the law were too close to government and affairs of state. Perhaps also, law and lawyers have never been viewed with the benevolence that medicine has enjoyed. In part, medicine has wanted law's status.[34] Law has coveted medicine's esteem. I shall argue in a moment that the prestige of law is declining. Medicine now stands alone.

It is useful here to compare changes in the practice of medicine with those of law during the last ten years. When this book was first published one had the feeling that medicine was about to be radically reorganized. After all, in Britain it was organized through the very bureaucratic procedures of the National Health Service. It was open to the latest fads and fashions of political and managerial life. There was much talk of performance-related contracts, medical audit, consumer power, and similar mechanisms that would upset the old ways of doing things. These devices did not eventually upset the core of medicine. On the other hand, ten years ago however, law appeared immune from the modern age. True, there had been changes in, for example, the way solicitors were paid for their work: they were charging on an hourly basis. The size of law firms had vastly increased.[35] There was significant use of technology but it was still in its infancy. The consequences of these other changes had not, and have not, been fully assessed. In a nutshell, we can now see it as the transformation from a profession to a restrained occupation organized about making a return on capital. If this is so, it is law, not medicine, that has mutated.

Before the last decade, it was common to compare the scheme of the health service with that of legal aid. The health service was created in 1948 and the legal aid and advice scheme in 1949. The health service was funded out of general taxation. It offered the whole population health care at the point of need without charge. Again, out of taxation, the legal aid scheme offered the legal skills of even the best lawyers to those who could satisfy the twin tests of merits and need. Over the last ten years, the legal universe has been replaced. In the 1980s and 1990s, the cost of litigation has risen beyond all reasonable forecasts. One suspects one reason for this is that in Britain now, as was not the case earlier, litigation is part of the global legal order. In effect, the best lawyers are working for organizations dealing in financial questions of a different order of magnitude from those in the mere domestic or national world. The money paid out under the legal aid scheme very largely has had to follow these global trends. The Courts and Legal Services Act 1990 made provision for lawyers performing certain kinds of work to be paid by results.[36]

The idea that a professional person should have a personal financial interest in the outcome of his or her skills contradicts the basis of professional practice. It was in a medical context that the law had held that practice on the basis of 'no cure, no fee' was quackery. That was the nineteenth century. As far as the law was concerned, such practices were regarded as maintenance or even champerty. These were made criminal offenses in 1275. The professional bodies themselves condemned such practice as unethical. The criminal nature of the activity was repealed as obsolete in 1967.[37] The professional condemnation remained until the 1990 Act. Now, whatever the cause, government has decided that it can no longer afford to underwrite the old legal aid arrangements. In the future, it is envisaged, plaintiffs with financial claims will only be able to pursue them if they can make arrangements, if necessary by 'conditional fee', with their lawyers.[38] Within thirty years what was once criminal has become the mode of practice. And it is less than ten years since this mode merited professional censure. The basis of legal practice has been changed not in any re-assertion of professional values but in timid acquiescence in the economic critique. The questions are: Why has law given up so easily? And, is medicine subject to the same threat?

The last decade has seen other major changes to both medicine and law. As we have seen, medicine is organized about giving each patient the right healing action. As it has become technically more accomplished so it has been able to treat more and more patients. In so doing it has been more difficult and at times impossible to make a fine variation of judgment for each individual. Modern medicine has become a mass commodity. Nevertheless, the ultimate value that we accord it is based on medicine being humanity's instrument for combating 'brute nature'. For all the successes of modern medical science and for all the intrusion of modern managerial techniques, the ethical kernel of medicine has not been changed. Indeed, the expansion of medicine by treating more people and with more success, tending, as we shall see to empiricism, might be having the effect of deepening the value we accord it. This is not to say that physicians are becoming more popular. The evidence is that complaints, both those that lead to litigation and those that are dealt with by other means, are rising rapidly. There is no contradiction in these two trends. We are learning to want more from medicine and we are accordingly disappointed in Hirschman's sense more often.[39]

Law, by contrast, has not just known major change. Its alterations are fundamental to its purposes and its method of delivery. We have seen the government has responded to the expansion of the legal aid budget by legalizing conditional fee arrangements. More importantly, litigation is no longer regarded as an evil.[40] It is now seen as one of a number of important ways to regulate public authorities and other large tortfeasors.[41] It is a weapon in the armory of the consumer movement. Proposals are now in place, too, to marginalize public settlement of private disputes. Britain is following the American example of introducing alternative dispute resolution mechanisms.[42] The public courts are increasingly being seen as being there to control public wrongs. But usually in doing this, they are adopting, again in the American style, mechanisms of case and caseload management.[43] The courts are as much concerned to give guidance to the world's future conduct as to justify particular decisions. Sometimes the guidance takes precedence over the justification.[44] As Murphy puts it:[45]

> Modern bureaucracies acquire and process and store and analyse information, in ever-increasing amounts. They become vehicles not just for decontextualization through rules . . . but for decontextualization through statistics and other forms of scientific knowledge. Unlike legal adjudication systems, which look back, such bureaucracies produce the future and are oriented to pro-

ducing the future. Whereas the primary task of adjudicators and of those working around them is to ascertain the law applicable to the matter in hand and apply it, the fundamental orientation of bureaucracy to law is instrumental and manipulative: activity is objective or goal-driven, and if there is a mismatch between goal and law, the law must be changed.

In general, a discipline means more than knowledge or even organized knowledge. That it is organized implies both that it has rigour and a sense of the relevant. It is knowledge organized for reasons beyond being merely instrumental. A discipline need not be useful. Indeed, it is more recognizable and more able to be easily appreciated if it is not. If one thinks of the disciplines in the social sciences (history, anthropology, sociology) one finds ways of thinking that do not have immediate utility. A discipline is a particular way of thinking about a topic, but a discipline need not make claims to universality. It is knowledge organized as part of a way of life. This implies that it must be akin to a vocation. It is not an occupation although an occupation may be organized about it. Medicine and law each claim to be disciplines but they also have direct relation to the practical world. Both have had centuries of competition with *empirics* who have offered the community the same skills as they but without the vocation.[46] The modern world has repeated some of the old and found new challenges to the insistence that practice ought to be on the basis of the discipline rather than on mere functional utility. There is repetition of the view that both should be practiced in the vernacular (in the modern world this has become the plain English movement)[47] and that they should be comprehensible to the lay mind. A new breed of lawyer was created in the form of licensed conveyancers.[48] These are specifically not fully qualified but are empowered to enter the field of work that had hitherto provided a considerable part of the total income of the profession. Empirics were legalized.

But some aspects of law and medicine are in contrast. The introduction of the licensed conveyancers was done deliberately to attack an economic monopoly held by lawyers. The rules about what drugs nurses can prescribe, and pharmacists dispense without prescription, have been relaxed.[49] This has been done partly in recognition of climbing professional status, partly because of the growth of team medicine and partly to free doctors from the routine to enable them better to fight man's battle with nature.

In all this, medicine has been able to keep its sense of discipline and purpose. Law, and again by contrast, has been losing it. Vilified as ever, but now by an increasingly powerful consumer movement, law no longer has respect for its own discipline. Its historic method was a reliance on tradition. Medicine, even at the highest level in the Royal College of Physicians, abandoned that more than a hundred years ago. To be sure, precedent is still applied in the courts but its voice is heard less easily as the competing sounds of policy (judicial commonsense) and legislative law reform gather volume.[50] Once, and not very long ago, law's purpose was concerned to do justice between man and man. Echoing medicine's right healing action, Lord Diplock once told us:[51] 'The primary duty of the Court of Appeal on an appeal in any case is to determine the matter actually in dispute between the parties'. But medicine was and is sustained by more than the right healing action. It carries humanity's hopes against nature. Law has no such enduring validation. It is sustained by the need not to maintain justice but to uphold order, any order. My *Republican Crown* argued that separation of powers is twofold between the legislative and executive branches rather than the threefold system supposed by many. Judging, I said, was part of the executive function separated no more from the administrative than are auditors. The collapse of law's profession, and discipline, re-enforces this conclusion. If we may talk in retrospect of the present, we may say that medicine is sanctioned by a stable value. Law, which has ever to be two-faced, is undermined by the ambiguities and vagueness of the concept of justice. In short, although we can imagine many reasons why medicine will change, there are too many differences between it and law to conclude that it must inevitably go the same way. The only remaining point to make, and perhaps it is one of threat to medicine, is that it will be the last of the professional beacons for civilized society.

Theme 3—What are the origins and force of the internal and external rules governing practice?

This book accepts Durkheim's view of the guild in two major respects.[52] First, they are the kernel of morality within an occupational group. It is 'collective discipline' and is based in 'mutual understanding'. It arises out of the facts that over time each member of the group faces similar problems, they learn from each other and find similar solutions. This morality is different from and cannot live with what Durkheim called 'workshop regulations'. We now call them charters, mission statements, codes of practice, and guidelines. These texts necessarily replace intuitive common understandings as the source of regulation. The more extensive they are, the less force that discipline can have.

The modern world is based on a rejection of collective action. It refuses to understand the results of group activity. Its universe is based in what this book variously calls 'the cult of the individual' and 'whiggery'.[53] It is the result of its rejection of historical and sociological insight. It follows that the modern world cannot accept Durkheim's view of guild morality. Having thus rejected morality as the means of group control it resorts to other ways of defining how people ought to behave. Besides, being based in an individualistic and democratic vision, the secret and private morality of Durkheim's guilds is simply unacceptable. The control devices must be seen to be open and accessible to all. The consequence is that the guild loses its self-confidence in its mutual understandings. The occupation becomes a job, and its morality must be visible and publicly accountable. The modern world is aided in this by the application of either the new discipline of *Regulation* (briefly discussed in a moment) or by conventional economics. All occupational groups, including medicine (and the NHS), are regarded as being in business. Commentators, then, are left to wonder why business methods are not applied.[54] To make Vico's point again, they look at the world as they want it to be. Then, when they find it is not like that they self-consciously reconstruct it. When they are successful, their work becomes a self-fulfilling prophecy.

These theoretical musings show themselves in relation to the practice of law and medicine. In both cases, statute has intervened to insert a lay input in the institutional bodies that govern 'professional ethics'. The difference between them is that, as I have previously suggested, medicine still maintains its self-confidence and is still accorded the high value based on its opposition on our behalf to the realities of nature. The consequence is, as far as medicine is concerned, that while there is opposition and even disgust when a doctor is found to have failed, medicine as a whole continues to maintain its public esteem. The perceived need to make medicine 'democratic' has led the General Medical Council to include lay people in its decision making and expand the range of conduct with which it is concerned. The outside world did not understand why professional incompetence was not regarded as 'infamous misconduct'.[55] Under pressure both from the government and the Monopolies and Mergers Commission (neither of which, for their own ideological reasons, could accept the distinction this book so firmly draws between a profession and a trade)[56] the GMC has relaxed its historic prohibition on advertising.[57] So also, it is clear that the volume of complaints to the General Medical Council, to the courts and to others is rising. Nevertheless, despite all this it would seem that failures by individuals within the profession lead to a public response of being appalled and not mere timid acquiescence or resignation. Despite everything, the medical profession still arouses our hopes and our expectations.

It is otherwise with law. This takes us to the second main idea that this book accepts about Durkheim's view of the guild. He said that it was an enduring social form. The lawyer's guilds have been broken by new external regulation. The profession's collective lack of confidence in its traditions opened the way. It is seen to have failed in the essential tests of the way it treats its own, for example, often in terms of race and sex discrimination, and the way it treats it clients. It is not just a matter of fees. It is also a matter of the profession being seen to be complacent about delay. The consequences have been the introduction of the Lord Chancellor's Advisory Committee on Legal Education and Conduct.[58] True, there are lawyers on the committee, but the regulation of entrance to the profession (including now the need for continuing education) and conduct within it, is outside the profession's control. Matters of individual discipline are ultimately under the jurisdiction of the non-lawyer, independent complaints commissioner. The laws' delays are to be dealt with by case management by the judges. Where an agreement to waive a time limit is made by lawyers the judge must sanction it, with the lay parties actually in court.[59] A lawyer's client is no longer allowed to trust his lawyer.

This book places a heavy emphasis on the link between professional behavior and gentlemanly conduct.[60] It suggests that, via Baldesar Castiglione's *Book of the Courtier*, the Renaissance made it possible for everybody to aspire to that status. Having examined, English literature, Philip Mason reflected on the effects of the French Revolution on the idea of class and rank in England. He says:[61] '[In Chaucer's England men] took it for granted that . . . things were arranged in an order of precedence. . . . After the French Revolution, people were by no means sure that there would be another world and it was openly proclaimed that there ought to be equality here and now.' Mason goes on:[62]

> Until the French Revolution everyone took for granted what Shakespeare called 'degree', the fact of social difference. . . . But the barriers were not clear cut. It was not always easy to tell who

was who. . . . Certain of inequality, even though not always quite clear who was who, the English of the 18th century lived in close physical proximity with their servants and made them confidants of the most intimate secrets. . . . but as the century wore on they came by little and little to insist on greater social distance. . . . That insistence on aloofness may stand to underline the growing stiffness of class barriers, which crept over the century as slowly, as intermittently but as inexorably as stiffness in the joints of an ageing man.

He argues:[63]

[By Victorian times there was] a swing to the country and away from the court. . . . Before the French Revolution and the proclamation of equality, [Squires of the 18th century] had known very well that because of their birth they were quite different from the common people. Therefore a gentleman could be familiar with his servants and talk bawdy to them. But once the great kingdom across the Channel had become a republic where all men were said to be equal, it became more necessary to insist on difference. . . . This need to be distinguished from the people was surely the reason for the growth of prudishness as well. Physical functions were something shared with the great mass of the people, so the privileged few who had to show they were different pretended that they did not exist. . . . Victorian prudishness was a remnant of the Manichaean heresy, the belief that matter was evil.

Mason suggests that, in Edwardian times,[64] 'The mental barriers were higher than they had ever been. This was partly because, since the French Revolution, the whole principle of stratification was threatened and therefore it was necessary to be persuaded that the barriers were not conventional but real'. Nevertheless, he says:[65]

Britain in 1914 was half way to being a democracy, but effective power was still in the hands of a ruling class. That class was not a closed caste but a body to whose ranks there was continual recruitment. . . . And the name for that ruling class carried moral overtones and stood for certain standards of behaviour. The paradox lay in the fact that while the rank had little point if it included everyone, almost everyone thought that it might one day include himself or at least his son, and almost everyone admired the ideal of conduct.

Today, we have moved on. The ruling class, in the old sense, has
gone. Rank, indeed, has little point. Standards of behaviour are governed now as much by written rules as intuitive understanding. We
live in an egalitarian, classless meritocracy that firmly rejects doing
things in the old ways because they used to work and even more
clearly rejects the old values that went with them. The gentleman has
become an anachronism. But as we have cast that status out, so we
have reduced the space, not only for the gentleman in law and medicine, but also for the *professional* in the precise sense that this book
uses the term, with all its overtones of Hippocratic practice. Indeed,
to compensate for this, we have transformed the meaning of *professional* from that ideal to a paid, competent, commonly economic
actor. Having done that, our language has lost the word to describe
the ideal. Not only does it not exist, it cannot. Despite this, the traditions of the occupation live on. The result is inevitable confusion.

We have gained external control of occupations in place of this
essentially intuitive self-regulation of the professions which used to
require the gentlemanly arts. The area of study concerned with these
new forms of control is an embryonic discipline to rank with the
others of the social sciences, sociology, economics, history, and the
rest. It has taken the name *regulation*. Because in one sense all life is
an economic activity, economics may be said to be have been the
elder child of sociology. But, in another sense, economic activity has
to be profit motivated. And since all life is manifestly not for profit, in
recent years this other child has been gaining maturity. *Regulation*
seeks to study the activity by which[66] 'the rules governing the exchange of goods and services are made and implemented'. It describes
how the rules that set standards, define accountability, and prescribe
efficiency are made. Like sociology and economics, it too tries to tell
us about the foundations of human intercourse; and, like them also,
out of its discrete assumptions, it is developing its own methods.
Given its genealogy, we should not be surprised that it shares things
with its parent, sociology, and with its elder sibling, economics. From
sociology it takes the idea that it can describe social organization;
from economics it takes the idea that:[67] 'The activity of regulation
can in turn be broken down into four separate tasks: the control of
market entry and exit, of competitive practices, of market organization and of remuneration'.

The subject assumes that, in their idealized form (which is what
rule-makers have to have in mind as they draft),[68] 'Doctors are busi-
nessmen, part of the real economic world, in need of money'. However, on the contrary, ideal typical doctors are treated by those who

create and apply professional ethics as if they have capacity to spend and consume rather than a need to earn. As the International Code of Medical Ethics puts it, 'A doctor must practice his profession uninfluenced by motives of profit'. We may grant that the profession has always been concerned with prestige. It does not follow that it is concerned with incomes, except in so far that it is either a measure of status or the means to have the ability to spend. To insist that medicine has to have a commercial base is to remove hope. It is a philosophy of the young and the fit, and of despair. There is no need for this. Medicine need not be seen to have a commercial base.

Because of its desire to develop tools for comparison between occupations, *regulation* minimizes the differences in their objectives. For example, they do not notice the differences we saw above, between the words *patient, client, consumer*. They are all the same economic actors. Hence, the subject can assert, in line with fashionable egalitarian and democratic views,[69] 'Professional autonomy has been granted to an excessive degree, and this cannot be said to be an outcome which is in the interests of patients'. But we may ask why? If the autonomy gives them confidence in what doctors do, maybe we can have a reflected trust in them. As Parsons and Freidson told us, the patient's knowledge of disease is necessarily different from the doctor's. More generally, regulation does not understand that trust may be, as I shall argue, either conditional or unconditional. An occupation that allows itself to be ensnared in this discourse rapidly loses that concept with all its associated power of social adhesion. Law has fallen for the new discipline. Medicine, so far, has been able to resist.

As a device rather than a subject, the method regulation uses is *audit*. Michael Power has traced the reasons for the growth of this device in general.[70] He says:[71] 'Auditing has become an article of regulatory faith'. In essence, he follows Mead:[72] that predictions of behavior can so alter behavior as to invalidate the predictions. Power variously refers to 'The Audit Society' and to the 'The Audit Explosion'. Among the reasons he identifies are the fiscal crisis in the West, which has led to[73] 'auditing, both for probity and programme effectiveness . . . [audits have] emerged as prominent instruments of administrative reform'. As a matter of principle there has been a political commitment to the idea of the reduction of the provision of state services. So also, 'institutional changes and regulatory responses . . . are being accomplished with more or less reliance on something called "auditing"'. And there have been changes in the nature of government from hierarchical command to self-regulation

backed by audit, quality assurance, beginning in standardization ini-
tiatives for technical products and recently to strategic management
imperatives. Taken together, he says, all these elements have fueled
the demand for auditing and auditors. As we shall see, the 1997 White
Paper on the New NHS, which charts the next ten years, relies heavily
on audit and measurement. It proposes the introduction of wider,
and possibly softer, ranges of indicators.

Power argues[74] 'auditing in all its guises has emerged as a popular
tool of control because it satisfies different features of the regulatory mood of the times . . . audits of all shapes and sizes seem to
make practices transparent and hence accountable even though they
also claim to leave everything as it is'. He points out that auditing
can look relatively neutral. But this is only so if there are no standards or such as there exist are ambiguous or indeterminate. In this
case,[75] 'the audit process cannot be separated from strategies of making organisations or individuals accountable'. In this sense audit is a
device tending to the proceduralization of occupations. The substance of what is done is supposed to remain the same. Audit insists
on measuring the way it is done. Here, it comes close to new public
law. That, too, does not seek directly to change things. On its face, it
merely requires that decisions be made only after commonly publicly stated procedures have been applied. The problem is that both
audit and new public law have nothing to bite on unless there are
proper procedures. Since we now insist that that these new regulatory devices must be fed, we also, if need be, change the decision-
making process so that there are indeed procedures that can be su-
pervised. Newdick says:[76] 'The development of guidelines is part of
a distinct cultural shift, a move away from unexamined reliance on
professional judgment to award more structured support for, and
accountability of, such judgment. The explosion of medical information and the increased complexity in today's health-care system has
made this support necessary.' The pity in this is twofold. It is the procedure not the substance that is controlled and the change in the
process may lead to even undesired change in the substance.

As Power argues the creation of external evaluation can cause
defensive mentalities. He says:[77]

Some studies show the impact of the audit process on the discourses of the auditee; it is as if a new subject of the audit process
is emerging from clinician stress, practitioner distrust, eroded professionalism and collegiality and the burdens of systems
formalisation as a bureaucratic surface for audit. . . . In short, au-

dits with quality as their objective may lead to unintended forms of mediocrity as games of 'creative compliance' develop around auditable information systems.

Power suggests[78] that 'auditable performance measures are *intended* to colonise and transform the audited domain'. Power suggests that there is some evidence of increased executive stress and 'loss of organisational loyalty'.[79] He says that the value for money auditing emphasizes auditable matters such as economy and efficiency at the expense of 'more problematic ideas of effectiveness'. Hence, he says, 'the effectiveness of complex organisations is redefined in financial terms'. As we shall see, the 1997 White Paper criticizes the reforms to the NHS of the late 1980s and early 1990s in precisely these terms.

This audit by colonisation might involve peer or expert review. Power suggests there is a separation between medical and financial audit. He says:[80] 'The former seem to be rich local forms of clinical accounting whose role is primarily heuristic and oriented towards diagnostic improvement: quality assurance for medicine. In contrast, the latter appear to be more standardised, with external funding audiences in mind, and more probative and results oriented in nature'. Power says, 'These audits occupied distinct realms with different projects'. With medical audit as with financial audit, there is hope in its reforming and revelatory power. So, too, there is some idea of accountability. The differences between financial and medical audit are that the latter is to be conducted by peer review.[81] In financial audit, outsiders set organizational goals. In medical audit, they are established by the brotherhood of the profession; medical audit represents an extension of epidemiological techniques for disease, through particular treatments, to the effectiveness of particular practitioners. The similarity between two types of audit is that both assume that to some degree the results of the activity are measurable. In the case of medicine, the assumption is that one doctor practices or ought to practice in the same way as another. In this vein the Department of Health once said, it looked forward to an[82] 'era of knowledge-based care [in which] diversity of approach in routine practice will be increasingly difficult to defend unless supported by a sustainable and convincing rationale'. The neutral, epidemiological tool of medical audit is in danger of being corrupted into a piece of management machinery. Early on the Department of Health and Social Services was attracted to the idea. It said it[83] 'can be defined as the systematic, critical analysis of the quality of medical care, including the procedures used for diagnosis and treatment, the use of resources and the resulting outcome and quality of life for the patient'.

One can perhaps see why the medical profession has embraced medical audit. It reinforces its claim to practice a science. To an extent, the profession itself has been misled by its own rhetoric. The rhetoric of audit and the rhetoric of science pretend to an objectivity which practice denies. It may be inevitable and even accurate for modern medicine to claim a scientific base. But the claim to objectivity is also a strategy that contradicts important elements of the art of medicine. It has, if only as a by-product, the effect of reducing its dependence on trust and thus increasing the prospect of complaints, including litigation, consequent on the creation of self-interested suspicion, if not distrust. As Power puts it,[84] 'the assumptions sustaining audits often deny the trust that exists between practitioners and those they serve. These assumptions can be self-fulfilling: the auditee is necessarily an isolatable, measurable and auditable object'.

And, thus, what the auditee does is transformed in the process. Put another way, the occupation is changed. It requires different personal attributes. The search for efficiency, giving it primacy, thus alters the attractiveness of the occupation: there is, then, no surprise that there are reports of fewer people entering the professions and of established practitioners leaving before retirement. Without being as critical, Marnoch points[85] to the fact that many clinicians, including many clinical directors, are developing new management skills and that 'this is reflected in the large numbers undertaking MBAs and other courses'. This involves not only reskilling, but also changing aspirations. More seriously, it reinforces the idea that the attractions of the job are being altered. Prospective practitioners are ceasing to have traditional motivations.

This is not all. Medicine faces another threat. It is to be found in attempts to measure quality of life and the application of these attempts in assessing the desirability of particular treatments through such means as 'quality adjusted life years'. Ann Bowling has discussed the former. She says:[86] 'One of the most common methods of assessing outcome of care in a broader sense is in terms of the people's ability to perform tasks of daily living. Disability measures are more meaningful to people's lives than objective biochemical measures or measures of timed walking or grip strength'. She acknowledges that the problem is that the majority of the population is healthy but, without asking why clinicians should require to know when a population is healthy, she says[87] a positive conception of health is difficult to measure because of the lack of agreement over its definition. Clinical judgments focus on the absence of disease; lay people too may hold a variety of concepts such as the ability to carry out normal everyday tasks, feeling strong, good, fit and so on. Without an operational definition it is not possible to determine if and when a state of health has been achieved by a population.

Bowling argues that:[88]

positive health could be described as the ability to cope with stressful situations, the maintenance of a strong social-support system, integrated into the community, high morale and life satisfaction, psychological well-being, and even levels of physical fitness as well as physical health. . . . It is composed of distinct components that must be measured and interpreted separately.

This body of knowledge then goes on to try to define 'social health' (social well-being).[89] Bowling discusses the concept of the quality of life. It is a broader concept than personal health status. She concedes at present there is no definition. Nevertheless, the attempt is to find one reflecting the qualities that made life and survival liable, so that they may be measured. She says:[90]

Whilst a plethora of quantitative tools exist which operationalize and attempt to measure aspects of quality of life which are regarded as pertinent to health status, such as life satisfaction, well-being and morale, functional ability, social interaction, stress and psychiatric disturbance attempts to combine them into a single tool have been less successful.

Newdick explains what I regard as the second aspect of this other threat to medicine—the idea behind the 'quality adjusted life year' (QALY):[91]

[It] attempts to evaluate healthcare outcomes according to a generic scale. It asks (i) to what extent, and how long, will a treatment improve the quality of the patient's life and (ii) how much does the treatment cost. . . . [T]here is a sliding scale . . . if the improvement in health after treatment is both significant and long-lasting, the patient . . . scores high on the quality of life measure. If the treatment is relatively inexpensive, then the cost per quality of unit is low. The theory favours treatments which achieve the greatest increase in the quality of life, over the longer period, for the least cost. Conversely, if the cost of medical intervention is high, and relative improvement in the condition of the patient is small, or capable of being enjoyed over a short period of time only, then the cost per QALY will be relatively high.

Newdick concedes that the scheme has had little practical impact.[92] How could it be when it is so dependent on the measurement of something on which, as Bowing tells us, there is little agreement? Newdick recognizes that democratic opinion is not easy to apply to the 'infinite degrees of severity' of illness or 'the infinite combination of diseases' that may be in the same patient. Nor, he says,[93] is it easy to see how such measures can accommodate 'the subtle shifts over time in social attitudes to the concepts of "health" and "illness"'. He recognizes, too, that the scheme disadvantages the disabled and the elderly. He suggests[94] 'a more sensitive measure of the benefits must be found'.

Newdick asks also to what extent the theory is ethically acceptable.[95] It is entirely egalitarian because it seeks only to maximize the number of QALYs and makes no attempt to say which categories of patient, or types of illness, ought to be given priority. The theory would have the advantage of preventing an unethical waste of money which may deprive patients of access to care. On the other hand, strictly applied, the theory would 'erode the traditional view of the relationship between doctor and patient'. The doctor would be promoting the interests of the group rather than the interests of the particular patient. He quotes Mooney as saying:[96] 'medical ethics, particularly in the form of clinical freedom, tends to breed inefficiency. Indeed, it seems it sometimes provides a convenient escape mechanism for the romantic member of the medical profession neither to pursue efficiency nor to attempt any rationalisation at all of the potential for pursuing efficiency in health care'. Newdick says that the ethical theory used in QALY dilutes concern for the individual.[97] 'Some for whom we might have great sympathy and compassion could score rather badly. . . . For example, pure economic logic does not see a return in treating pain . . . particularly if there is little chance of that patient being cured'. 'More broadly', he says,[98] 'outcome measurements equate the idea of health 'need' with the ability to benefit from treatment'. He concludes by arguing that:[99] 'the concept of the outcome measurement has the most value when it forms one of the many clinical, moral, and compassionate considerations which motivate medical care. It informs, but does not decide, how money ought to be spent.'

This is an advance but it does not answer the central critiques of these approaches. As McKeown tells us, among the determinants of health, clinical medicine ranks a poor fourth, a long way behind nutrition, the environment, and behaviour. Much of clinical medicine is always inefficient when compared with these. As we shall see, the government's 1997 White Paper on the *New NHS* as well as the forthcoming Green Paper *Our Healthier Nation* recognize this. Second, both the attempt to measure quality of life and to adjust it for life expectancy are examples of the age-old search for a single truth which the Enlightenment pioneered and which Vico showed to be false. The problem is with the imposition of either one's own sense of right or of some majoritarian values, however derived. The former is not as silly or uncommon as it seems when one 'means well'. The latter belies the experience that the hopes, aspirations, fears, concerns of individuals are too secret, too unknown, too various, too unpredictable to be defined by mere voting. A minority, even a minority of one, is entitled to think or believe it is right. At bottom, the uniqueness of each individual member of human kind prevents any of us being accurately represented as a statistic.

It is not just an intellectual error to ignore these dimensions. It is a delusion of essentially selfish arrogance to believe we can measure what causes the pleasure and pain of others. Of that, we can have knowledge by conviction, but not by causes. The arrogance becomes unforgivable when this error is used to determine who shall and who shall not receive treatment. Doctors, however, do not search for this uniqueness of the individual. In their ideal, they work not on that, but on the conception of us that their art teaches them. If their art becomes a science, as the search for quality of life measurement assumes it can, it has to be the expense of our humanity and of their profession. We are diminished when we are treated as a number. Their profession is imperiled if it replaces *knowledge by conviction* with *knowledge by causes*.

Theme 4—What do the rules governing practice teach about social cohesion in general?

One of the curiosities, and greatest changes, of the last decade (and maybe more) is the growth of emphasis on what is often called *new public management*. The main characteristic of this approach is that it has been applied throughout the public sector, irrespective of what tasks were being organized.[100] Jorgenson called it[101] 'the spirit of the times'. It is the application of 'little box' theories to which I referred in the Prelude at the start of this chapter. This style of management includes much that it has borrowed from accountancy such as performance indicators, performance-related pay and measures of quality of service. It has also included decentralization and ostensible or real contracting out. This section sets out what this style involves and then assesses the possible counter-revolution in the government's White Paper of December 1997. It concludes by relating these changes to the central argument of this book.

Hood[102] has described what he calls the 'doctrinal components' of this mechanism of management. They are sevenfold. The first requires that the individuals who were responsible for any action are visible by name to the members of the public who deal with them. His second component, and perhaps it is the most important of them all, is that there shall be explicit standards and measures of performance. There should be definitions of goals, targets, indicators of success, all preferably expressed in quantitative terms. This is especially true of delivery of professional services. It explains the *Citizens Charter* and its progeny, including the *Patient's Charter*. Again, these techniques are designed to improve accountability and efficiency. They require a reassessment of objectives, and, thus, what is done. In essence, generally they consist of rather vague promises. The third component is that there shall be a greater emphasis on 'output controls'. This is based on the need to stress results rather than procedures. It is manifested in changes in resource allocation methods so that rewards are linked to measured performance, there is a break-up of centralized bureaucracy and of wide personnel management. Most importantly, it points to use of performance-related contracts. At least in my argument, to a large extent the rhetoric of results rather than procedures is belied by its own technique. Possibly arising out of the ethical problems associated with payment by results (to Hippocrates it was, as we have seen, quackery) the shift is incomprehensible to traditional professional practice.

Hood's fourth component is linked to the third. There should be disaggregation of units in the public sector. The broken-up units should deal with each other on an arms-length basis, as in the creation of the *Next Step Agencies* and, specifically, the *NHS trusts*. The need here is to create manageable units and to gain efficiency advantages by the use of contract and franchise arrangements both by units within the public sector and outside. In general, but whether now the NHS will become an exception is yet to be seen, it also separates the determination of requirements from their supply: both sides, amongst others, will be party to the planning. The disaggregated units will be required to cooperate.

Linked to this is Hood's fifth component that there must be greater competition in the public sector. This was introduced on the belief that competition always lowers costs and improves standards. Large elements of the public sector now use fixed-term contracts, public tendering procedures, and compulsory competitive tendering. As Marnoch remarked:[103]

> the market dynamic outlined in Working for Patients certainly equated well with the radical third-term programme for privatisation and de-regulation embarked on by the Conservatives. . . . Underpinning the introduction of the internal market was the belief that choice, efficiency and quality . . . would be encouraged by competition between provider units for contracts from purchasers.

Hood's sixth component is that private sector styles of management should be applied. There is a move away from the old rank-based, public service ethic towards greater flexibility in the hiring and the rewarding of staff. So also, there has to be a greater use of public relations techniques. This component is justified on the basis that private sector management tools have been seen to work. This needs to be expanded on later.

Hood's last component is that there must be stress on greater discipline and parsimony in the use of resources. This is based on a new emphasis to check resource demands within the public sector and to do more with less. It involves cutting direct costs, increasing discipline within the workforce, and limiting the costs of compliance.

It was to be expected the NHS would not be exempt from *new public management*. The idea was driven by equating management in the public with that in the private sector. As the Griffiths Report said:[104]

> The NHS does not have the profit motive, but it is, of course, enormously concerned with the control of expenditure. Surprisingly, however, it still lacks any real continuous evaluation of its performance against criteria. . . . Businessmen have a keen sense of how well they are looking after their customers. Whether the NHS is

meeting the need to the patient, and the community, and can prove it is doing so, is open to question.

That was in 1983. We have seen already the growth of audit and its associated auditable standards. The previous government established a measure known as the Purchaser Efficiency Index. It was much concerned with financial efficiency in a very narrow sense. But certainly, combined with medical audit and the *Citizens Charter*, it was part of Hood's second component. His third component was to be found in the career patterns of the administrators who ran them. They at least were given performance-related and often short-term contracts. Hood's fourth component as regards the NHS was the creation of the NHS trusts, which now provide all secondary care. It is also to be found in the split between the purchasers and suppliers of medical care. The suppliers were these trusts. The purchasers were either general practitioners organized as 'fundholders' or District Health Authorities. The fifth component, that there must be greater competition, was to be found in the need for the suppliers, the NHS trusts, to compete amongst themselves for the business of the purchasers. The sixth component rejected the old rank-based public service ethic. Accordingly, the ethic of the ideal-typical doctor was placed in doubt by the introduction of a new breed of manager from outside both the health service and the public sector. So also, this sixth component requires a greater use of public relations techniques. This is to be seen in such diverse matters as limitations on staff contacts with the press and the use of attitude surveys of patients.

The White Paper, *The New NHS*, expressly says that it does not wish to abolish things that are working. Accordingly, in the future there will be a revised *Patients Charter*. Something of gap between supplier and purchaser will remain. The Purchaser Efficiency Index will be replaced by[105] 'a new framework which will look at six factors: health improvement; equality of access; effective delivery of appropriate care; efficiency, in terms of value for money; patient care experience; and, health outcomes of NHS care'. So also re-emphasising the point,[106] 'there will be a new national survey of patient and user experience'.

On the other hand, the government is promising a 'third way'. Purchasers and suppliers, and more particularly the medical staff, who work for them will be required to plan health care delivery within a locality.[107] The White Paper tells us that the new emphasis will be on cooperation not competition, even between suppliers of health care.The White Paper places emphasis on what it calls[108] 'clinical governance'. In some sense, this restores something of the old ethic. But it is the ethic much modified. Henceforth, clinicians will have to have regard not only to the clinical efficacy of what they do but also to its cost. Both Newdick[109] and Marnoch[110] have suggested that the traditional idea of clinical freedom may be jeopardized.The ethic is also modified because clinical governance is no longer to be ruled by doctors only.The White Paper recognizes the clinical skills of midwives, nurses, and pharmacists.The old hierarchies of medicine are under challenge.

This idea of empowering staff is at one with the late 1990s. Marnoch pointed out:[111]

> the message to be drawn from the writers on management is that the successful organisations of the 1990s will be those who succeed in empowering employees at every grade enabling them to contribute to the general management process at strategic and operational levels. The strategic managers at the peak level will have to realize their new dependency on the expertise of those at the operational end. . . . The age of managing by uniformity and standardization is apparently over.

The mechanism used in the White Paper to bridge the gap between doctor and manager is to make the doctor financially aware. Of itself, this is neutral.This book insists that doctors are not interested in their own incomes (however much they might be in the capacity to spend, which is a completely different thing). The emphasis on making doctors aware of the cost of treatment need not affect their personal conduct. On the other hand, it seems most likely that if one is aware of cost some of the time and that money becomes part of the culture, then it is likely to shift doctors' attitudes to their own positions.

The White Paper makes a further radical shift. Having accepted the idea of cooperation, it then goes on to envisage this cooperation taking place not just between units within the health service but also in the whole range of other activities that have effects on health.The planning at local level will thus include local authorities and those concerned with social services, housing, education, and employment. What this means for the thesis of this book and the nature of strictly professional activity for doctors is that they would have to become aware of the concerns of these other agencies. McKeown would be pleased.

It is possible, but too early to be certain, that the 1997 White Paper may distinguish the future of health administration from forms of management generally in the public sector. If this is so, history will repeat itself and it is just as likely that the health service will remain misunderstood even by those who work in it and who study it. When the health service came fully into the public sector in 1948 (as Titmuss said, 'The most unsordid act of British social policy in the twentieth century'),[112] it was under the direct and accountable control of the secretary of state. Other areas of the public sector were run by non-accountable boards or by local democracy. Now the old nationalized industries are almost entirely under the control of private companies regulated by officials acting under some semi-independent mandates from their secretaries of state. Even as late as 1979, the Royal Commission misunderstood the structure of the old health service. It, and it alone, of the large public corporations established in the 1940s, was headed by a minister who was responsible to Parliament for the whole of its operation. It, and it alone, was old-style British democratic socialism in action.[113] The failure to understand this led the Royal Commission to suggest other forms of accountability.[114] And, from a different direction, it probably led to the reforms of the 1980s and 1990s. As we have seen, the White Paper is proposing a different structure from that envisaged in *new public management*. As it is implemented, the bulk of medical practice (that is, in the NHS) will be organized in a way sharply contrasting both with the rest of the public service and the other old-style learned professions. In the 1940s, it was different because the minister in charge had a different vision. Under this White Paper, it is different because the new Labour government is without an overarching ideology. Rather, it seems to have an attitude that free markets can provide but that, on occasions, the state must apply criteria other than the exclusively financial. In the absence of any other overriding theory, medicine has been able to re-infuse its enduring value into its own organization. Medicine, unlike for example law, is no longer to be organized about making a return on capital.

The new organizational form will be unique. Properly understood, this could be justified. As I suggest, the probabilities, however, are that neither medicine nor its organization will be understood. A range of difficulties is outstanding. First, as we have seen, medicine is the last of the learned professions to hold to the professional ideal this book describes, including the specific responsibilities of being a professional. Secondly, however, that ideal is predicated on a concept of rank that has gone. The ideal will have to be modified in ways yet to be found.Thirdly, there is the notion that good medicine is only science and has no art. Leaving aside its practice, this leads to the emphasis on management through audit. Fourthly, practice itself is to be infused with ideas of resource management.The consequence is that the individual patient can no longer be given the same priority as hitherto.This changes clinical freedom but does not necessary abolish it. If this resource management becomes infused with the same guild-like, private ethic as medicine in its pure form already is, no harm will come of it. If, on the other hand, this new form practice becomes adopts the techniques and goals of ordinary management, genuine clinical freedom will undoubtedly suffer.

Fifthly, it is increasingly common to talk of doctors as having *careers*.There is danger in this.True, they have careers so long as they are in training grades.True also, these training grades last longer than in most other occupations.When applied to those doctors, who have won their consultancies in their hospitals and their fellowships of their royal colleges, the guild-like structures of medicine require the equality implicit in collegiality. How far there can be co-existence between this equality and professional self-management is an open question. It certainly did exist, and might have been accentuated, when lay managers were making resource allocations:there was something the guild could unite about. Under the new arrangements, as with the notion of clinical freedom, the question is whether collegiate practice or hierarchical bureaucratic management will have priority.[115]

Conclusion

This book is about more than medical practice and its organization.Throughout this book,I have been worried about ways of knowing.I have been concerned with the distinction between liberty and freedom and with the possibility of social cohesion. Medicine has been studied to find what it teaches about these things.As I discussed Vico's distinction between *knowledge by causes* and *knowledge by conviction*, I suggested that, in public life at least, the former was more fashionable but led to fragmentation.We are following fashion and abandoning *knowledge by conviction*. In this, we can only return to a primeval solitude.The consequence, as I argue in chapter 7, is that:[116] 'Increasingly, the reality of whole ranges of human experience—all those feelings which are other related (love, sorrow, compassion, pity)—are rejected or reconstructed'.This is not all. In its hegemony, individualism, whiggery (call it what you will), 'has

appropriated . . . the judgement of what is good for society', and it
has to reject honesty and truth telling because they are other regarding virtues. 'Lies', I said, 'are blameworthy only if they are found out,
but not always even then, for individualism is more concerned with
purposes and results than with means. Thus, by a perversion, trust
itself has become anti-social'.[117] This argument is at one with the world
of audited measurement of which power spoke. None of the writers
of the Enlightenment would have welcomed this. Nevertheless, it is
part of its final victory which I spoke of earlier. It is a complex route
and one where, it is fair to assume, the navigators have meant well.
But, for all that, it contains the making of social disaster. And, as Penty
says:[118]

> A belief in the possibility of social catastrophe is . . . essential to
> the integrity of sociology [he does not use the term as it is now
> be used in the academy]. . . . Deny the possibility of
> catastrophe . . . and morality and intellectual integrity are com-
> pletely undermined, while history itself becomes meaningless, for
> with catastrophe history abounds. Right and wrong cease to have
> meaning because apart from revelation, the only final test of right
> is that it tends to promote social cohesion, and wrong that it leads
> to social disruption. If right and wrong cease to have meaning,
> everything becomes a matter of opinion. Social restraints disap-
> pear. Thus, paradoxically it will happen that the denial of the pos-
> sibility of catastrophe operates to encourage the growth of those
> very evils which make catastrophe inevitable.

Looking ever at the world as they want it to be, our times disregard this possibility of social catastrophe. Discussing complaints procedures and informed by the commonsense of our day, one writer
says:[119] 'when things have gone wrong then is a need for more, not
less, candour between the parties. It would foster the relationship of
trust about which judges speak so often. It might also tend to defuse
situations which do not warrant litigation by encouraging atmosphere
of reconciliation and settlement.' This trust is born out of the individualism and *knowledge by causes* endemic in the modern world.
The trust that requires candor is the conditional trust of the market-
place. It is this, and only this sort of trust, that *regulation* can understand. In medicine, it is bolstered by informed consent. This is all very
well but a different form of trust can exist between people whether
they are in a relationship of equality as friends or lovers or spouses,
or they are in a relationship of inequality as between parent and

child, teacher and pupil, or doctor and patient. It is a trust not built by giving or needing accounts. Where it exists, accountability and justification do not arise. The trust that should, and as far as I can see does, apply between the ideal typical doctor and the patient rests on their asymmetrical relationship. This sort of trust is born out of social engagement and *knowledge by conviction*. The idea of rank that this book argues for underpins the professional ideal that was part of the cause of this trust. If it is not replaced by something equally effective then the trust that came with it will be transformed. If this is so, medicine will move from unconditional to conditional trust and in doing so restructure its whole self. Earlier, I suggested that there is a distinction between peace on terms and an unconditional sort of peace, closer to tranquillity. This is the same distinction as between these conditional and unconditional ways of trusting.

The concerns of this book are rooted in something beyond these considerations. They are means, not ends. Fundamentally, my concern has been to achieve a better world (I have not forgotten my youthful dream) and in that better world, humanity is contented. There cannot be such contentment, unless there is also the possibility of tranquillity.

Notes

1. Hobson, 1898:91-2.
2. Said, 1994:xv, 9, and 17.
3. Ruskin, 1988:67, *The Lamp of Truth*, §xxviii.
4. Penty, 1920:73ff.
5. Titmuss, 1997:60.
6. Taylor, 1967. There is a vast theoretical and empirical literature flowing out of this, see e.g. Pollitt, 1993.
7. Ruskin, 1988:170, *The Lamp of Life,* §XXI. His emphasis.
8. Arnold, 1993: 107.
9. Ruskin, 1988:200-1, *The Lamp of Obedience* §II. 10 The word is taken from Arnold, 1993:2-3. The idea is discussed in Jacob, 1996.
11. Kiernan, 1941:51.
12. Vico lived from 1668 to 1744. See Adams, 1935 and Berlin, 1998. His main work was *la Scienza Nuova*, 1725. It is translated at Vico, 1968. For assessments see Vaughan, 1972 and Berlin, 1998:326-58, 'The Divorce between the Sciences and Humanities'. As to Vico's importance, see Tagliacozzo, 1981. There is an English language journal, *New Vico Studies*, produced by the Institute for Vico Studies, New York. It began in 1983.

Vico himself was rejected for a chair of civil law. His response was *la Scienza Nuova* and he was scarcely modest about it. He said:

Providence be for ever praised, since what appeared severe justice has turned out the supreme benefaction. For this work has invested me with a new manhood. No longer do I lament without reservation my adverse fortune and the corrupt mind of the age. That fortune and that mind have strengthened and aided me to accomplish this work. Thus (and if it be not true I wish it to be true) my work has filled me with a certain spirit of heroism, so that I am no longer shaken by any fear of death, nor have I any mind to speak of rivals. In fine, the judgment of God has set my feet as it were upon a rock of adamant, for he causes works of the mind to be judged by the esteem of the wise, who are always and everywhere few. (Adams, 1935:146)

13. Adams, 1935:117.

14. Adams, 1935: 89.

15. But see, for example, Jacob, 1990. As I argue above at pp.22 and 129, professional medical ethics, as I define it, has little to contribute to the rights and wrongs of biomedical technologies.

16. Berlin, 1998:352-3, 354, and 356.

17. He cites Edgeworth, 1881:8. Emphasis in original.

18. Titmuss, 1997:290.

19. Atkin, 1932:580.

20. Titmuss, 1997:290-1. Le Grand at ibid., 333-7 has a different and narrower interpretation.

21. Bagehot, 1966:251: 'A people never hears censure of itself', and the individuals who choose particular newspapers are never criticized there for doing so.

22. See: *Bolam*, 1957; *Maynard*, 1984. But now see *Bolitho*, 1993.

23. See: Bennet, 1979; Cassell, 1978; and, Jacob, 1983, reviewing *inter alia* Beauchamp and Childress, 1981.

24. See Underwood and Bailey, 1993. But more authoritatively, see General Medical Council, 1993b:para.7, 'It is . . . unethical for a doctor to withhold treatment from any patient on the basis of a moral judgment that the patient's activities or lifestyle might have contributed to the condition to which treatment was being sought'.

25. Above p.171.

26. But see Chadwick, 1975.

27. Above p.59.

28. Adams, 1935:149.

29. For an account of this mainly British made catastrophe of CJD, see Ratzan, 1998.

30. Parsons, 1964, cited above pp.29-30.

31. Hughes, 1958:84. 32 Lloyd, 1978, cited above pp.41.

33. Burrage, forthcoming.

34. See above p.105.

35. See Baldwin, 1997:54 and reference there cited.

36. Courts and Legal Services Act 1990, s.58.

37. Criminal Law Act 1967, s.13, sch.4.
38. Yarrow, 1997.
39. Hirschman, 1982 , cited above pp.73-4.
40. The Government's White Paper, *The NHS Modern • Dependable*, spoke of clinical quality standards. A Health Minister has now said they will be enforceable though the courts, April 13, 1998.
41. See: Harlow and Rawlings, 1992; and, Harlow and Rawlings, 1997.
42. Woolf, 1995 and Woolf, 1996.
43. Woolf, 1996:sect.II.
44. Jacob, 1998.
45. Murphy, 1997:58.
46. As regards law, see Burrage forthcoming.
47. Woolf, 1996:272.
48. Courts and Legal Services Act 1990, ss.34-53.
49. Eg, Medicinal Products: Prescription by Nurses Etc. Act 1992.
50. Jacob, 1998.
51. *Roberts Petroleum Ltd* v. *Bernard Kenny*, [1983] 2 A.C. 192, 201.
52. Above p.123ff.
53. Above p.182.
54. Department of Health and Social Security, 1983:10; Brazier, 1992:207.
55. It has now added professional incompetence to what it may condemn as serious professional misconduct, General Medical Council, 1993a:para.38.
56. For example, above p.42.
57. General Medical Council, 1993a:paras.97-106.
58. Courts and Legal Services Act 1990, ss.19-20.
59. Woolf, 1996:84.
60. Above p.117ff.
61. Mason, 1982:34-5.
62. Mason, 1982:69.
63. Mason, 1982:144-5.
64. Mason, 1982:197.
65. Mason, 1982:200-1.
66. Moran and Wood, 1993:17.
67. Moran and Wood, 1993:17
68. Moran and Wood, 1993:3.
69. Moran and Wood, 1993:112.
70. Power, 1994; Power, 1997a; Power, 1997b; and see McSweeney, 1988.
71. Power, 1997a:8.
72. See Merton, 1957:421-36.
73. Power, 1997a:1.
74. Power, 1997a:4.
75. Power, 1997a:4-5.
76. Newdick, 1995:174. He cites CASPE Research, 1994:94 and App. C.
77. Power, 1997a:8.

78. Power, 1997a:7. His emphasis.
79. He cites Hecksher, 1995.
80. Power, 1997a:8.
81. Department of Health and Social Security, 1989; J. Hughes and C. Humphrey (1990) *Medical Audit in General Practice:A Practical Guide to the Literature;* R. Baker and P. Presley, 1990; Irvine, 1990.The Royal College of General Practitioners has established an 'Audit Programme'.The Royal College of General Practitioners, 1995.The Royal College of Physicians is similarly attached to 'medical audit'. See: Craig *et al.*, 1990; Jacob, 1991; and Kogan and Redfern, 1995.
82. Department of Health, 1993:1.
83. Department of Health and Social Security, 1989, 3.
84. Power, 1997a:9.
85. Marnoch 1996:56. He cites Mark, 1991:6-12.
86. Bowling, 1997:3.
87. Bowling, 1997:4.
88. Bowling, 1997:5.
89. See Bowling, 1997:6.
90. Bowling, 1997:7; Bowling, 1997:111.
91. Newdick, 1995:22. He cites:Williams, 1985; Maynard, 1987; Gudex, 1986; and, generally, Mooney, 1992.
92. Newdick, 1995:25.
93. He cites Carr-Hill, 1989.
94. Newdick, 1995:27.
95. He cites Williams, 1992.
96. Newdick, 1995:28, Mooney, 1992:84.
97. Newdick, 1995:29.
98. Newdick, 1995:29.
99. Newdick, 1995:30.
100. See also Marnoch 1996:116.
101. Jorgenson, 1993.
102. C. Hood, 1991:3-19, and especially his table at 4-5. See also: Osborne and Gaebler, 1992; Drewry, 1993; Lewis, 1993; and, Jacob, 1996:213-21.
103. Marnoch 1996:27-8. He cites Le Grand and Bartlett, 1993.
104. Department of Health and Social Security, 1983:10.
105. Department of Health, 1997:para.8.9.
106. Department of Health, 1997:para.8.10
107. Newdick anticipated this, Newdick, 1995:222. He cites:Audit Commission, 1993; and, Graffy and Williams, 1994.
108. Department of Health, 1997:para.6.12 et seq.
109. Newdick, 1995:276.
110. Marnoch 1996:62.
111. Marnoch 1996:9.
112. Titmuss, 1997:292.
113. Bevan, 1961.

114. Royal Commission, 1979:para.19.33.
115. Marnoch 1996:57-8; Newdick, 1995:168. Packwood, Keen and Buxton, 1991.
116. Above, p.188.
117. I cited Shetreet, 1976.
118. Penty, 1930, quoted by Reckitt, 1934:266.
119. Newdick, 1995:247.

References

Access to Health Records Act 1990.

H.P.Adams (1935) *The Life and Writings of Giambattista Vico*. London:Allen & Unwin.

Matthew Arnold (1993) *Culture and Anarchy and Other Writings*, (including *The Function of Criticism at the Present Time*, 1864, and *An Essay in Political and Social Criticism*, 1867-9) edited by Stefan Collini, Cambridge and New York: Cambridge University Press.

Atkin (1932) *Donoghue* v. *Stevenson* [1932] A.C. 562.

Audit Commission (1993) *Practises Make Perfect: the Role of the Family Health Services Authority*, London:Audit Commission.

Walter Bagehot (1966) *The English Constitution*, first published in 1867, with an introduction by R.H.S. Crossman, Ithaca, N.Y.: Cornell University Press.

J. Baker and P. Presley (1990) *Medical Audit in General Practice: A Practical Guide to the Literature*.

R. Baker and P. Presley (1990) *The Practice Audit Plan: A Handbook of Medical Audit for Primary Care Teams*.

Robert Baldwin (1997) *Regulating Legal Services*, Research Programme, London: Lord Chancellor's Department.

Burrage (forthcoming) *Revolution and the Making of the Legal Profession in France, the United States, Russia and England*.

Tom L. Beauchamp and James F. Childress (1981) *Principles of Biomedical Ethics*, New York: O.U.P.

Glin Bennet (1979) *Patients and Their Doctors, The Journey through Medical Care*, London: Baillière Tindall.

Sir Isaiah Berlin (1998) *The Proper Study of Mankind: an Anthology of Essays*, eds Henry Hardy and Roger Hausheer, London: Pimlico.

Bolitho v. *City and Hackney HA* (1993) 13 BMLR.

Bolam v. *Friern Hospital Management Committee* [1957] 1 W.L.R. 582.

Ann Bowling (1997) *Measuring Health, a Review of Quality of Life Measurements Scales*, 2nd ed, Buckingham: Open University Press.

M. Brazier (1992) *Medicine, Patients and the Law*, Harmondsworth: Penguin Books.

British Medical Association (1993) *Medical Ethics Today*.

R. Carr-Hill (1989) 'Assumptions of the QALY Procedure', 29 *Social Science and Medicine* 469.

CASPE Research (1994) *Evaluating Audit: the Development of Audit*, London: CASPE Research.

Eric J. Cassell (1978) *The Healer's Art, A New Approach to the Doctor-Patient Relationship*, 1976, Harmondsworth: Penguin Books.

Owen Chadwick, *The Secularization of the European Mind in the Nineteenth Century*, Cambridge: Cambridge University Press.

Courts and Legal Services Act 1990.

M. Craig *et al.* (1990) 'Medical Audit and Resource Management: Lessons from Hip Fracture', 6 *Financial Accountability and Management* 285.

Criminal Law Act 1967.

Data Protection Act 1984.

Department of Health and Social Security (1983) *National Health Service Management Inquiry* ('the Griffiths' Report).

Department of Health and Social Security (1989) *Working for Patients: Medical Audit* (Working Paper 6).

Department of Health (1993) *Research for Health*.

Department of Health (1997) White Paper, *The NHS: Modern • Dependable*, Cm 3807.

Department of Health (1998) *NHS to Have Legal Duty of Ensuring Quality for First Time*, Press Notice 98/141.

Department of Health (forthcoming 1998) Green Paper, *Our Healthier Nation*.

G. Drewry (1993) 'Mr. Major's Charter: empowering the consumer', *Public Law*, 248-256.

F.Y. Edgeworth (1881) *Mathematical Physics*, London: Kegan Paul, cited in Titmuss, 1997.

General Medical Council (1992) *Contractual Arrangements in Health Care: Professional Responsibilities in Relation to the Clinical Needs of Patients*.

General Medical Council (1993a) *Professional Conduct and Discipline: Fitness to Practice*, 'The Blue Book', cited in Newdick, 1995. It is frequently updated.

General Medical Council (1993b) *HIV Infection and AIDS: the Ethical Considerations*.

J. Graffy and J. Williams (1994) 'Purchasing for All: An Alternative to Fundholding', 308 *British Medical Journal* 391.

C. Gudex (1986) *QALYs and Their Use by the Health Service*, Centre for Health Economics, University of York.

C. Harlow and R.W. Rawlings (1992) *Pressure Through Law*, London: Routledge.

C. Harlow and R.W. Rawlings (1997) *Law and Administration*, 2nd ed. London: Butterworths.

Charles Hecksher (1995) *White Collar Blues: Management Loyalties in an Age of Corporate Restructuring*, New York: Harper Collins.

A.O. Hirschman (1982) *Shifting Involvements, Private Interest and Public Action*, Oxford: Martin Roberston.

J.A. Hobson (1898) *John Ruskin, Social Reformer*, London: James Nisbet & Co.

C. Hood (1991) 'A Public Management for All Seasons', 69 *Public Administration*, 3-19.

E.C. Hughes (ed.) (1958) *Men and Their Work*. Chicago: The Free Press of Glencoe.

D.H. Irvine (1990) *Managing for Quality in General Practice*.

Joseph M. Jacob (1983) 'Biomedical Law: Lost Horizons Regained', 46 *Modern Law Review*, 21-38.

Joseph M. Jacob, (1990) 'Annotations to the Human Fertilisation and Embryology Act', *Current Law Statutes*, London: Sweet and Maxwell.

Joseph M. Jacob (1991) 'Lawyers Go To Hospital', *Public Law*, Summer, 255-281.

Joseph M. Jacob (1996) *The Republican Crown: Lawyers and the Making of the State in Twentieth Century Britain*, Ashford: Dartmouth.

Joseph M. Jacob (1998) 'The Bowman Report', 61 *Modern Law Review*, 390.

T. Jorgenson (1993) 'Modes of governance and administrative change', in Kooiman, 1993.

E.J. Kiernan (1941) *Arthur J Penty: His Contribution to Social Thought*, Washington: The Catholic University of America.

J. Kooiman (1993) *Modern Governance*, London: Sage.

Maurice Kogan and Sally Redfern with Anémone Kober (1995) *Making use of Clinical Audit: A Guide to Practice in the Health Professions*, Buckingham and Philadelphia: Open University Press.

J. Le Grand and W. Bartlett (1993) *Quasi-Markets and Social Policy*, London: Macmillan.

N. Lewis (1993) 'The Citizen's Charter and Next Steps: A New Way of Governing?', *Political Quarterly*, 316.

G.E.R. Lloyd (1978) *Hippocratic Writings* (first published 1950) Harmondsworth: Penguin.

A. Mark (1991) 'Where are the medical managers?' *Journal of Management in Medicine*, 5(4): 6-12.

Gordon Marnoch (1996) *Doctors and Management in The National Health Service*, Buckingham: Open University Press.

Philip Mason (1982) *The English Gentleman: the Rise and Fall of an Ideal*, London: André Deutsch.

A. Maynard (1987) 'Logic in Medicine', 295 *British Medical Journal* 1537.

Maynard West Midlands Regional Health Authority [1984] 1 W.L.R. 635.

McSweeney (1988) 'Accounting for the Audit Commission', 59 *Political Quarterly* 28.

Medicinal Products: Prescription by Nurses Etc. Act 1992.

Robert K. Merton (1957) 'The Self-Fulfilling Prophecy', *Social Theory and Social Structure*, New York: The Free Press.

G. Mooney, *Economics, Medicine and Health Care*, (1992) Harvester Wheatsheaf, 2nd ed.

Michael Moran and Bruce Wood (1993) *States, Regulation and the Medical Profession*, Open University Press.

Tim Murphy (1997) *The Oldest Social Science? Configurations of Law and Modernity*, Oxford: OUP.

Christopher Newdick (1995) *Who Should We Treat? Law, Patients and Resources in the N.H.S.*, Oxford: Clarendon Press.

D. Osborne and T. Gaebler (1992) *Reinventing Government: How the Entrepreneurial Spirit is Transforming the Public Sector*, Reading, Mass.: Addison Wesley.

T. Packwood, J. Keen, and M. Buxton (1991) *Hospitals in Transition—the Resource Management Experiment*, Buckingham: Open University Press.

T. Parsons (1964), *The Social System* (first published 1951) London: Routledge & Kegan Paul.

A.J. Penty (1930) 'Industry in a Revived Christendom', *Green Quarterly* VII (Summer) 140.

Christopher Pollitt (1993) *Managerialism and the Public Service: Cuts or Cultural Change in the 1990s?* 2nd ed., Oxford: Blackwell.

Michael Power (1994) *Audit Explosion*, Demos Paper No. 7, London: Demos.

Michael Power (1997a) *The Perils of the Audit Society*, London: Public Policy Group.

Michael Power (1997b) *The Audit Society: Rituals of Verification*, Oxford: Clarendon Press.

Scott C. Ratzan (1998) *The Mad Cow Crisis, Health and the Public Good*, Basingstoke: UCL Press, Taylor and Francis Group.

M.B. Reckitt (1934) *A Christian Sociology for To-day*, New York: Longmans, Green & Co.

Roberts Petroleum Ltd v. Bernard Kenny [1983] 2 A.C. 192.

The Royal College of General Practitioners (1995) *Guidelines Working Party*.

Royal Commission on the National Health Service, 1979 Cmnd. 7615.

J. Ruskin (1988) *The Seven Lamps of Architecture*, first published 1848 with 3rd edition, 1880. Introduction by A. Saint, this edition, London: Century Hutchinson Ltd.

Edward W. Said (1994) *Representations of the Intellectual*, London: Vintage.

Giorgio Tagliacozzo, ed. (1981) *Vico, Past and Present*, Atlantic Highlands, N.J.: Humanities Press.

Frederick W. Taylor (1967) *The Principles of Scientific Management*, New York: W.W. Norton. First published 1911.

Richard M. Titmuss (1997) *The Gift Relationship: From Human Blood to Social Policy*, ed. Ann Oakley and John Ashton, expanded and updated edition, London: LSE Books; United States edition, New York: The New Press. First published, 1970, London: Allen and Unwin.

M. Underwood and J. Bailey (1993) 'Coronary Bypass Surgery Should Not Be Offered to Smokers', 306 *British Medical Journal* 1047.

F. Vaughan, (1972) *The Political Philosophy of Giambattista Vico: An Introduction to La Scienza Nuova*, The Hague.

G.Vico [1744] *The New Science of Giambattista Vico*, trans. from the 1744 ed. by Thomas Goddard Bergin and Max Harold Fisch, (1968) Ithaca, N.Y.: Cornell University Press, revised ed. First published, 1948.

A.Williams (1985) 'The Economics of Coronary Artery Bypass Grafting', 291 *British Medical Journal* 326.A.Williams (1992) 'Cost-Effectiveness Analysis: Is It Ethical?' 18 *Journal of Medical Ethics* 18.

Woolf (1996) *Access to Justice—Final Report.*

Woolf (1995) *Access to Justice—Interim Report.* For this, *The Final Report, Draft Rules* and *Consultation Papers*, see the World Wide Web at http://www.open.gov.uk/lcd/justice/cjdnet.htm.

Stella Yarrow (1997) *The Price of Success: Lawyers, Clients and Conditional Fees*, London: Policy Studies Institute.

Notes

Preface

1 Foucault, 1981b.
2 Barlow, 1958:132–3.

1 An Introduction

1 Hughes, 'Licence and Mandate' in Hughes, 1958:85.
2 In this it is similar to Freidson, 1970b.
3 Freidson, 1970b:4–5.
4 Freidson, 1970b:160.
5 Davies and Jacob, 1987: Introduction. The edition of 1987 was written alongside this work and in some measure each rests on the other. That is a description of legal forms. This explains their underlying basis.
6 Russell, 1925. It was an attempt at a layman's guide to the Theory of Relativity.
7 Russell, 1925: 2f. Russell's general position prevented him from seeing any philosophical implications in the Theory of Relativity. But see Foucault, 1981a, where he does to discourse what Einstein did to matter and energy: one by one he steps outside the constraints of everyday language. At one and the same time he leaves it more bound and less firm. Rajchman, 1985, variously describes Foucault as a 'skeptic' involved in 'self-disengagement'.
8 Weber, cited in Runciman, 1978:75.
9 A 'norm' is a rule or authoritative standard. It is an Anglicized form of the Latin *norma* – a carpenter's square. It seems possible that there is a link between this imperative meaning and Christianity through the fact that the husband of the mother of Christ was a carpenter. The word therefore may have spiritual or mystical overtones. In this work 'norm' carries this imperative meaning.
10 Leake, 1927:1ff, Introduction.

11 Hyde, 1983.
12 Parsons, 1951; Parsons, 1964; and Parsons, 1975.
13 Foucault, 1963.
14 Pellegrino and Thomasma, 1981.
15 Davey, 1957:xlii.
16 Compare the use of the term 'polycentric' by: Polanyi, 1951; Weiler, 1968; Jowell, 1973:213. With these authors it concerns the criteria to be used in problem resolution. It is reasonable to use the same term to describe the distribution of power.
17 In Popper, 1961:27ff.
18 Freidson, 1986:xi.
19 Freidson, 1986:3f.
20 Popper, 1979:106ff.
21 Freidson, 1986:215f.
22 Freidson, 1986:219.
23 Freidson, 1986:227. He made the same point earlier: Freidson, 1970a: 86, where he argues in effect that clinical experience prevails over basic science.
24 See Epstein, 1982:1717.
25 Popper, 1961:77.
26 I hope I will not be taken to have adopted the approach so fully condemned by Butterfield, 1931.
27 Mandrou, 1978:17
28 The issue is approached from a slightly different position by Hirschman, 1982, discussed in a later chapter. And see Oppenheimer, 1954.
29 Montesquieu, *The Spirit of the Laws* quoted in Althusser, 1972. See also: Butterfield, 1931; Hawthorn, 1987: Preface.
30 See Popper, 1961, on the one hand and Carr, 1964, on the other. See also Hirschman, 1982:72, where it is argued that history is the unfolding of both precipitating events and expressions of volition.
31 Churchill, 1944. And see Wolf, 1970:783–92.
32 Hawthorn, 1987:192–6.
33 See Wilson and Levy, 1938; Gittings, 1984.
34 For a study of one example, see Prior, 1985. A special issue of *Annals of the AAPSS*, 447, in January 1980 was devoted to this.
35 This in part explains the contemporary North American interest in death. In addition to the previous note, see e.g., Law Reform Commission of Canada, 1979.
36 Freidson, 1986:21ff, esp. at 35.
37 Bevan, 1961:34.
38 Clark, 1964:602f, says that at the end of the eighteenth century 'the total number of medical practitioners of all branches ... [was] well over 4,000 in England and Wales ... this is in the region of 1 to every 2,000 [members of the population], whereas in the twentieth century the proportion has run at about 1,400 or 1,500'. Even if the figures are

correct, they give no idea of what was expected of any of the branches of medicine. As to this last see: Porter, 1987a; and Porter, 1987b.

39 See, e.g. Freidson, 1970b:168 and 266ff. He cites Shapiro, 1960:109–35. But see also Porter 1987a and Porter 1987b cited in the previous note.

40 Cartwright, 1977:2.

41 Cartwright, 1977:3. And see Aristotle, 1928: Book 3, 983b(7)–984b(23).

42 See Azouri, 1979:112.

43 Lloyd, 1978: Introduction.

44 Finucane, 1975.

45 Finucane, 1975:6. He cites: Robertson, 1875–85:444.

46 Finucane, 1975:7.

47 Finucane, 1975:8.

48 Cellini, 1558–66:55, and see also 250.

49 *Hupe* v *Phelps*, 1819:481.

50 Finucane, 1975:10.

51 Rousseau, 1957:421–2, quoted in Althusser, 1972:29–30.

52 Foucault, 1963: Preface, xix.

53 See Jonas, 1973. His point is general. It starts in Sophocles' *Antigone* with the need for man's morality and nature's power. But now, he says, nature is vulnerable to technological intervention.

54 See, e.g. Phillips and Dawson, 1985.

55 See Murphy and Rawlings, 1981 and 1982.

56 James, 1963:150 and 157, says that writers who seek to describe social events and ideas refuse to take any account of popular thinking about sport. As he says, it was otherwise for Plato and Aristotle. Weber, 1930, argues that the parvenu bourgeoisie of the early seventeenth century rejected all modes of impulsive enjoyment of life. It seems that many modern scholars have not rid themselves of this asceticism. But see now Elias and Dunning, 1986.

57 Goldstein, 1982:xvii. And see: Reich, 1978; and Reich, 1983. These works provide more than a useful starting point for any enquiry.

58 Pellegrino and Thomasma, 1981:170.

59 Giesen, 1981:150.

60 Meynell, 1981, is of some comparative interest. So also popularizers transmit ideas.

61 See Lorber, 1985.

2 Medical Practice

1 Parsons, 1964:Ch.10.

2 Parsons has been subjected to many other criticisms. See, e.g.: Freid-

son, 1970b:228–43 and 170–1; Freidson, 1970a; Berlant, 1975; and McCormack, 1981:30ff. In the main, they are refutations of his claim that his ideal model is a realistic description.

3 Parsons, 1964:430.

4 Parsons, 1964:444 and 448. Compare Smith, 1779:Bk.1, Ch.x (pp. 209ff) discussing participation in lotteries. And see below for a discussion of the role of disappointment.

5 Parsons, 1964:467 and see: Tuckett, 1976:197ff; Freidson, 1970b:244ff; Dowling, 1963; Scheff, 1963.

6 Compare Foucault, 1963:Ch.8, 'Open up a few corpses', and Ch.9, 'The visible invisible', on what he calls the trinity of life/disease/death; and, see Mainland, 1967:127 for a sociologist's call for 'studies of the total process of seeking health care'.

7 Berlant, 1975, draws a distinction between social and individual utilitarianism, which, he says, Parsons does not make. This distinction is similar to that which I elaborate on below between medicine and health. Contrary to Berlant, I think Parsons is correct in not confusing the two, although of course it might have helped if he had said so. Berlant is himself right to point to problems relating to palliative treatment.

8 Parsons 1964:431.

9 Parsons 1964:436.

10 Parsons 1964:462. His footnote adds that this 'has sometimes been called the "art of medicine"'. See Pellegrino and Thomasma, 1981:156, discussed below, p.xx.

11 Parsons 1964:432.

12 Parsons 1964:456.

13 Parsons 1964:435.

14 Parsons 1964:464f.

15 Parsons 1964:464ff.

16 Parsons 1964:347f.

17 Parsons 1964:471.

18 Freidson, 1970b:158.

19 Laymen must know they are ill, Freidson, 1970b:278.

20 Apple, 1960, cited in Freidson, 1970b:283.

21 Freidson, 1970b:285.

22 Zola, 1966. See also Twaddle, 1969, cited in Freidson, 1970b:281.

23 Freidson, 1970b:279–80. And see Zborowski, 1958:256–68.

24 Black, 1980:43.

25 In specifically legal terms the issue was faced by the Court of Appeal in *Minister of Health* v. *General Committee of The Royal Midland Counties Home of Incurables at Leamington Spa*, 1954, where it had to decide whether the home was a hospital within the meaning of the take over under the National Health Service. And see: *Tendring Union* v. *Woolwich Union*, 1923.

26 Foucault, 1963:58ff.

27 See Chappell and Colvill, 1981; Fox, 1957; and Olmstead and Sheffrin, 1981.

28 Quoted in Richardson, 1901:656.

29 Corvisart, 1825:174, quoted in Foucault, 1963:120.

30 Foucault, 1963:121.

31 But see, e.g., Stanway, 1979, discussed below, and Easthope, 1986.

32 For early examples, see Bright, 1827 and Bright, 1831. *The Lancet* (founded in 1823) also provided reports of hospital cases but, it would seem, a part of its objective was to expose, as well as describe, the internal mysteries of the London hospitals. See Sprigge, 1897:73ff.

33 See below for a resumé of the passage of the Act.

34 Foucault, 1963:83.

35 Foucault, 1963:84f and the references there cited.

36 Much of this section, particularly the discussion of the second and third of these categories, rests on Pellegrino and Thomasma, 1981. For reasons to be noted, I depart from their principal conclusion.

37 It therefore rejects almost the whole argument in Faulder, 1985. The critique advanced there, although ostensibly feminist, owes little to the relation of medicine and the female but rests instead on ideas of individualism and consumerism.

38 Sherwood Taylor, 1943:4.

39 Popper, 1961:131ff.

40 Barlow, 1958:84.

41 Sherwood Taylor, 1943:310.

42 Bernard, 1865.

43 Huxley, 'Agnosticism'. Quoted in Clark, 1968:107.

44 Letter to Dyster, quoted in Clark, 1968:110.

45 Russell, 1985:480ff.

46 As regards a somewhat later period see: Friedman and Donley, 1985. They argue that science has an influence over other aspects of culture.

47 See further: Bronowski, 1964; Holton, 1960.

48 Cassell, 1976, produced an analysis of tape-recordings of the way patients speak of illness. The recordings were of those who existed in socio-culture of the west. In other cultures, it would be reasonable to expect incommensurable results. Thus, for example, those who live under the regime of ayureda medicine in India might well not distinguish self and disease. For a more sophisticated view of disease as an 'it', see Pellegrino and Thomasma, 1981:76, discussed below.

49 Matthews, 1983, argues that, although there is much legal authority for the view that bodies are not capable of being owned, it tends to be circular and without foundation. He argues also that there can be an ownership of parts, whether renewable or not, of living people. The argument thus reflects the idea that 'I' can be separated from each part of 'me' and the sum of the parts. In short, that my body is an 'it'. This view, I suggest, is contemporary in its conception and reflects the growth of scientism.

50 Black, 1980:41.
51 See Gilson, 1938. Cited in Pellegrino and Thomasma, 1981.
52 How much of the *Corpus* is his own work and how much that of others is uncertain but irrelevant for the current purpose; it is clear that different sections were inspired by different philosophies. The emphasis on justice and fairness in *The Physician* is Aristotelian. The stress on gentleness and kindness in *The Precepts* is Epicurean. In *Decorum*, there is a stoic highlighting of duty and *Law* is Democritian. See: Edelstein, 1967a cited in Pellegrino and Thomasma, 1981:195.
53 Guthrie, 1945:36, says that independent of a knowledge of Hippocrates, in China, Chang Chung-King (AD 195) developed the twin idea of study of disease by bedside observation and the 'noble aims and high ideals' of the physician.
54 McCullough, in Reich, 1978:962, suggests that medical ethics in the Enlightenment broke with 'the earlier Hippocratic tradition'. This may be so as regards medicine, but I argue otherwise as regards its ethics.
   Nutton, 1981:211 suggests that 'its spirit influences much of the ethics of health care ... and it is frequently invoked as normative by the layman'. It is reprinted in numerous works on medical ethics, including the British Medical Association, 1981. Teff, 1985, in criticizing the influence accepts the existence of the tradition.
55 See: Nittis, 1942; Edelstein, 1967b.
56 Lloyd, 1978: *Aphorisms*, Sect. 1 No.1.
57 Lloyd, 1978: *Epidemics*, Bk.1 Ch.11.
58 Hughes, 1958:84.
59 Hughes, 1951b:95.
60 Thus, e.g., *Royal College of Nursing* v. *Department of Health and Social Security*, 1981, or, e.g., in the bureaucracy for the delivery of health care, discussed below, which underlies coercive public health.
61 See: Edelstein, 1943; Edelstein, 1967a; and Jones, 1924.
62 In the modern age, the prohibitions on abortion and mercy-killing are so heavily qualified with subtle refinements that hardly more than a shell of their earlier clarity is left.
63 See Dubos, 1960:109. Aesculapius was deified.
64 The statement is sometimes taken in a wider sense as a prohibition on surgery in general, see Webb-Peploe, 1979:21. But in Lloyd, 1978: *Aphorisms*, Sect.VII, No.87, there is approval of the use of the knife. In Lloyd, 1978: *The Corpus* there is a whole treatise devoted to Fractures. To be sure, this does not recommend any cutting but the treatment of fractures was a part of the surgeon's craft throughout the Middle Ages and later. It seems unlikely that Hippocratic physicians would have found it necessary wholly to exclude themselves from such work. Plato, *The Republic*, talks of Aesculapius using 'the knife'.
65 Pellegrino and Thomasma, 1981:52. See also Freidson, 1970b:122.
66 Edelstein, 1976a.
67 See Cornford, 1912.

68 Russell, 1985:54.
69 M. Weber, *Economy and Society*, cited in Runciman, 1978:7f.
70 Gregory, 1958.
71 Burnet, 1930:108.

3 Theories of medicine

1 Pellegrino and Thomasma, 1981:10.
2 Pellegrino and Thomasma, 1981:227.
3 Pellegrino and Thomasma, 1981:10.
4 Pellegrino and Thomasma, 1981:23-4.
5 Pellegrino and Thomasma, 1981:23.
6 Pellegrino and Thomasma, 1981:50.
7 See: James, 1909; James, 1955; and Husserl, 1954:130, on what he calls *Lebenswelt* (lifeworld). See also: Zaner, 1970; and Gurwitsch, 1973:esp. 36f.
8 Pellegrino and Thomasma, 1981:53.
9 Pellegrino and Thomasma, 1981:63. They cite Lain-Entralgo, 1950:8.
10 Pellegrino and Thomasma, 1981:65f.
11 Pellegrino and Thomasma, 1981:66. Compare Parsons, 1964:471.
12 Seneca, 1896:VI 16. Seneca lived circa 3 BC to AD 65.
13 Pellegrino and Thomasma, 1981:73ff. They cite: Marcel, 1608.
14 Pellegrino and Thomasma, 1981:76.
15 Pellegrino and Thomasma, 1981:74. Ruthschuh, 1972.
16 Pellegrino and Thomasma, 1981:84.
17 Erasmus, 1511:Ch.33, satirizes this aspect: 'medicine as it is practised now by so many, is really only one aspect of flattery, just as rhetoric is'.
18 Pellegrino and Thomasma, 1981:177.
19 Pellegrino and Thomasma, 1981:105ff. Canguilheim, 1966:73 and 143.
20 Pellegrino and Thomasma, 1981:107.
21 Pellegrino and Thomasma, 1981:110-11.
22 Pellegrino and Thomasma, 1981:107.
23 Pellegrino and Thomasma, 1981:112f.
24 Pellegrino and Thomasma, 1981:114. Cassirer, 1970:25.
25 Pellegrino and Thomasma, 1981:115.
26 Pellegrino and Thomasma, 1981:173.
27 Thus by implication, the argument rejects, e.g., much of Beauchamp and Childress, 1979, not because that thesis advances the wrong conclusions but because it does not start with 'the body'. Of course in so far as it informs itself by reference to the 'healing act' or 'the body', it becomes acceptable. Because that work starts elsewhere, admirable as it is, it shifts the emphasis from what is to what should be.
28 Pellegrino and Thomasma, 1981:177.

29 Lloyd, 1978: *Epidemics*, Bk.1 Ch.11.
30 Pellegrino and Thomasma, 1981:185.
31 Pellegrino and Thomasma, 1981:186.
32 Pellegrino and Thomasma, 1981:175.
33 Pellegrino and Thomasma, 1981:209.
34 Pellegrino and Thomasma, 1981:207.
35 Marcovitch, 1982:14.
36 Berlant, 1975:38. He concedes that 'time-consuming simple services' are intellectually unrewarding.
37 Pellegrino and Thomasma, 1981:209.
38 Pellegrino and Thomasma, 1981:212f. Their emphasis.
39 Similarly that of the British Medical Association. Childress, 1982:41f, while arguing in similar vein notes the restrictions on paternalism contained in recent American Medical Association codes, see, e.g., American Medical Association, 1980: Principles II and IV.
40 Pellegrino and Thomasma, 1981:203.
41 Pellegrino and Thomasma, 1981:122f.
42 Pellegrino and Thomasma, 1981:123. They cite MacIntyre, 1977.
43 Pellegrino and Thomasma, 1981:126.
44 Pellegrino and Thomasma, 1981:128.
45 Pellegrino and Thomasma, 1981:131.
46 Pellegrino and Thomasma, 1981:132ff. Their emphasis.
47 Pellegrino and Thomasma, 1981:144ff.
48 Pellegrino and Thomasma, 1981:156. Compare Parsons, 1964:462, discussed above, p.xx.
49 Pellegrino and Thomasma, 1981:159ff.
50 Pellegrino and Thomasma, 1981:161ff.
51 McKeown, 1979.
52 McKeown, 1979:192.
53 McKeown, 1979:190. And see also: Callahan, 1973; and Vuori, 1983.
54 See also: Winter, 1982; and more generally, Eyles, 1987.
55 McKeown, 1979:47, and also 25 and 77.
56 He cites Magill, 1955:47.
57 McKeown, 1979:120.
58 McKeown, 1979:78.
59 McKeown, 1979:123. For a recent application of this idea, see: Melville and Johnson, 1983.
60 Mackenzie, 1957:342. See to the contrary, e.g., Zaridze and Peto, 1986. For a more balanced view see Ashton and Stepney, 1983.
61 Mackenzie, 1957:324.
62 Elias, 1939.
63 McKeown, 1979:131f. McDermott, 1977.
64 McKeown, 1979:132.
65 McKeown, 1979:132ff.
66 McKeown, 1979:xii.

67 See further, Calabresi and Bobbitt, 1978, on the difference between expenditure on prevention and rescue.
68 Bloor and Horobin, 1975:271.
69 This expression is used by Tudor Hart, 1981.
70 Szasz, 1979:xivf.
71 Erasmus, 1511:ch.29. And see Castiglione, 1528:109f. He attributes it to Socrates via Plato.
72 Szasz, 1979:xv.
73 Szasz, 1979:xv. Szasz himself provides no evidence for this but for some corroboration, with a different but more sensitive interpretation, see Donzelot, 1977:12ff.
74 Dubos, 1968:85. See also Dubos, 1960.
75 Time and again the radical critique returns to what it sees as the false optimism of technological medicine, perhaps particularly as represented by drug therapy. See Melville and Johnson, 1983.
76 Illich, 1977.
77 Kennedy, 1981.
78 Johnson, 1972.
79 Cain, 1983.
80 Kennedy, 1984.
81 Berlinguer, 1981:57.
82 Berlinguer 1981:60.
83 Foucault, 1963:35.
84 The word *whisky* is derived from the Gaelic *uisge beatha*, water of life. The Middle Ages saw the invention and production of various spirits to be used first as medicines and then later for pleasure. See Daiches, 1969:3.
85 Thevet, 1568: 'it is very wholesome to cleanse and consume the superfluous humours of the brain'. And Burton, 1925: II §4 memb.2.1 'Tobacco ... which goes far beyond all ... panaceas ... a sovereign remedy to all diseases ... But as it is commonly abused ... the ruin and overthrow of body and soul.' See also Cartier, *Brief Recit*, 1545. See generally: Apperson, 1914; Corti, 1931; and Mackenzie, 1957.
86 Harding, 1987.
87 For 'modern' views see: Royal College of Physicians, 1987; and Royal College of Psychiatrists, 1987.
88 It is significant that the British Medical Association was much involved in opposing it at the turn of this century, see British Medical Association, 1911 and British Medical Association, 1912. Among other things, the Association was critical of profit margins and of the use of certain types of ingredient such as opiates.
89 Stanway, 1979:23ff. And see: Salmon, 1985; Easthope, 1986.
90 Foucault, 1976:139ff, suggests that there was a power over life which took two forms: (1) a mechanistic view of the body, and (2) a bio-politics of the population.

91 Ham, 1986, and more generally Ham, 1985. Hill, 1972:80, says that to regard the similar use of lay people in tribunals as 'representative' 'drains almost all meaning' from the term.

92 For example, Sigerist, 1961:3–101.

93 Lakoff and Johnson, 1980.

94 Childress, 1982:5ff. In addition to Lakoff and Johnson, he cites Ortony, 1979; Black, 1962; Ricoeur, 1978; Vaisrub, 1977; and, Sontag, 1979.

95 This has in effect been done by Navarro, 1986.

96 Burt, 1979:48ff.

97 Burt, 1979:91.

98 Hirschman, 1982. He says the work is a partly autobiographical, conceptual novel. Be that as it may, the biography is not only of him, but also of others including myself.

99 See Arendt, 1958.

100 Hirschman, 1982:12. The emphasis is in the original in all the quotations taken from Hirschman.

101 Hirschman, 1982:16ff. He is also, more for his purpose than mine, concerned with whether what he says about the micro level is also applicable to the macro.

102 He cites Festinger, 1957.

103 Hirschman, 1982:16.

104 Hirschman, 1982:20.

105 See: Lane, 1978; and Posner, 1977:1 and Ch.5.

106 Hirschman, 1982:21.

107 He cites Inglehart, 1977.

108 Freidson, 1970b:302ff.

109 Simmel, 1907:246.

110 Scitovsky, 1977.

111 Hirschman, 1982:27.

112 Hirschman, 1982:32f.

113 Lloyd, 1978: *Aphorisms*, section 1, 3.

114 See Seneca, 1896, cited above.

115 See Lockwood, 1966:16ff, esp. 23.

116 Smith, 1779:Bk.III Ch.4.

117 Hirschman, 1982:53.

118 Hirschman, 1982:57.

119 Hirschman, 1982:58.

120 Compare Dubos, 1968.

121 Hirsch, 1978.

122 Hirschman, 1982:66.

123 Hirschman, 1982:67.

124 Frankfurt, 1971; see also Sen, 1977.

125 Hirschman, 1982:69.

126 Margolis, 1982. See also Mueller, ⁷9.

127 Hirschman, 1982:79.

128 Olson, 1965.

129 Hirschman, 1982:80.

130 See Hughes, 1951a:48ff.

131 Hirschman, 1982:85f.

132 See Williams, 1958:30ff.

133 Hirschman, 1982:99.

134 Hirschman, 1982:100. He cites Walzer, 1973.

135 See, e.g., Elshtain, 1982. Perhaps, one may speculate, this was another cause of the difficulty that women have had in gaining established respect for their medical practice; see, e.g., The Preamble to the first Medical Act in 1511.

136 Ouida was the pen name of Marie Louise de la Ramée. Her attack came in Ouida, 1893; Shaw's in Shaw, 1911. And see also: Pitt, 1703; and Discriminator, 1790.

137 Hirschman, 1982:126.

138 Benichou, 1948:155.

139 Foucault, 1977:193. And see Foucault, 1976:73, 79.

140 Hirschman, 1982:128.

141 Hirschman, 1982:128f.

142 Hirschman, 1982:129.

143 Khayyám, 1859: Fitzgerald, 1st Translation Verses 27–28, 1859 (see also 2nd Translation Verses 30–31).

144 See Milsom, 1969. For a detailed account of the change in the epistemology of law, see Siegal, 1981.

145 See generally: Wolf, 1935.

146 St Germain, 1969 and see Coke's *Reports*.

147 Bacon, 1604. And see Bacon, *New Atlantis*, 1627. Vickers, 1987, argues that he was influential on writers up to the foundation of the Royal Academy a century or so later.

148 Saint-Simon had sought to create science as religion and despite their differences had a marked influence over Comte and J.S. Mill (see Hawthorn, 1987:69ff). Between them they articulated a basis for positivism.

149 Quoted, without citation, in Gellner, 1974:37.

150 See Dvorak, 1984.

151 Shelley, 1821:270.

152 Foucault, 1963.

153 And see Liebenhau, 1983.

154 Letter to R. Hooke 5 February 1675 or 1676. It is an immodest paraphrase, but characteristic of him, from Bernard of Chartres quoted in John of Salisbury, 1159:bk.III ch.iv. See also Merton, 1965.

155 For a brief account of the reception of the theory, see Clark, 1964:297f and references there cited.

156 The change may be attributed to Copernicus (1473–1543), Galileo, Kepler (c.1620), Newton, Herschel (1738–1822), Laplace (1749–1822) and others.

157 Lyle, 1833.

158 Virchow, 1858.

159 Foucault, 1963:135f attributes something like this new idea to studies of pathological anatomy at a rather earlier date, namely between 1801 and 1818 but at Foucault, 1976:149ff he returns to the tissue orientated theories as applying at that time, and see generally Foucault, 1976:Ch.10, 'Crisis in fevers'.

160 See e.g.: Young, 1985; Himmelfarb, 1959; and Cheesman, 1953.

161 Bernard, 1865.

162 Darwin, 1958:123f.

163 Darwin, 1958:152.

164 Darwin was himself influenced by Malthus. Hawthorn, 1987:91 argues, contrary to much popular agreement, that Spencer owed nothing to Darwin. But see Hawthorn, 1987:198ff where he discusses the effects of the fact that they were received together in the United States.

165 Hawthorn, 1987:97 and 101.

166 See Foucault, 1963:115.

167 Spring Rice, 1832.

168 Southwood Smith, 1828.

169 The other illegal source was 'grave robbery'. See Select Committee, 1828, which cites *R* v. *Lynn* (1788). It was said to be *contra bonos mores*. And also see: Adams, 1972; Barzun, 1975; and Ross and Ross, 1979. On 'grave robbery' see Matthews, 1983.

170 Royal College of Surgeons, 1831.

171 Robinson, 1832.

172 As to the rivalry between the Webb Street School and the more establishment United Hospitals (of St Thomas's and Guy's) see Sprigge, 1897:13ff.

173 Lewis, 1898:46f.

4 The profession of medicine: some more history

1 Pliny, 1887–98:Bk.29.

2 Daremberg, 1865:65.

3 Justinian:9,2,7,pr.

4 For a review of his efficacy in modern terms see Brain, 1986.

5 See Browne, 1921:28.

6 See Corner, 1933.

7 See Lain-Entralgo, 1969:55ff. And also Lain-Entralgo, 1955.

8 Fletcher, 1912.

9 Erasmus, 1511:chs.40–1.

10 For a fourteenth-century view of the physician and 'Old Ypocras' (Hippocrates), see Chaucer, 1986: 'The Physician's Tale'.

11 Copeman, 1960:30f.

12 Freidson, 1970b:72.

13 Freidson, 1970b:18ff.

14 Durkheim, 1938:II 115, cited in Lukes, 1973:385.

15 For a fascinating account, see MacLean, 1987: esp. 28–46.

16 Copeman, 1960. And Hibbert, 1979:29 but see 108.

17 See, e.g., Chase, 1985.

18 Pagel, 1968.

19 Webster, 1979.

20 For accounts of his influence, his work and of the things which influenced him, see: Temkin, 1952.

21 Medical Act 1511–12. Much of this account relies on Clark, 1964, but the interpretation is mine.

22 Cartwright, 1977:45.

23 Copeman, 1960:15.

24 Company of Physicians Act 1523. No mention was made of the 1511 Act. The Act of 1523 also contained provision for extra-licentiates. In this book I do not discuss them and the extra-licentiates. There were occasions in later centuries when these groups might have been fully organized in a separate institution (see e.g. *R.* v. *Askew*, 1768). This did not happen and Fellowship remained the aspiration.

25 Clark, 1964.

26 The concentration of medicine in London is exampled by the discussion as late as *Davies* v. *Makuna*, 1885, but not there decided, as to whether the 1511 Act was subject to an implied repeal by the 1518 Act. But see *D'Allex* v. *Jones*, 1856. It would appear that until this litigation, it was thought that Bishops of London assumed their powers were either abrogated or only to be exercised in favour of decisions of the College, see Clark, 1964:60.

27 Mandrou, 1978:62, attributes the foundation to Cuthbert Tunstall's persuading Henry VIII to set up 'a sort of medical university ... in the form of readings of learned papers'. He says it was part of the Renaissance trend to establish new colleges. There was a Tunstall who was Bishop of Durham but since his name does not appear in any of the histories of medicine, it may be assumed that Mandrou has inadvertently confused him with Linacre.

28 See Clark, 1964:88ff for the Charter and statutes.

29 Clark, 1964:161.

30 *Allison* v. *Haydon*, 1827. Wilcox, 1830.

31 Medical Act 1542–3.

32 Clark, 1964:263f.

33 Barber-Surgeons Act, 1540. Immediately prior to 1540 in London there was a Barber-Surgeons' Guild as well as a Surgeons' Guild. This Act amalgamated them.

34 As to a knowledge of Latin, see *R.* v. *Master and Wardens of the Company of Surgeons*, 1766.

35 See Parker, 1920. These Companies existed in London and some other towns. See also Cope, 1959.

36 For a copy of the Charter, see British Parliamentary Papers, 1844.

37 Clark, 1964:240f, notes that one of the charges supporting the indictment for treason against Francis Bacon in 1621 was that he took a bribe in connection with the grant of the Charter. More generally, see Wall and Cameron, 1963.

38 It would appear that one reason was the curious judgment of Coke CJ in *Bonham*, 1610.

39 Clark, 1964:437.

40 Clark, 1964:431 and 480ff.

41 *Rose* v. *College of Physicians*, 1703.

42 Clark, 1964:476ff.

43 *Fuller* v. *Executors of the Duke of Queensbury*, 1811. This was confirmed by the Apothecaries Act 1815. And see *Handey* v. *Henson*, 1830.

44 *Davies* v. *Makuna*, 1885:606 *per* Cotton L.J. The remark is similar to the description of the role of the apothecary offered by Smith, 1779:214, Bk.1xpt.I.

45 *Apothecaries Society* v. *Gregory*, 1908.

46 *Apothecaries Company* v. *Allen*, 1833; *Batty* v. *Monks*, 1865.

47 *Apothecaries Company* v. *Greenough*, 1841; *Apothecaries Company* v. *Nottingham*, 1876. It was necessary to distinguish practice as an apothecary from practice as a surgeon or accoucheur, *Woodward* v. *Ball*, 1834; *Apothecaries Society* v. *Gregory* (1908).

48 See: *Boots* v. *Pharmaceutical Society*, 1953; Klass, 1975.

49 Abel-Smith, 1964:5 and Clark, 1964:3.

50 Abel-Smith, 1964.

51 Donzelot, 1977:55. See also Hay, 1976.

52 Donzelot, 1977:66. See also Outka, 1972. A special issue of *Daedalus*, 1987, was devoted to the topic.

53 *Royal College of Surgeons* v. *National Provincial Bank*, 1952, where the status of both the College and the nationalization of the Middlesex Hospital are discussed.

54 As to the relationship between property, philanthropy and religion among the English ruling class see Tawney, 1926:261ff.

55 Baker, 1980.

56 The statute was repealed in 1703/4. Clark, 1964:461.

57 Compare *Allison* v. *General Medical Council*, 1894, discussed below.

58 Holloway, 1966:114f.

59 Forbes, 1955:285.

60 And by the American Medical Association in 1847, see: Konold, 1978; and Leake, 1927:33ff.

61 Apothecaries Act, 1815. I have omitted an account of the formalization of pharmacy.

62 Abel-Smith, 1964:22.

63 Peterson, 1978.
64 See Jewson, 1974.
65 Foucault, 1963:26ff. See also Mitchell, 1981.
66 Foucault, 1963:28.
67 E.g. the first and London based British Medical Association or the London College of Medicine.
68 Poisons Act 1972 sch.1; Misuse of Drugs Act 1971 sch.3 pt.I; Hairdressers Registration Act 1964 sch.1 pt.I (one is tempted to regard this as a return to the Barbers Company, but whereas then manipulative skills were joined, now the involvement is a matter of iatrocracy).
69 There were 17 medical reform Bills between 1840 and 1858. See generally Waddington, 1984.
70 Clark, 1964:705.
71 See *A.G.* v. *Royal College of Physicians*, 1861 and *Gibbon* v. *Budd*, 1863.
72 The Act was not passed without difficulty. There were 23 amendment Bills between 1858 and 1886.
73 Crossman, 1883, Cook, 1976, and Johnston, 1977. It is of interest that the Bar was trying to copy the doctors.
74 *British Medical Journal*, 1878, 9 February, p.197. As to consultants in the 1840s see Waddington, 1984:17.
75 Abel-Smith, 1964:19. See above for Foucault's discussion of economic liberalism in *The Clinic*.
76 *BMJ Supplement*, 1921. The Committee was established to inquire into the finances of voluntary hospitals.
77 Wilson, 1928.
78 E.g. Outdoor Relief Regulation Order, 1852.
79 Poor Law Commissioners, 1836:17f.
80 See the acknowledgement by Hardy, 1867:col.153 but it is probable that Florence Nightingale and her associates were also influential.
81 Abel-Smith, 1964:82.
82 Abel-Smith, 1964:205ff.
83 Bynum and Porter, 1987; Green, 1985.

5 Professionalism

1 Clarke, 1964:623 reports that the College of Surgeons consulted the Royal College of Physicians regarding its charter of 1800.
2 Freidson, 1986:9ff.
3 Freidson, 1970b:370f. His emphasis.
4 Most notably of Larson, 1977 and Durman, 1979.
5 For example, Berlant, 1975.
6 Holmes, 1982. Note, as regards lawyers, Duman, 1982.
7 See Berlant 1975:xxff.
8 Plumb, 1964:313. In the early seventeenth century the common law

provided new means to preserve its utility and to enable an occupier to recover possession. See: Smith, 1779:492, Bk.3 Ch.II.

9 Berlant, 1975:51ff.
10 Berlant, 1975:58.
11 Freidson, 1986:200.
12 Freidson, 1986:185.
13 Freidson, 1986:63.
14 Freidson, 1986:69.
15 Freidson, 1986:76. He cites Finkin, 1973.
16 Freidson, 1970a:176.
17 Freidson, 1970b:81–2.
18 Freidson, 1986:166–7.
19 Freidson, 1970a:119. His emphasis.
20 Freidson, 1970a:143. See also Freidson, 1970b:ch.8.
21 Freidson, 1970a:154.
22 Freidson, 1970a:155.
23 Freidson, 1970b:43.
24 Freidson, 1970b:45.
25 Freidson, 1970b:200.
26 Freidson, 1970a:155–6.
27 Freidson, 1970b:369ff.
28 Freidson, 1970b:89ff.
29 Freidson, 1970b:172–4.
30 Freidson, 1970b:192ff. He also cites Hall, 1946.
31 Freidson, 1986:48.
32 Freidson, 1986:59.
33 Rueschemeyer, 1983.
34 Rueschemeyer, 1983:41.
35 Rueschemeyer, 1983:42.
36 Rueschemeyer, 1983:44f.
37 Freidson, 1970b:71.
38 See Rueschemeyer, 1983:46.
39 Larson, 1977.
40 Rueschemeyer, 1983:52.
41 See Eckstein, 1959.
42 Compare St Matthew, *Gospel*, 19,24 'It is easier for a camel to go through the eye of a needle than for a rich man to enter into the Kingdom of God'.
43 Horobin, 1983.
44 Horobin, 1983:89.
45 Horobin, 1983:101.
46 Horobin, 1983:90.
47 Ladd, 1981:39ff.
48 Castiglione, 1528.
49 Della Casa, 1558. It has been through many English translations. The first was that of Peterson in 1576. In a note to the 1958 translation

Pine-Coffin describes the mutation of such books through manners into etiquette where apparently quite trivially one might learn that a barrister's wife would be led into dinner before a doctor's.

50 Elias, 1978.

51 See Cartwright, 1908.

52 See further Coleman, 1973. This also contains useful references to other and later influential books of manners.

53 Hay, 1961:197. Manners were the subject of comment and praise by Chaucer, 1986: Prologue, describing the Knight and the Prioress. It was the Renaissance which made them an aspiration. See also Elias, 1939:53ff.

54 Ostensibly for other reasons, the book was placed on the Papal Index in Spain.

55 Castiglione, 1528:141.

56 Castiglione, 1528:141.

57 Castiglione, 1528:54, 56.

58 Coleman, 1973:105.

59 Castiglione, 1528:61 and 115ff.

60 Castiglione, 1528:60f.

61 Castiglione, 1528:134.

62 Castiglione, 1528:135.

63 Castiglione, 1528:58f.

64 Castiglione, 1528:296.

65 Castiglione, 1528:64. At Castiglione, 1528:157ff there is a long discourse on humour.

66 Castiglione, 1528:147.

67 Castiglione, 1528:155.

68 Castiglione, 1528:59f.

69 Castiglione, 1528:129.

70 Castiglione, 1528:67.

71 Castiglione, 1528:89f.

72 Castiglione, 1528:114.

73 Castiglione, 1528:118.

74 Castiglione, 1528:147.

75 Castiglione, 1528:147f.

76 Peterson, 1978:204, exaggerates the significance of the Royal Warrant of 1884. It did not in one blow render medical men officers. For example, even afterwards many were excluded from the Officers' Mess.

77 Peterson, 1978:204

78 Coleman, 1973:96.

79 Coleman, 1973;101.

80 In Elias and Dunning, 1986, Elias's thesis of the 'civilising process' has been applied to sport. And see also Hargreaves, 1986.

81 See Sprigge 1895:103.

82 James, 1963:160.

83 Compare Richards, 1926:20 on the social function of art.
84 See Warner, 1950.
85 Mandle, 1973.
86 Graves, 1900.
87 James, 1963:190.
88 Mandle, 1981:361. And see further: Darwin, 1934;131f.
89 *Cf* the involvement of Dr Roger Bannister with ASH (Action on Smoking and Health). As to iatrocratic power, see Haley, 1978.
90 Mandle, 1981:360.
91 Freidson, 1970a:220. And see Blau and Scott, 1963.
92 E.g. Penty, 1920. See also: Tawney, 1982:117; Williams, 1958:186ff citing Belloc 1927, Penty, 1917 and Penty, 1919; and Cole, 1950.
93 Durkheim, 1957.
94 Hawthorn, 1987:31-2.
95 Hawthorn, 1987:135.
96 Penty, 1920:38.
97 Penty, 1920:39.
98 See further Smith, 1987.
99 Penty, 1920:73ff.
100 Freidson, 1970a:136.
101 Durkheim, 1957:19, Lecture II.
102 Durkheim, 1957:17. He argues that they were well established by the time of the earliest records. *Per contra*, Davis, 1957:28ff, suggests that they were the creation of the late Roman Empire. This view is best confined to the imposition of the hereditary principle to be found in many medieval guilds.
103 Durkheim, 1957:2, Lecture I.
104 Durkheim, 1957:3, Lecture I.
105 Durkheim, 1957:3, Lecture I.
106 Durkheim, 1957:4f, Lecture I.
107 Durkheim, 1957:5f, Lecture I.
108 Durkheim, 1957:6, Lecture I.
109 Hawthorn, 1987:158, from M. Weber, *Economy and Society*.
110 Pellegrino and Thomasma, 1981:227.
111 Pellegrino and Thomasma, 1981:101ff.
112 Foucault, 1963:28.
113 Durkheim, 1957:7f, Lecture I.
114 Durkheim, 1957:9, Lecture I.
115 Durkheim, 1957:10.
116 Durkheim, 1957:12, Lecture I.
117 Durkheim, 1957:15, Lecture II.
118 Durkheim, 1957:14, Lecture II.
119 Popper, 1961:82.
120 Durkheim, 1957:25, Lecture III.
121 Durkheim, 1957:25, Lecture II.
122 Durkheim, 1957:26, Lecture II.

123 Durkheim, 1957:28f, Lecture III.
124 Durkheim, 1957:29, Lecture III.
125 Hughes, 1951a:47.
126 Kennedy, 1981:128–30; Grubb, 1987:264–6; Brazier, 1987:191–2.
127 E.g. Scorer and Wing, 1979:vii.
128 Pellegrino and Thomasma, 1981:228.
129 Kennedy, 1981:123ff.
130 The evidence is necessarily scanty but, for example, in Ancient Greece, Democedes of Croton is said to have earned some 16 times the normal wage. On this see Lloyd, 1978: Introduction. For other periods see: Pliny, 1887–98:Bk.29, and Copeman, 1960:49ff; Waddington, 1984:32f and 146f as regards the early and late nineteenth century respectively.
131 Berlant, 1975:41.
132 Clark, 1964, e.g. 138, 321, and 335.
133 May, 1980.
134 Merrison, 1975: para.4.
135 Freidson, 1970b:23f.
136 *British Medical Association* v. *Marsh*, 1931; *General Council and Register of Osteopaths* v. *Guild of Naturopaths and Osteopaths*, 1960; *General Council and Register of Osteopaths* v. *Register of Osteotherapists and Naturopaths*, 1968; but contrast *Society of Architects* v. *Kendrick*, 1910. Note also *Whitwell* v. *Shakesby*, 1932.
137 Merrison, 1975: para.379.
138 Freidson 1970b:192.
139 Freidson, 1970b:81.
140 Freidson, 1986:201.
141 Lloyd, 1978: *The Canon*, cited at the head of Chapter 1.
142 Davies and Jacob, 1987.
143 Davies and Jacob, 1987: Introduction.
144 *Leeson* v. *General Medical Council*, 1887. And see: *Allbutt* v. *General Medical Council*, 1889.
145 Here the expression is loose. A more precise account is given in Davies and Jacob, 1987.
146 See also: on the 1858 Act, *R.* v. *General Medical Council ex parte Organ*, 1861 and *Hunter* v. *Clare*, 1899; on dentists, *A.G.* v. *Weeks*, 1932. And also note *Hughes* v. *Architects Registration Council*, 1957.
147 *McCoan* v. *General Medical Council*, 1964.
148 *de Gregory* v. *General Medical Council*, 1961:965–6.
149 *Allison* v. *General Medical Council*, 1894.
150 *Marten* v. *Royal College of Veterinary Disciplinary Committee*, 1966:6 and 9.
151 See *Allison* v. *General Medical Council*, 1894:761 *per* Lord Esher M.R.
152 *R.* v. *General Medical Council ex parte Kynaston*, 1930:569.

153 *Chorley* v. *Bolcot*, 1791. See also 3 Bl.Com 28.9.
154 *Gibbon* v. *Budd*, 1863.
155 *Tuson* v. *Batting*, 1800 and see *Handey* v. *Henson*, 1830.
156 See *Re Palmer, ex parte Crabb*, 1856, construing the Bankruptcy Laws Consolidation Act 1849, s.69.
157 Hughes, 1951a:52.
158 Freidson, 1970b:16.
159 Freidson, 1970b:107 and see 306f.
160 *Hupe* v. *Phelps*, 1819, and *Thompson* v. *Lewis*, 1828.

6 Administration and medicine

1 But see Carmichael, 1986.
2 Clark, 1964.
3 See the Vaccination Acts 1840 and 1841.
4 Morris, 1976.
5 Cartwright, 1977:99ff.
6 British Parliamentary Papers, 1831.
7 *Hansard*, 1831–2.
8 Cited in Vaughan, 1959:36. And see also Cartwright, 1977:99.
9 Lewis, 1952.
10 See Southwood-Smith, 1830.
11 Chadwick, 1828. See also *Annales d'hygiene publique et de medecine legale*, Preface to vol.1 (1827) cited in Donzelot, 1977:56.
12 Midwinter, 1968:11.
13 See Seymour, 1854.
14 See also Anonymous, 1856.
15 Cabanis, 1799:12ff, cited in Foucault, 1963:79f.
16 Freidson, 1986:162.
17 *R.* v. *Secretary of State for Social Services et al., ex parte Hincks et al.*, 1980.
18 Cameron, *et al.*, 1982. And see Winslow, 1982.
19 See: *R.* v. *East Berkshire H.A. ex parte Walsh*, 1984; and *Nelson* v. *Cookson*, 1940; *Bullard* v. *Croydon H.M.C.*, 1953; *Higgins* v. *N.W. Metropolitan H.B.*, 1954; *Razzel* v. *Snowball*, 1954.
20 For example, the older cases are never cited.
21 *O'Reilly* v. *Hull Board of Prison Visitors*, 1982 and *Cocks* v. *Thanet D.C.*, 1982.
22 See Jacob, forthcoming.
23 Mommsen, 1974:81.
24 Weber, 1947:329ff.
25 See generally, Hill, 1972.
26 Hill, 1972:35ff. Selznick, 1957:7f.
27 Thompson, 1977:6.

28 See Glasser, 1983.

29 Presthus, 1962:123.

30 Thompson, 1977:120.

31 Hill, 1972:117ff.

32 E.g. Cartwright and Zander, 1968:305.

33 E.g. Miller, 1955:271ff.

34 Etzioni, 1965:696.

35 Hill, 1972:124ff.

36 Etzioni, 1964:31.

37 *Royal College of Nursing* v. *DHSS*, 1981. And see *Davis* v. *Morris*, 1923.

38 Abel-Smith, 1964:498–501.

39 See National Assistance Act 1948 s.47.

40 The duties in primary care are defined by the National Health Service (General Medical and Pharmaceutical) Regulations and those in secondary care by 'collective agreements' between the National Health Service on the one side and consultants and other grades of staff (known as junior doctors) on the other.

41 British Medical Association, 1981.

42 See Abel-Smith, 1960.

43 Freidson, 1986:175.

44 Freidson, 1986;191ff.

45 For a review of classifications, see Harlow and Rawlings, 1984.

46 Birkinshaw, 1985:1.

47 Birkinshaw, 1985:185. His emphasis.

48 Stein, 1984:3ff.

49 Stein 1984:33.

50 Roberts, 1979.

51 Roberts, 1979:25.

52 For a more sophisticated articulation and critique of the theory, see Calabresi, 1970.

53 Posner, 1977.

54 Posner, 1977:157ff.

55 Calabresi and Bobbitt, 1978.

56 For an exposition of health care on such a basis, see Navarro, 1978, and Navarro, 1986.

57 Davis, 1971. For a recent assessment, see Hawkins and Baldwin, 1984.

58 Abel, 1982:267.

59 Abel, 1982:308.

60 Pearson, 1978.

61 For a United States example, see *Wyatt* v. *Stickney*, 1972.

62 E.g. the Rampton Hospital Enquiry.

63 E.g. the Stafford Hospital Enquiry, 1985.

64 National Health Service Act 1977 s.84.

65 Griffith, 1985:34ff. The phenomena are not new, see Havinghurst, 1950.

66 Compare Aristotle, 1928: *Poetics* 6.
67 E.g. the Normansfield Hospital Enquiry, 1977.
68 Kennedy, 1986:8.
69 Canguilheim, 1978, cited in Pellegrino and Thomasma, 1981, above.
70 In *Latter* v. *Braddell*, 1891, Lindley J. distinguished consent from acquiescence or submission but Lopes J. disagreed holding that there may be a lack of consent although the will is not 'overpowered by force or fear of violence'. The one judge looked at the surrounding circumstances; the other was concerned only with the state of mind regarding the touching.
71 Ramsey, 1970:5f.
72 Giesen, 1981.
73 Mill, 1859:Ch.IV.
74 Mill, 1971.
75 *Slater* v. *Baker*, 1767:862, emphasis added.
76 Tennyson, 1854.
77 See Lidz *et al.*, 1984:Ch.3 for a survey of the literature and later chapters for their own later evidence. See also the authorities cited by Kennedy, 1984:466f and notes thereto. In *Sidaway*, 1985:652, the paper was cited by Lord Scarman with approval. Earlier in the Court of Appeal, *Sidaway*, 1984:1034, Browne-Wilkinson L.J. adopted some of this idea. It corresponds to Parsons' application of Malinowski's description of magic, see above.
78 Kennedy, 1984:461.
79 Kennedy, 1984:468. His emphasis.

7 Conclusion

1 The word is used by Pellegrino and Thomasma, 1981:247f.
2 Burt, 1979.
3 The tape, 'Please let me die', is available from the Department of Psychiatry, University of Texas, Medical Board, Galveston, Texas. The transcript is set out in Burt, 1979:174ff. See also White, 1975. The case is also discussed in Childress, 1982:xx.
4 *Lake* v. *Cameron*, 1966. For a comparable English case see *Re V.E.*, 1973, where however the case came before the court on narrower and more technical grounds.
5 He cites: Goffman, 1963:84f and Goffman, 1971; and Foucault, 1977:290ff.
6 Burt, 1979:37.
7 Burt, 1979:44.
8 Milgram, 1974.
9 Burt, 1979:48.
10 Burt, 1979:50f.
11 Freud, 1933: 'where id is, there ego shall come into being'; Burt adds

(citing Loewald, 1978:16) 'where ego is, there id shall come into being again'.

12 Burt, 1979:54.

13 Burt, 1979:65.

14 Burt, 1979:67.

15 Burt, 1979:92.

16 Burt, 1979:94. He cites Waitztein and Stoectcle, 1972:196.

17 Burt, 1979:98.

18 Burt, 1979:99f.

19 Santarcangeli, 1979:28. And see; Billington, 1987; and Powell and Paton, 1987.

20 Santarcangeli, 1979:30, Schlegel, 1876:117.

21 As a matter of legal history, Burt, 1979:102ff, argues that the nineteenth-century cases upon which the courts relied were not concerned with whether a doctor had given enough information to justify his treatment but merely whether it could truly be said there was a doctor–patient relationship at all. He cites: Katz, 1977 and *Slater* v. *Baker*, 1767; *State* v. *Housekeeper* 1889; *Pratt* v. *Davis*, 1905; *Mohr* v. *Williams*, 1905; in contrast to: *Canterbury* v. *Spence*, 1972; *Cobbs* v. *Grant* 1972; *Natanson* v. *Kline*, 1960.

22 Burt, 1979:103.

23 Burt, 1979:112.

24 Burt, 1979:112f.

25 Burt, 1979:114.

26 Burt, 1979:115f.

27 Burt, 1979:120. Similarly, Lord Scarman sought to impose on Mrs Sidaway (*Sidaway*, 1985:495) an implied acceptance of her lawyer's advice and conduct.

28 Burt, 1979:137.

29 See Williams, 1958, on the effect that the change from patronage to a wider public had on writers, and see also Eco, 1983.

30 Foucault, 1963, especially 84f discussed above.

31 Pellegrino and Thomasma, 1981, especially at 66 discussed above.

32 Durkheim, 1938:II 115, cited in Lukes, 1973:385.

33 'Why beholdest thou the mote that is in thy brother's eye, but considerest not the beam that is in thine own eye?' St Matthew, *Gospel*, 7.3.

34 Freidson, 1986:103.

35 Oakeshott, 1962:1ff.

36 See Shakespeare, 1955:I, i *per* Menenius.

37 Hawthorn, 1987:85f. And see also Hawthorn, 1987:13.

38 Hawthorn, 1987:10–11. And see Hawthorn, 1987:27.

39 Alexander, 1985.

40 Bentham, 1834:vol.1, 300.

41 Freidson, 1970a:64.

42 Compare Shetreet, 1976.

43 Shakespeare, 1946:II vii, 139.
44 See further: Turner, 1984; Dingwall, 1977.
45 For an attempt to apply this idea to medical practice, see Dossey, 1982.
46 This explains the link between the debates concerning the claim for privacy and the protection of personal information held by others. So also as Loizou, 1986, argues, the future exists in our present and as Castoriadis, 1987, implies so also does the past. Truly as William James says 'a man has as many selves as there are individuals who recognise him and carry an image of him in their mind', cited in Hawthorn, 1987:207.
47 Tawney, 1926:26. It is to be observed that this was written at a time of relative stability when change within generations was less apparent.
48 Dahrendorf, 1985.

Appendix: The Hippocratic Oath

1 Duncan, *et al.*, 1981.

Bibliography

This bibliography includes only those works mentioned in the text and notes, including those cited by authors whom I have in turn cited.

R.L. Abel (ed.) (1982) 'The contradictions of informal justice', *The Politics of Informal Justice*, vol. 1 *The American Experience*, New York: Academic Press.

B. Abel-Smith (1964) *The Hospitals*, Cambridge, Mass: Harvard University Press.

B. Abel-Smith (1960) *The Nurses. A History of the Nursing Profession*, London: Heinemann.

N. Adams (1972) *Dead and Buried? The Horrible History of Body Snatching*, Aberdeen: Impulse Publication.

A.G. v. Weeks [1932] 1 Ch. 211.

A.G. v. Royal College of Physicians (1861) 1 J. and H. 561.

P. Alexander (1985) *Ideas, Qualities and Corpuscles: Locke and Boyle on the External World*, Cambridge: Cambridge University Press.

Allbutt v. General Medical Council (1889) 23 Q.B.D. 400.

Allison v. General Medical Council [1894] 1 Q.B. 750.

Allison v. Haydon (1827) 3 Car. and P. 246 at 248–50; 172 E.R. 406 at 407. It is also, but less fully reported at (1828) 4 Bing. 619; 130 E.R. 907.

L. Althusser (1972) *Montesquieu, Rousseau, and Marx*, trans. B. Brewster, 1982 ed. republished London: Verso.

American Medical Association (1980) *Principles of Medical Ethics*, 1980 revision.

Annales d'hygiene publique et de medecine legale (1827) Preface to vol.1 cited in J. Donzelot (1979) *The Policing of Families, Welfare versus the State*, trans. R. Hurley, London: Hutchinson.

Annals of the AAPSS, (1980) 447, January.

Anonymous (1856) *Engineers and Officials*, 1856, quoted in R.A. Lewis (1952) *Edwin Chadwick and the Public Health Movement, 1832–54*, London: Longman, Green:369.

Apothecaries Act 1815 55 Geo.3, c.194.

268 *Doctors and Rules*

Apothecaries Company v. *Greenough* (1841) 1 Q.B. 799.

Apothecaries Company v. *Nottingham* (1876) 34 L.T. 76.

Apothecaries Society v. *Gregory* (1908) 25 T.L.R. 37.

Apothecaries Company v. *Allen* (1833) 4 B. and Ad. 625, 110 E.R. 591.

G.L. Apperson (1914) *The Social History of Smoking*, London: Martin Secker.

D. Apple (1960) 'How laymen define illness', *Journal of Health and Human Behavior*, I 219–25.

H. Arendt (1958) *The Human Condition*, Chicago: University of Chicago Press.

Aristotle *The Works*, ed. and trans. W.D. Ross (1928) Vol. VIII, *Metaphysics*, 2nd ed., Oxford: Clarendon.

H. Ashton and R. Stepney (1983) *Smoking: Pharmacology and Psychology*, London: Tavistock.

P. Atiyah (1979) *The Rise and Fall of Freedom of Contract*, Oxford: Oxford University Press.

F. Azouri (1979) 'The Plague, Melancholy and the Devil', trans. J. Ferguson *Diogenes* 108:112.

F. Bacon (1604) *The Advancement of Learning*, A. Johnston (ed.) (1974) Oxford: Clarendon Press.

F. Bacon (1627) *New Atlantis*, in B. Vickers (ed.) (1987) *English Science, Bacon to Newton*, Cambridge: Cambridge University Press.

J. Baker (1980) 43 *Modern Law Review* 467.

Bankruptcy Laws Consolidation Act 1849.

Barber-Surgeons Act 1540, 32 Hen.8 c.42 (see also 5 Car.1 recited in 18 Geo.2 c.15).

N. Barlow (ed.) (1958) C. Darwin, *Autobiography*, London: Collins.

J. Barzun (ed.) (1975) *Burke and Hare: The Resurrection Men*, New York Academy of Sciences, Metuchen NJ: Scarecrow.

Batty v. *Monks* (1865) 12 L.T. 852.

T.L. Beauchamp and E.F. Childress (1979) *The Principles of Biomedical Ethics*, New York: Oxford University Press.

H. Belloc (1927) *The Servile State*, 3rd ed. London: Constable.

P. Benichou (1948) *Morale du grand siècle*, Paris: Gallimard.

J. Bentham (1834) *Deontology*, London: Longman.

J.L. Berlant (1975) *Profession and Monopoly: A Study of Medicine in the United States and Great Britain*, Berkeley: University of California Press.

G. Berlinguer (1981) 'Life-styles and health: alternative patterns', *International Journal of Health Services* vol.11:53–61.

C. Bernard (1865) *An Introduction to Experimental Medicine* trans. H.C. Green, (1927) 1957 ed., New York: Macmillan.

Bernard of Chartres quoted in John of Salisbury (1195) *Metalogician* bk.III ch.iv.

A. Bevan (1961) *In Place of Fear*, (first published, 1952) London: Macgibbon & Kee.

X. Bichat (1825) *Anatomie pathologique*, Paris.

S. Billington (1987) *A Social History of the Fool*, Brighton: Harvester Press.

P. Birkinshaw (1985) *Grievances, Remedies and the State*, London: Sweet & Maxwell.

Sir D. Black (Chairman) (1980) *The Report of the Working Group in Inequalities and Health*, reprinted as *Inequalities in Health: the Black Report* P. Townsend and N. Davidson (eds) (1982) Harmondsworth: Penguin.

M. Black (1962) *Models and Metaphors: Studies in Language and Philosophy*, Ithaca, NY: Cornell University Press.

Blackstone Commentaries.

P.M. Blau and R.W. Scott (1963) *Formal Organizations*, London: Routledge & Kegan Paul.

G.W. Bloor and M.J. Horobin (1975) 'Conflict and conflict resolution in doctor/patient relationship' in C. Cox and A. Mead (eds) *A Sociology of Medical Practice*, London: Cassell and Collier Macmillan.

Bonham's Case (1610) 8 Co. Rep. 114a.

Boots v. *Pharmaceutical Society* [1953] 1 Q.B. 401.

P. Brain (1986) *Galen on Bloodletting*, Cambridge: Cambridge University Press.

M. Brazier (1987) 'Patient autonomy and consent to treatment: the role of law?' *Legal Studies* 169–93.

R. Bright (1827 and 1831) *Reports of Medical Cases*.

British Medical Association v. *Marsh* (1931) 48 R.P.C. 565.

British Medical Association (1911) *Secret Remedies*, London: British Medical Association.

British Medical Association (1912) *More Secret Remedies*, London: British Medical Association.

British Medical Association (1980) *Handbook of Medical Ethics*, London: British Medical Association.

British Medical Association (1981) *Handbook of Medical Ethics*, London: British Medical Association.

British Medical Journal Supplement 20 July 1921:72.

British Parliamentary Papers, 1831, xvii:20–3.

British Parliamentary Papers, 1844, XL.

J. Bronowski (1964) *Science and Human Value*, Harmondsworth: Penguin.

E.G. Browne (1921) *Arabian Medicine*, being the Fitzpatrick Lectures at the College of Physicians 1919 and 1920, Cambridge: Cambridge University Press.

Bullard v. *Croydon H.M.C.* [1953] 1 All E.R. 596.

J. Burnet (1930) *Early Greek Philosophy*, London: A & C Black.

R.A. Burt (1979) *Taking Care of Strangers*, London: Macmillan.

R. Burton (1925) *Anatomy of Melancholy*, 1651, rep. Nonesuch, New York: Harcourt.

H.R. Butterfield (1931) *The Whig Interpretation of History*, (reprinted 1951) London: G. Bell & Sons.

W.F. Bynum and R. Porter (eds) (1987) *Medical Fringe and Medical Orthodoxy 1750–1850*, Beckenham: Croom Helm.

Cabanis (1799) *Rapport du Conseil des cinq cent sur un mode provisoire de police medicale*, cited in M. Foucault (1963) *The Birth of The Clinic, An Archaeology of Medical Perception*, trans. A.M. Sheridan (1973) 1976 ed. London: Tavistock:79f.

M. Cain (1983) 'The general practice lawyer and the client' in R. Dingwall and P. Lewis (eds) *The Sociology of the Professions: Lawyers, Doctors and Others*, London: Macmillan.

G. Calabresi (1970) *The Costs of Accidents: A Legal and Economic Analysis*, New Haven and London: Yale University Press.

G. Calabresi and P. Bobbitt (1978) *Tragic Choices*, New York: W.W. Norton.

D. Callahan (1973) 'The WHO Definition of Health', *Hastings Center Studies*, 1, no.3, Hastings and Hudson NY:77–87.

J. Cameron, C. Ogg, and D.G. Williams *The Lancet* 19 November 1982.

G. Canguilheim (1966) *On the Normal and the Pathological*, trans. C.R. Fawcett, (1978) Boston: Deidel.

Canterbury v. *Spence* (1972) 464 F. 2d 772.

A.G. Carmichael (1986) *Plague and the Poor in Renaissance Florence*, Cambridge: Cambridge University Press.

E.H. Carr (1964) *What is History?* (first published, 1961) Harmondsworth: Penguin.

J. Cartier (1545) *Brief Recit*, trans. J. Florio (1580).

J. Cartwright (1908) *Baldassare Castiglione, The Perfect Courtier: His Life and Letters*, London: Murray.

D. Cartwright and A. Zander (eds) (1968) *Group Dynamics; Research and Theory* 3rd ed. London: Tavistock.

F.F. Cartwright (1977) *A Social History of Medicine*, London: Longman.

E. Cassell (1976) 'Disease as an it', *Social Science and Medicine*, vol.10: 143–6.

E. Cassirer (1970) *An Essay on Man: An Introduction to a Philosophy of Human Culture*, New York and London: Bantam.

B. Castiglione (1528) *The Book of the Courtier*, published 1972, Milan: Mursia. The modern translation is by G. Bull (1967) (rev.1976) Harmondsworth: Penguin.

C. Castoriadis (1987) *The Imaginary Institution of Society: Creativity and autonomy in the Social-Historical World*, Oxford: Polity Press.

Benvenuto Cellini (1558–66) *Autobiography* first printed 1728 ed. and trans. G. Bull, (1956) reprinted London: Folio Society, 1966.

E. Chadwick (1828) *Westminster Review*, February vol.ix:85 and 413.

N. Chappell and N. Colvill (1981) *Canadian Review of Sociology and Anthropology* (18):67–81.

M.P. Chase (1985) 'Fevers, poisons, and apostemes: authority and experience in Montpellier plague treatises' in P.O. Long (ed.) *Science and Technology in Medieval Society, Annals of the New York Academy of Sciences*, vol.441.

G. Chaucer *Canterbury Tales*, D. Wright (ed.) (1986) Oxford: Oxford University Press.

E. Cheesman (1953) *Charles Darwin and his Problems*, London: Bell & Sons.

J.F. Childress (1982) *Who Should Decide? Paternalism in Health Care*, New York: Oxford University Press.

Chorley v. *Bolcot* (1791) 4 T.R. 317.

W.C. Churchill (1944) Address to the Royal College of Physicians.

Sir G. Clark (1964) *A History of the Royal College of Physicians of London*, Oxford: Clarendon.

R.W. Clark (1968) *The Huxleys*, London: Heinemann.

Cobbs v. *Grant* 502 P. 2d 1 (Cal., 1972).

Cocks v. *Thanet District Council* [1982] 3 W.L.R. 1121.

G.D.H. Cole (1950) *Essays in Social Theory*, London: Macmillan.

D.C. Coleman (1973) 'Gentlemen and Players' *Economic History Review* 26:92–116.

Company of Physicians Act 1523, 14 and 15 Hen.8, c.5.

R. Cook (1976) 92 *Law Quarterly Review* 512.

Sir Z. Cope (1959) *History of the Royal College of Surgeons of England*, London: Anthony Blond.

W.S.C. Copeman (1960) *Doctors and Disease in Tudor Times* (Society of Apothecaries of London) London: Wm Dawson & Sons.

G.W. Corner (1933) 'The rise of medicine at Salerno in the twelfth century', in *Lectures on the History of Medicine, 1926–32*, Philadelphia: Saunders.

F.M. Cornford (1912) *From Religion to Philosophy: a study in the origins of Western Speculations*, London: Edward Arnold.

Count Corti *A History of Smoking*, trans. P. England (1931) London: G.G. Harrap.

J.-N. Corvisart (1808) Preface to Auenbrugger, *Nouvelle methode pour reconnaître les maladies internes de la poitrine*, Paris.

E. Crossman (1883) *British Medical Journal*, 14 July:63.

Daedalus, (1987) 'Philanthropy, patronage and politics', vol.116, no.1.

R. Dahrendorf (1985) *Law and Order*, London: Stevens.

D. Daiches (1969) *Scotch Whisky, Its Past and Present*, London: André Deutsch.

D'Allex v. *Jones* (1856) 26 L.J. (Ex.) 79.

Dalton (1808–10) *New System of Chemical Philosophy*, Bickerstaff.

C.V. Daremberg (1865) *La Medicine, Histoire et Doctrines*, 2nd ed., Paris: Didier.

B. Darwin (1934) *W.G. Grace*, London: Duckworth.

C. Darwin *Autobiography*, N. Barlow (ed.) (1958) London: Collins.

C. Darwin (1859) *Origin of Species*, J.W. Burrow (ed.) (1982) Harmondsworth: Penguin.

C. Darwin (1871) *The Descent of Man*, London: Murray.

G. Davey (1957) 'Introduction' in E. Durkheim, *Professional Ethics and Civic Morals*, trans. C. Brookfield, London: Routledge & Kegan Paul.

J. Davies and J. Jacob (eds) (1987) (looseleaf) *Encyclopedia of Health Services and Medical Law*, London: Sweet & Maxwell.

Davies v. Makuna (1885) 29 Ch.D 596.

K.C. Davis (1971) *Discretionary Justice. A Preliminary Inquiry*, London: University of Illinois Press.

R.H.C. Davis (1957) *A History of Medieval Europe from Constantine to Saint Louis*, London: Longman and Green.

Davis v. Morris [1923] 508.

de Gregory v. General Medical Council [1961] A.C. 957.

Della Casa (1558) *Galetio*, trans. R.S. Pine-Coffin, (1958) Harmondsworth: Penguin.

R. Dingwall (1977) *Aspects of Illness*, London: Martin Robertson.

R. Dingwall and P. Lewis (eds) (1983) *The Sociology of the Professions: Lawyers, Doctors and Others*, London: Macmillan.

Discriminator (1790) *The Apothecaries' Mirror, or the present state of pharmacy exploded*.

J. Donne *Devotions*, J. Sparrow, ed. (1923) reprinted Cambridge: Cambridge University Press 1977.

J. Donzelot (1977) *The Policing of Families, Welfare versus the State*, trans. R. Hurley, (1979) London: Hutchinson.

Dorland's American Illustrated Medical Dictionary (1974) 25th ed., Philadelphia: Saunders.

L. Dossey (1982) *Space, Time and Medicine*, London: Routledge & Kegan Paul.

H.F. Dowling (1963) 'How do practicing physicians use new drugs', *Journal of American Medical Association* cixxxv:233ff.

R. Dubos (1960) *Mirage of Health: Utopias, Progress and Biological Change*, London: Allen & Unwin.

R. Dubos (1968) *Man, Medicine, and Environment*, London: Pall Mall.

D. Duman (1982) *The Judicial Bench in England 1727–1875*, London: Royal Historical Society.

A.S. Duncan, G.R. Dunston, and R.B. Welbourn (eds) (1981) *Dictionary of Medical Ethics*, London: Danton, Longman & Todd.

E. Durkheim (1922) *Education and Sociology*, trans. S.D. Fox, (1956) Chicago: Free Press of Glencoe.

E. Durkheim (1938) *L'Évolution pedéagogique en France*, Introduction by M. Halbwachs, vol. II: *De la renaissance à nos jours*, Paris: Alcan.

E. Durkheim (1957) *Professional Ethics and Civic Morals*, trans. C. Brookfield, London: Tavistock.

D. Durman (1979) 'The creation and diffusion of a professional ideology in nineteenth century England', *Sociological Review*:113–38.

M. Dvorak (1984) *The History of Art as History of Ideas*, trans. J. Hardy, London: Routledge & Kegan Paul.

G. Easthope (1986) *Healers and Alternative Medicine: A Sociological Examination*, Aldershot: Gower.

H. Eckstein (1959) *The English Health Service*, Cambridge, Mass.: Harvard University Press.

U. Eco (1983) *Reflections on the Name of the Rose*, trans. E. Weaver, (1985) London: Martin Secker & Warburg.

L. Edelstein (1943) 'The Hippocratic Oath: text, translation, and interpretation', *Supplement to the Bulletin of the History of Medicine* No.1.

L. Edelstein (1967a) 'The professional ethics of the Greek physician' in O. Temkin and C.L. Temkin (eds) *Ancient Medicine, Selected Papers*.

L. Edelstein (1967b) 'Hippocrates of Cos' in P. Edwards, (ed.) *The Encyclopedia of Philosophy*, vol.III, New York: Macmillan.

N. Elias (1939) *The Civilizing Process vol.1, A History of Manners*, trans. E. Jephcott (1978) Oxford: Blackwell.

N. Elias and E. Dunning (1986) *Quest for Excitement: Sport and Leisure in the Civilising Process*, Oxford: Basil Blackwell.

J.B. Elshtain (1982) *Public Man, Private Woman: Women in Social and Political Thought* Oxford: Martin Robertson.

H.L. Engelhardt and S. Spricker (eds) (1977) *Philosophical Medical Ethics: Its Nature and Significance*, Dordrecht, Netherlands: Reidel.

R.A. Epstein (1982) 'Social consequences of common law rules' 95 *Harvard Law Review* 1717.

D. Erasmus (1511) *Praise of Folly*, trans. B. Radice (1971) Harmondsworth: Penguin.

D. Erasmus (1530) *On Civility in Children*.

A. Etzioni (1964) *A Comparative Analysis of Complex Organizations*, London: Collier Macmillan.

A Etzioni (1965) 'Dual leadership in complex organizations', *American Sociological Review*, 30:696.

J. Eyles (1987) *The Geography of the National Health*, Beckenham: Croom Helm.

C. Faulder (1985) *Whose Body Is It? The Troubling Issue of Informed Consent*, London: Virago.

L. Festinger (1957) *A Theory of Cognitive Dissonance*, New York: Harper & Row.

M.W. Finkin (1973) 'Federal reliance on voluntary accreditation: The power to recognize as the power to regulate', *Journal of Law and Education* 2:339–67.

R.C. Finucane (1975) 'The use and abuse of medieval miracles', *History* (Journal of the Historical Association), vol. 60:1–10.

R. Fletcher (1912) 'Some diseases bearing the names of saints', *Bristol Medical-Chirical. Journal* vol.xxx:289.

R.A. Forbes (1955) 'A historical survey of medical ethics', *St Bartholomew's Hospital Journal* 59:284–6, 316–19.

M. Foucault (1963) *The Birth of The Clinic, An Archaeology of Medical Perception*, trans. A.M. Sheridan (1973) 1976 ed. London: Tavistock.

M. Foucault (1974) *The Order of Things: An Archaeology of the Human Sciences*, London: Tavistock.

M. Foucault (1976) *The History of Sexuality vol.1*, trans. R. Hurley, (1979) (first trans. 1978) Harmondsworth: Pelican Books.

M. Foucault (1977) *Discipline and Punish: The Birth of the Prison*, trans. A.M. Sheridan, New York: Pantheon Books.

M. Foucault (1981a) 'The order of discourse', (first published 1971) Paris in R. Young (ed.) *Untying the Text*, London: Routledge & Kegan Paul.

M. Foucault (1981b) 'Est-il donc important de penser?', *Libération*, Paris, May 30–31, quoted in J. Rajchman (1985) *Michel Foucault: The Freedom of Philosophy*, New York: Columbia University Press.

R.C. Fox (1957) 'Training for uncertainty' in R.K. Merton, G.G. Reader and P.L. Kendall (eds) *The Student Physician*, Cambridge, Mass.: Harvard University Press.

H.G. Frankfurt (1971) 'Freedom of the will and the concept of a person', *Journal of Philosophy* 68:5–20.

E. Freidson (1970a) *Professional Dominance*, New York: Atherton.

E. Freidson (1970b) *Profession of Medicine: A Study of the Sociology of Applied Knowledge*, New York: Dodd, Mead & Co.

E. Freidson (1986) *Professional Powers: A Study of the Institutionalization of Formal Knowledge*, Chicago: University of Chicago Press.

S. Freud (1933) *New Introductory Lectures on Psychoanalysis*, trans. J.M. Sprott (1937) New York: Norton.

A.J. Friedman and C. Donley (1985) *Einstein as Myth and Muse*, Cambridge: Cambridge University Press.

Fuller v. *Executors of the Duke of Queensbury*, 1811, referred to in Sir G. Clark (1964) *A History of the Royal College of Physicians of London*, Oxford: Clarendon:649.

E. Gellner (1974) *Legitimation of Belief*, Cambridge: Cambridge University Press.

General Council and Register of Osteopaths v. *Guild of Naturopaths and Osteopaths, The Times* 27 July, 1960.

General Council and Register of Osteopaths v. *Register of Osteotherapists and Naturopaths*, (1968) 112 Sol.Jo. 443.

Gibbon v. *Budd* (1863) 2 H.C. 91.

I.D. Giesen (1981) *Medical Malpractice Law: A Comparative Law Study of Civil Responsibility arising from Medical Care. Arzthaftungsrecht: Die zivilrechtliche Verantwortlichkeit des Arztes in rechtsvergleichender Sicht*, Bielefeld: Gieseking.

Gilbert (1600) *De Magnete.*

E. Gilson (1938) *The Unity of Philosophical Experience*, London: Sheed.

C. Gittings (1984) *Death, Burial and the Individual in Early Modern England*, Beckenham, Kent: Croom Helm.

C. Glasser (1983) reviewing *The Reform of Civil Procedural Law*, Sir Jack I.H. Jacob [1983] *Public Law.*

E. Goffman (1963) *Behaviour in Public Places*, London: Macmillan.

E. Goffman (1971) *Relations in Public: Microstudies of the Public Order*, London: Basic Books.

D.M. Goldstein (1982) *Bioethics, A Guide to Information Sources*, vol.8 in the Gale Research Health Affairs Information Guide Series, Detroit: Gale Research.

H. Graves (1900) 'A philosophy of sport', *Contemporary Review*, vol.LXXVII:890.

D.G. Green (1985) *Working-Class Patients and the Medical Establishment: Self-help in Britain from the Mid-nineteenth Century to 1948*, Aldershot: Gower.

J. Gregory (1958) 'Lectures on the duties and qualifications of a physician', quoted in L.S. King, *The Medical World of the Eighteenth Century*, Chicago: University of Chicago Press, 1958 and in J.K. Mason and R.A. McCall-Smith (1987) *Law and Medical Ethics* 2nd ed., London: Butterworths.

J.A.G. Griffith (1985) *The Politics of the Judiciary*, 3rd ed., London: Fontana.

A. Grubb (1987) 'The emergence and rise of medical law and ethics', 50 *Modern Law Review* 241–67.

A. Gurwitsch (1973) 'Problems of the life-world', in M. Natanson (ed.) *Phenomenology and the Social Sciences*, Evanston: Northwestern Press.

D. Guthrie (1945) *A History of Medicine*, London: Nelson.

Hairdressers Registration Act 1964.

B. Haley (1978) *The Healthy Body and Victorian Culture*, Cambridge, Mass.: Harvard University Press.

O. Hall (1946) 'The informal organization of the medical profession', *Canadian Journal of Economics and Political Science*, XII:33.

C. Ham (1985) *Health Policy in Britain: The Organisation and Politics of the NHS*, 2nd ed. London: Macmillan.

C. Ham (1986) *Managing Health Services: Health Authority Members in Search of a Role*, Bristol: University of Bristol, School for Advanced Urban Studies.

Handey v. Henson (1830) 4 Car. & P. 110.

Hansard, xi, 1831–32, cols.308–311.

G. Harding (1987) *Opiate Addiction. From Moral Illness to Pathological Disease* London: Macmillan.

G. Hardy (1867) President of the Poor Law Board moving the Metropolitan Poor Bill at 1st Reading *Hansard* February 8th cols 150–175 at col.153.

J. Hargreaves (1986) *Sport, Power and Culture: A Social and Historical Analysis of Popular Sports in Britain*, Oxford: Polity Press.

C. Harlow and R. Rawlings (1984) *Law and Administration*, London: Weidenfeld & Nicolson.

A.F. Havinghurst (1950) 'The judiciary and politics in the reign of Charles II' 66 *Law Quarterly Review* 62ff and 229ff.

K. Hawkins and R. Baldwin (1984) 'Discretionary justice: Davis reconsidered' [1984] *Public Law* 570–99.

G. Hawthorn (1987) *Enlightenment and Despair: A History of Social Theory*, 2nd ed. Cambridge: Cambridge University Press.

D. Hay (1961) *The Italian Renaissance in its Historical Background*, Cambridge: Cambridge University Press.

D. Hay (1976) *Albian's Fatal Tree*, London: Allen Lane.

C. Hibbert (1979) *The Rise and Fall of the House of Medici*, (first published 1974) Harmondsworth: Penguin.

Higgins v. North Western Metropolitan Hospital Board [1954] 1 W.L.R. 411.

M.J. Hill (1972) *The Sociology of Public Administration*, London: Weidenfeld.

G. Himmelfarb (1959) *Darwin and the Darwinian Revolution*, London: Chatto & Windus.

F. Hirsch (1978) *Social Limits to Growth*, London: Routledge.

A.O. Hirschman (1982) *Shifting Involvements, Private Interest and Public Action*, Oxford: Martin Robertson and Princeton: Princeton University Press. (Quotations reprinted with permission.)

History of Thomas Becket (RS, 1875–85) i, 444.

S.W.F. Holloway (1966) 'The Apothecaries Act 1815: A reinterpretation', *Medical History*:107–29, 221–36.

G. Holmes (1982) *Augustan England: Professions, State and Society 1680–1730*, London: Allen & Co.

G. Holton (1960) 'Modern science and the intellectual tradition', *Science*:131 1187–93.

G. Horobin (1983) 'Professional mystery: the maintenance of charisma in general medical practice', in R. Dingwall and P. Lewis (eds) *The Sociology of the Professions: Lawyers, Doctors and Others*, London: Macmillan:84ff.

Hughes v. Architects Registration Council [1957] 2 Q.B. 550; [1957] 2 All E.R. 436.

E.C. Hughes (1951a) 'Work and the self' in E.C. Hughes (ed.) (1958) *Men and Their Work*, Chicago: The Free Press of Glencoe and reprinted from J.H. Rohrer and M. Sherif (eds) *Social Psychology at the Crossroads*, New York.

E.C. Hughes (1951b) 'Mistakes at work' in E.C. Hughes (ed.) (1958) *Men and Their Work*, Chicago: The Free Press of Glencoe, reprinted from *The Canadian Journal of Economics and Political Science*, vol. X–VIII.

E.C. Hughes (ed.) (1958) *Men and Their Work*, Chicago: The Free Press of Glencoe.

Hunter v. Clare [1899] 1 Q.B. 635.

Hupe v. Phelps (1819) 2 Stark 480.

E. Husserl (1954) *Die Krisis der Europaischen Wissenschaften*, Haag: M. Nijhoff.

A. Hyde (1983) 'The concept of legitimation in the sociology of law', [1983] *Wisconsin Law Review* 379.

I. Illich (1977) *Limits to Medicine. Medical Nemesis: the Expropriation of Health* (first published in 1976) Harmondsworth: Penguin Books.

R. Inglehart (1977) *The Silent Revolution: Changing Values and Political Styles among Western Publics*, Princeton NJ: University of Princeton Press.

Inquiry into the outbreak of legionnaires' disease (1985) Press Release, 85/132, May, Department of Health and Social Security.

J. Jacob *The Talk of Parliament*, forthcoming.

C.L.R. James (1963) *Beyond the Boundary*, London: Stanley Paul.

W. James (1909) *The Meaning of Truth, a Sequel to Pragmatism*, reprinted in 1976 the *Works of William James*, vol.2, Cambridge, Mass.: Harvard University Press.

W. James (1955) *Varieties of Religious Experiences*, reprinted 1982, Harmondsworth: Penguin.

N. Jewson (1974) 'Medical knowledge and the patronage system in 18th century England' *Sociology* 8:369–85.

John of Salisbury (1159) *Metalogician*.

T.J. Johnson (1972) *Professions and Power*, London: Macmillan.

R. Johnston (1977) 'History of the two counsel rule in the nineteenth century' 93 *Law Quarterly Review* 190.

H. Jonas (1973) 'Technology and responsibility: reflections on the new tasks of ethics', *Social Research*:31–54.

W.H.S. Jones (1924) *The Doctor's Oath*, Cambridge: Cambridge University Press.

J. Jowell (1973) 'The legal control of administrative discretion' [1973] *Public Law* 178.

Justinian Digest.

J. Katz (1977) 'Informed consent – a fairy tale? Law's vision', *University of Pittsburgh Law Review* 39:137.

I. Kennedy (1981) *The Unmasking of Medicine*, London: George Allen & Unwin.

I. Kennedy (1984) 'The patient on the Clapham omnibus', 47 *Modern Law Review* 454–71.

I. Kennedy (1986) 'A survey of the year: 1. The doctor-patient relationship', in P. Byrne (ed.) *Rights and Wrongs in Medicine: King's College Studies, 1985–6*, King Edward's Hospital Fund, Oxford: Oxford University Press.

Omar Khayyám *Rubáiyát*, E. Fitzgerald's first translation 1859 verses 27–28, (see also second translation verses 30–31).

A. Klass (1975) *There's Gold in Them Thar Pills: An inquiry into the medical-industrial complex*, Harmondsworth: Penguin.

D.E. Konold 'History of the codes of ethics' in W.T. Reich (ed.) (1978) *Encyclopedia of Bioethics* 4 vols, Chicago: The Free Press of Glencoe.

J. Ladd (1981) 'Physicians and society: tribulations of power and responsibility' in S.F. Spiker, J.M. Healey and H.T. Engelhardt (eds), *The law-medicine relation: a philosophical exploration*, Boston: Reidel.

P. Lain-Entralgo (1950) *La Historia Clinica*, Madrid.

P. Lain-Entralgo (1955) *Mind and Body* London: Harvill.

P. Lain-Entralgo (1969) *Doctor and Patient*, London: World University Library.

Lake v. *Cameron* 364 F. 2d 657 (D.C. Cir., 1966).

M. Lakoff and G. Johnson (1980) *Metaphors We Live By*, London: University of Chicago Press.

R.E. Lane (1978) 'Markets and the satisfaction of human wants,' *Journal of Economic Issues* 12:815.

M.S. Larson (1977) *The Rise of Professionalism: A Sociological Analysis*, Berkeley: University of California Press.

Latter v. *Braddell* (1891) 50 Law Journal Q.B. 448.

Law Reform Commission of Canada (1979) *Criteria for the Determination of Death*, Working Paper 23.

C.D. Leake (ed.) (1927) *Percival's Medical Ethics*, Baltimore: Williams & Wilkins.

Leeson v. *General Medical Council* (1887) 43 Ch. 362.

G.M. Lewis (1898) *Dr Southwood-Smith – A Retrospect*, Edinburgh: Blackwood.

R.A. Lewis (1952) *Edwin Chadwick and the Public Health Movement, 1832–54*, London: Longmans, Green.

C.W. Lidz *et al.* (1984) *Informed Consent: A Study in Decision-Making in Psychiatry*, New York: Guilford Press.

J. Liebenhau (1983) 'Medicine and technology', *Perpectives in Biology and Medicine* 27:76–92.

G.E.R. Lloyd (1978) *Hippocratic Writings* (first published 1950) Harmondsworth: Penguin.

D. Lockwood (1966) 'Sources of variation in working-class images of society' *Sociological Review* 14:249–67 reprinted in M. Bulmer (ed.) (1975) *Working Class Images of Society*, London: Routledge & Kegan Paul.

H.W. Loewald (1978) *Psychoanalysis and the History of the Individual*, New Haven: Yale University Press.

A. Loizou (1986) *The Reality of Time*, Aldershot: Gower Publishing.

J. Lorber (1985) *Women Physicians: Careers, Status, and Power*, London: Tavistock.

S. Lukes (1973) *Émile Durkheim. His Life and Work: A Historical and Critical Study*, Harmondsworth: Penguin.

C. Lyle (1833) *Principles of Geology*.

N. Machiavelli *The Prince*, trans. H.C. Mansfield (1985) Chicago: University of Chicago Press.

A. MacIntyre (1977) 'Patients as agents', in H.L. Engelhardt and S. Spricker (eds) (1977) *Philosophical Medical Ethics: Its Nature and Significance*, Dordrecht, Netherlands: Reidel:147–212.

C. Mackenzie (1957) *Sublime Tobacco*, London: Chatto & Windus.

I. MacLean (1987) *The Renaissance Notion of Woman: A Study in the fortunes of scholasticism and medical science in European intellectual life*, (first published 1980, this edition first published 1983) Cambridge: Cambridge University Press.

T.P. Magill (1955) 'The immunologist and evil spirits', *Journal of Immunology*, 74:1, quoting M. Greenwood (1936) 'English death rates, past, present and future', *Journal of the Royal Statistical Society*, 99.

D. Mainland (1967) *Health Services Research* 127.

W.F. Mandle (1973) 'Games people played: cricket and football in England and Victoria in the late 19th century', *Historical Studies*, vol.15:514.

W.F. Mandle (1981) 'W.G. Grace as a Victorian hero', *Historical Studies*, vol.19 No.76:353.

R. Mandrou (1978) *From Humanism to Science, 1480–1700*, trans. B Pearce, (1973) Harmondsworth: Pelican.

G. Marcel (1608) *Canon Medicianae*.

H. Marcovitch (1982) 'Higher premiums and cold sweat', *The Health Services*, 26 November:14.

H. Margolis (1982) *Selfishness, Altruism and Rationality, A Theory of Social Choice*, Cambridge: Cambridge University Press.

Marten v. Royal College of Veterinary Disciplinary Committee [1966] 1 Q.B.1.

J.K. Mason and R.A. McCall-Smith (1987) *Law and Medical Ethics* 2nd ed., London: Butterworths.

P. Matthews (1983) 'Whose body? People as property', [1983] *Current Legal Problems* 193–240.

W.F. May (1980) 'Professional ethics', in D. Callahan and S. Bok (eds) *Ethics Teaching in Higher Education*, New York: Plenum Press:205–241.

McCoan v. General Medical Council [1964] 3 All E.R. 143.

T. McCormack (1981) 'The new criticism and the sick role' *Canadian Review of Sociology and Anthropology* 18:30–47.

L.B. McCullough in W.T. Reich (ed.) (1978) *Encyclopedia of Bioethics* 4 vols, Chicago: The Free Press of Glencoe.

W. McDermott (1977) 'Evaluating the physician and his technology', *Daedalus*, 106, No.1:155.

T. McKeown (1979) *The Role of Medicine: Dream, Mirage or Nemesis?*, (first published 1976, Nuffield Provincial Hospitals Trust) Oxford: Blackwell.

Medical Act 1542–3, 34 & 35 Henry 8, c.8.

Medical Act 1511–12, 3 Hen.8, c.11.

C. Melville and A. Johnson (1983) *Cured to Death: The Effects of Prescription Drugs*, London: Secker & Warburg.

A.W. Merrison, (1975) (Chairman) *The Report of the Committee of Inquiry into the Regulation of the Medical Profession* (Cmnd.6018).

R.K. Merton (1965) *On the Shoulders of Giants*, London: Macmillan.

H.A. Meynell (1981) 'Freud translated: an historical and bibliographical note' *Journal of the Royal Society of Medicine* vol 74:306–9.

E.C. Midwinter (1968) *Victorian Social Reform*, London: Longmans.

S. Milgram (1974) *Obedience to Authority*, London: Tavistock.

J.S. Mill (1859) *On Liberty*, C.V. Shields (ed.) (1956) New York: Bobbs-Merrill.

J.S. Mill (1971) *Autobiography*, J. Stillinger (ed.) New York: Oxford University Press.

W.B. Miller (1955) 'Two concepts of authority', *American Anthropologist*, 57:271ff.

S.C.F. Milsom (1969) *The Historical Foundations of the Common Law*, London: Butterworths.

Minister of Health v. *General Committee of The Royal Midland Counties Home of Incurables at Leamington Spa* [1954] 1 Ch. 530.

Misuse of Drugs Act 1971.

H. Mitchell (1981) 'Politics in the service of knowledge: the debate over the administration of medicine in late 18th century France' *Social History* 6:185–207.

Mohr v. *Williams* 104 N.W. 12 (1905).

W.J. Mommsen (1974) *The Age of Bureaucracy: Perspectives on the Political Sociology of Max Weber*, Oxford: Blackwell.

C.L. Montesquieu *The Spirit of the Laws* cited in L. Althusser (1972) *Montesquieu, Rousseau, and Marx*, trans. B. Brewster, 1982 ed. republished London: Verso.

R.J. Morris (1976) *Cholera 1832*, London: Croom Helm.

D. Mueller (1979) *Public Choice*, Cambridge: Cambridge University Press.

W.T. Murphy and R. Rawlings (1981 and 1982) 'After the Ancien Regime', 44 *Modern Law Review*: 617–57 and 45 *Modern Law Review*:34–61.

Natanson v. *Kline* (1960) 186 Kan. 393.

National Assistance Act 1948 s.47.

National Health Service Act 1977.

National Health Service (General Medical and Pharmaceutical) Regulations.

V. Navarro (1978) *Class Struggle, The State and Medicine: An Historical and Contemporary Analysis of the Medical Sector in Great Britain*, Oxford: Martin Robertson.

V. Navarro (1986) *Crisis, Health, and Medicine: A Social Critique*, London: Tavistock.

Nelson v. *Cookson* [1940] 1 KB 100.

I. Newton, (1675/6) Letter to R. Hooke 5 February.

S. Nittis (1942) 'Hippocratic ethics and present-day trends in medicine' *Bulletin of the History of Medicine*. vol.xii:336.

The Normansfield Hospital Enquiry, Department of Health and Social Services (Cmnd 7357, 1977).

V. Nutton (1981) in A.S. Duncan, G.R. Dunston, and R.B. Welbourn (eds) (1981) *Dictionary of Medical Ethics*, London: Darton Longman, & Todd:210–12.

M. Oakeshott (1962) 'Rationalism in politics', *Rationalism in Politics and other Essays*, London: Methuen.

A. Olmstead and S. Sheffrin (1981) 'The medical school admission process: an empirical investigation', *The Journal of Human Resources*, vol.XVI:459–67.

M. Olson (1965) *The Logic of Collective Action*, Cambridge, Mass.: Harvard University Press.

J.R. Oppenheimer (1954) Reith Lectures (1953) 'Science and the common understanding', London: Oxford University Press.

O'Reilly v. *Hull Board of Prison Visitors* [1982] 3 W.L.R. 1092.

A. Ortony (ed.) (1979) *Metaphor and Thought*, Cambridge: Cambridge University Press.

Ouida (Marie Louise de la Ramée) (1893) *The New Priesthood*, London: Chatto.

Outdoor Relief Regulation Order 1852, printed at British Parliamentary Papers 1852–53 LXXXIV.

G. Outka (1972) *Agape: An Ethical Analysis*, New Haven: Yale University Press.

W. Pagel (1968) 'Paracelsus: tradition and medieval sources' in L.G. Stevenson and R.P. Multhauf (eds) *Medicine, Science and Culture*, Baltimore: Johns Hopkins University Press: 51–75.

G. Parker (1920) *The Early History of Surgery in Great Britain*, London: Black.

T. Parsons (1951) 'Personality and social structure', in A. Stranton and S. Perry (eds) Chicago: Free Press of Glencoe.

T. Parsons (1964) *The Social System* (first published 1951) London: Routledge & Kegan Paul.

T. Parsons (1975) 'The sick role and the role of the physician reconsidered', *Milbank Memorial Fund Quarterly* 53.

Lord Pearson (Chairman) (1978) *The Report of the Royal Commission on Civil Liability and Compensation for Personal Injury* (Cmnd 7054).

Edmund Pellegrino and David Thomasma (1981) *A Philosophical Basis of Medical Practice: Toward a Philosophy and Ethic of the Healing Professions*, New York: Oxford University Press.

A.J. Penty (1917) *Old Worlds for New, a Study of the post-Industrial State*, London: Allen & Unwin.

A.J. Penty (1919) *Guilds and the Social Crisis*, London: Allen & Unwin.

A.J. Penty (1920) *A Guildsman's Interpretation of History*, London: George Allen & Unwin.

M. Peterson (1978) *The Medical Profession in Mid-Victorian London*, Berkeley: University of California Press.

M. Phillips and J. Dawson (1985) *Doctors' Dilemmas: Medical Ethics and Contemporary Science*, Brighton: Harvester.

R. Pitt (1703) *The Crafts and Frauds of Physic Expos'd*.

Plato *The Republic*, trans. F. MacDonald Cornford (1955) Oxford: Clarendon.

Pliny *Natural History*, trans. J. Bostock and M.T. Riley (1887–98) London: Bell.

J.H. Plumb (1964) *The Pelican Book of the Renaissance* (first published 1961) Harmondsworth: Pelican.

Poisons Act 1972.

M. Polanyi (1951) *The Logic of Liberty*, London: Routledge.

Poor Law Commissioners, (1836) *6th Annual Report, PLB 1839–40*.

K.R. Popper (1961) *The Poverty of Historicism*, (second ed. first published 1960) London: Routledge & Kegan Paul.

K.R. Popper (1979) *Objective Knowledge: An Evolutionary Approach* (rev. ed) Oxford: Clarendon Press.

R. Porter (1987a) *In Sickness and In Health: Experiences of the Body and Illness in Eighteenth-Century England*, Oxford: Polity Press.

R. Porter (ed.) (1987b) *Patients and Practitioners: Lay Perceptions of Medicine in Pre-Industrial Society*, Cambridge: Cambridge University Press.

R. Posner (1977) *Economic Analysis of Law*, (2nd ed.) Boston: Little, Brown & Co.

C. Powell and G.E.C. Paton (eds) (1987) *Humour in Society: Resistance and Control*, London: Macmillan.

Pratt v. *Davis* (1905) 128 Ill.App.161.

R.V. Presthus (1962) 'Authority in organizations' in *Concepts and Issues in Administrative Behaviour*, S. Mailick and E.H. van Ness (ed.) Englewood Cliffs, NJ: Prentice-Hall.

L. Prior (1985) 'The social organization of death: medical discourses and social practices in Belfast', Unpublished Ph.D, University of Aberdeen.

R. v. *General Medical Council ex parte Organ* (1861) 3 El. & El.524.

R. v. *General Medical Council ex parte Kynaston* [1930] 1 K.B. 562.

R. v. *Askew* (1768) 4 Burr.2168.

R. v. *Secretary of State for Social Services et al., ex parte Hincks et al.* (1980) Transcript, 18 March, Court of Appeal.

R. v. *East Berkshire Health Authority ex parte Walsh* (1984) *The Times* 15 May 1984.

R. v. *Master and Wardens of the Company of Surgeons* (1766) 2 Burr. 892.

R. v. *Lynn* (1788) cited in Select Committee Report (1828) *British Parliamentry Papers* vii p.6.

J. Rajchman (1985) *Michel Foucault: The Freedom of Philosophy*, New York, Columbia University Press.

The Rampton Hospital Enquiry, 1979–80 (Cmnd. 8073).

P. Ramsey (1970) *The Patient as Person – Exploration in Medical Ethics*, New Haven: Yale University Press.

Razzel v. *Snowball* [1954] 1 W.L.R. 1382.

Re Palmer, ex parte Crabb (1856) 8 De G.M. & G. 277; 44 E.R. 397.

Re V.E. [1973] 1 Q.B. 452.

W.T. Reich (ed.in chief) (1978) *Encyclopedia of Bioethics* 4 vols, Chicago: The Free Press of Glencoe.

W.T. Reich (ed.) (1983) *Encyclopedia of Bioethics*, 2 vols, London: Collier Macmillan.

I.A. Richards (1926) *Science and Poetry*, London: K Paul.

Sir B.W. Richardson (1901) *The Disciples of Aesculapius*, London: Hutchinson.

P. Ricoeur (1978) *The Rule of Metaphor*, trans. R. Czerny (1986) London: Routledge & Kegan Paul cited in J.F. Childress (1982) *Who Should Decide? Paternalism in Health Care*, New York: Oxford University Press:5ff.

S. Roberts (1979) *Order and Dispute: An Introduction to Legal Anthropology*, Harmondsworth, Pelican.

J. Robertson (ed.) (1975) *Materials for the History of Thomas Becket*, 1875–85, cited in R.C. Finucane (1975) 'The use and abuse of medieval miracles', *History* (Journal of the Historical Association), vol. 60:1–10.

Robinson, (1832) *Hansard*, xii col.318.

Rose v. *College of Physicians* (1703) 5 Bro. Parl. Cas. 553.

I. Ross and C.U. Ross (1979) 'Body snatching in nineteenth century Britain: from exhumation to murder', *British Journal of Law and Society* 108.

J.J. Rousseau (1957) *Émile*, trans. B. Foxley, London: Dent.

Royal College of Nursing v. *Department of Health and Social Security* [1981] 1 All E.R. 545.

Royal College of Physicians (1987) *A Great and Growing Evil: The Medical Consequences of Alcohol Abuse*, London: Tavistock.

Royal College of Psychiatrists (1987) *Alcohol: Our Favourite Drug*, London: Tavistock.

Royal College of Surgeons *British Parliamentry Papers*, 1831–2 xlv, 29–31, dated 10 December, 1831.

Royal College of Surgeons v. *National Provincial Bank* [1952] A.C. 631.

The Royal Commission on Civil Liability and Compensation for Personal Injury (Cmnd 7054, 1978).

D. Rueschemeyer (1983) 'Professional autonomy and the social control of expertise' in R. Dingwall and P. Lewis (eds) *The Sociology of the Professions: Lawyers, Doctors and Others*, London: Macmillan: 38ff.

W.G. Runciman (1978) *Max Weber – Selections in Translation*, Cambridge: Cambridge University Press.

B. Russell (1925) *ABC of Relativity*, London: Unwin.

B. Russell (1985) *A History of Western Philosophy* (first published 1945, 1961 ed.) Cambridge: Cambridge University Press.

K.E. Ruthschuh (1972) 'Der Krankheitsbegriff', *Hippokrates*, vol.43:3–17.

St Germain (1969) *Doctor and Student*, cited in S.C.F. Milsom (1969) *The Historical Foundations of the Common Law*, London: Butterworths: 382.

St Matthew *Gospel*

J.W. Salmon (1985) *Alternative Medicines: Popular and Policy Perspectives*, London: Tavistock.

P. Santarcangeli (1979) 'The jester and the madman, heralds of liberty and truth', *Diogenes* 101:28.

J.–P. Sartre *Dirty Hands* cited in A.O. Hirschman (1982) *Shifting Involvements, Private Interest and Public Action*, Oxford: Martin Robertson.

T. Scheff (1963) 'Decision rules, types of error, and their consequences', *Behavioural Science* 8:7–107.

F. Schlegel (1876) *Lucinde*, trans. R. Firchow, (1971) *F. Schlegel, Lucinde and Fragments*, Duluth, Minn: University of Minnesota Press.

T. Scitovsky (1977) *The Joyless Economy; An Inquiry into Human Satisfaction, and Consumer Dissatisfaction*, New York: Oxford University Press.

G. Scorer and A. Wing (eds) (1979) *Decision Making in Medicine*, London: Edward Arnold.

Select Committee, Report, (1828) *British Parliamentry Papers* vii 6.

P. Selznick (1957) *Leadership in Administration*, Evanston, Ill.: Row, Peterson.

A. Sen (1977) 'Rational fools: a critique of the behavioural foundations of economic theory', *Philosophy and Public Affairs* 6:336.

Seneca *de Beneficiis*, trans. T. Lodge, W.H.D. Rouse (ed.) (1896), London: Dent.

Lord Seymour in the Board's Supply Vote on 6 July, 1854, *Hansard*, vol.cxxxiv 1298–1300 and on the Second Reading of the Amendment Bill on 31 July, 1854 *Hansard*, vol.cxxxv 980–94.

W. Shakespeare (1946) *As You Like It*, Harmondsworth: Penguin.

W. Shakespeare (1955) *The Tragedy of Coriolanus*, Harmondsworth: Penguin.

A.K. Shapiro (1960) 'A contribution to history of the placebo effect', *Behavioral Science*, v:109–35.

G.B. Shaw (1911) *The Doctor's Dilemma*, (this edition 1930) London: Constable & Co.

P.B. Shelley (1819) 'Love's Philosophy', T. Hutchinson (ed.) *Shelley's Poetical Works* (1919) Oxford: Oxford University Press.

P.B. Shelley (1821) *A Defence of Poetry*, published 1840 and reprinted in R.A. Duerksen (ed.) (1970) *Political Writings*, New York: Appleton-Century-Crofts.

F. Sherwood Taylor (1943) *A Short History of Science*, London: Heinemann.

S. Shetreet (1976) *Judges on Trial*, Amsterdam: North-Holland.

Shorter Oxford English Dictionary.

Sidaway v. *Bethlem Royal Hospital Governors and Others* [1984] 1 All E.R. 1018 (Court of Appeal).

Sidaway v. *Bethlem Royal Hospital Governors and Others* [1985] 1 All E.R. 643 (House of Lords).

S.A. Siegal (1981) 'The Aristotelian basis of English law, 1450–1800', 56 *New York University Law Review* 18.

H.E. Sigerist (1961) *A History of Medicine*, vol.1, *Primitive and Archaic Medicine*, New York: Oxford University Press.

G. Simmel (1907) *Philosophie des Geldes*, 2nd ed. Leipzig: Duncker und Humblot.

Slater v. Baker (1767) 95 E.R. 860.

Adam Smith (1779) *An Inquiry into the Nature and Causes of the Wealth of Nations* Skinner A. (ed.) (1974, 1982 rev.) Harmondsworth, Penguin.

R.J. Smith (1987) *The Gothic Bequest: Medieval Institutions in British Thought, 1688–1863*, Cambridge: Cambridge University Press.

Society of Architects v. Kendrick (1910) 26 T.L.R. 433.

S. Sontag (1979) *Illness as Metaphor*, New York: Random House.

Sophocles (1954) *Antigone*, trans. George Murray, London: Allen & Unwin.

T. Southwood-Smith (1828) *On the uses of the Dead to the Living*, reprinted from the Westminster Review 1825.

T. Southwood-Smith (1830) *Treatise on Fever*. And see *Westminster Review* 1825:519.

S.S. Sprigge (1895) *The Life and Times of Thomas Wakley*, London: Longmans.

Spring Rice, *Hansard*, xii (1832) col.311.

The Stafford Hospital Enquiry, 1985.

A. Stanway (1979) *Alternative Medicine, A Guide to Natural Therapies*, Harmondsworth: Pelican.

State v. Housekeeper 16 A. 328 (1889).

P. Stein (1984) *Legal Institutions: The Development of Dispute Settlement*, London: Butterworth.

T. Szasz (1979) *The Theology of Medicine: The Political-Philosophical Foundations of Medical Ethics* Oxford: Oxford University Press.

R.H. Tawney (1926) *Religion and the Rise of Capitalism*, reprinted 1969, Harmondsworth: Pelican.

R.H. Tawney (1982) *The Acquisitive Society*, Brighton and London: Harvester.

H. Teff (1985) 'Consent to medical procedures: paternalism, self-determination or therapeutic alliance', vol.101 *Law Quarterly Review* 432–53.

O. Temkin (1952) 'The elusiveness of Paracelsus', *Bulletin of the History of Medicine* 26:201–17.

Tendring Union v. Woolwich Union [1923] 1 K.B. 121.

Tennyson, Alfred Lord, (1854) *The Charge of the Light Brigade*.

A. Thevet (1558) *The New Found Worlde*, trans. T. Hacket 1568.

V.A. Thompson (1977) *Modern Organization*, 2nd ed., Alabama: University of Alabama Press.

Thompson v. Lewis (1828) 3 C. & P. 483.

D. Tuckett (ed.) (1976) *An Introduction to Medical Sociology*, London: Tavistock.

J. Tudor Hart (1981) 'A new kind of doctor', *Journal of the Royal Society of Medicine*, 74:871–82.

B. Turner (1984) *The Body and Society, Explorations in Social Theory*, Oxford: Blackwell.

Tuson v. Batting 1800 3 Esp. 192.

A.C. Twaddle (1969) 'Health decisions and sick role variations: An Exploration', *Journal of Health and Social Behavior*, X:108.

Vaccination Act 1840 3 & 4 Vict. c.29.

Vaccination Act 1841 4 & 5 Vict. c.32.

S. Vaisrub (1977) *Medicine's Metaphors: Messages and Menaces*, Oradell, NJ: Medical Economics.

P. Vaughan (1959) *Doctors' Commons, A Short History of the British Medical Association*, London: Heinemann.

B. Vickers (ed.) (1987) *English Science, Bacon to Newton*, Cambridge: Cambridge University Press.

R. Virchow, (1858) *Cellular Pathology*, trans. F. Chance, (1865) New York: R.M. de Witt.

H. Vuori (1983) 'Medicalization of social phenomena', *Scandinavian Journal of Social Medicine* (S31):95–110.

I. Waddington (1984) *The Medical Profession in the Industrial Revolution*, London: Gill & Macmillan.

H. Waitztein and J. Stoectcle (1972) 'The communication of information about illness' *Advances in Psychosomatic Medicine* 8:180.

C. Wall and H.C. Cameron (1963) *History of the Worshipful Society of Apothecaries*, New York: Oxford University Press.

M. Walzer 'Political action: the problem of dirty hands', (1973) *Philosophy and Public Affairs* 2:160–80.

Sir Pelham Warner (1950) *Gentlemen v. Players 1806–1949* cited in D.C. Coleman (1973) 'Gentlemen and Players', *Economic History Review* 26:92–116.

M. Webb-Peploe (1979) 'The medical profession' in G. Scorer and A. Wing (eds), *Decision Making in Medicine*, London: Edward Arnold.

M. Weber (1946) 'Politics as a vocation', in H. Gerth and C.W. Mills (ed. and trans.) *From Max Weber*, New York and Oxford.

M. Weber (1947) *The Theory of Social and Economic Organization*, (trans.) A.M. Henderson and T. Parsons, reprinted 1964, Chicago: The Free Press of Glencoe.

M. Weber (1930) *The Protestant Ethic and the Spirit of Capitalism*, trans. T. Parsons and published in this edition 1985 London: Unwin.

C. Webster (1979) (ed.) 'Alchemical and Paracelsian medicine' in *Health, Medicine and Mortality in the Sixteenth Century*, Cambridge: Cambridge University Press.

P. Weiler (1968) 'Two models of judicial decision-making' 46 *Canadian Bar Review* 406.

White (1975) *The Hastings Center Report* 5 no.3:9.

Whitwell v. Shakesby (1932) 48 T.L.R. 489.

J.W. Wilcox (1830) *The Laws Relating to the Medical Profession*.

R. Williams (1958) *Culture and Society*, London: Chatto & Windus.

Sir A. Wilson and H. Levy (1938) *Burial Reform and Funeral Costs*, Oxford: Oxford University Press.

C.M. Wilson later Lord Moran (1928) Pay beds and the future of the voluntary hospitals' *British Medical Journal* 17 March:85.

G.R. Winslow (1982) *Triage and Justice: The Ethics of Rationing Life-Saving Medical Resources*, London: University of California Press.

J.M. Winter (1982) in T. Barker and M. Drake (eds) *Population and Society in Britain 1850–1950*, London: Batsford.

A. Wolf (1935) *A History of Science, Technology and Philosophy in the Sixteenth and Seventeenth Centuries*, London: George Allen & Unwin.

C. Wolf (1970) 'The present value of the past', *Journal of Political Economy* 78:783–92.

Woodward v. *Ball* (1834) 6 C. & P.571, 172 E.R. 1372.

Wyatt v. *Stickney* 344 F. Supp. 387 (MD Ala.1972) discussed in Note, 'The *Wyatt* case: implementation of a judicial decree ordering institutional change', (1985) 84 *Yale Law Journal* 1338.

R.M. Young (1985) *Darwin's Metaphor: Nature's Place in Victorian Culture*, Cambridge: Cambridge University Press.

R.M. Zaner (1970) *The Way of Phenomenology*, New York: Pegasus.

D. Zaridze and R. Peto (eds) (1986) *Tobacco: A Major International Health Hazard*, Oxford: Oxford University Press.

M. Zborowski (1958) 'Cultural components in response to pain' in E.G. Jaco (ed.) *Patients, Physicians and Illness*, New York: Free Press.

I.K. Zola (1966) 'Culture and symptoms: an analysis of patients presenting complaints', *American Sociological Review*, 31.

Index

Abel, R.L., 162–3, 164
Abel-Smith, B., 97, 102, 108, 153
abortion, 23, 153, 192, 198
academic training, 142; *see also*
  hospitals; medical schools;
  universities
acute illness, 32
administration and medicine, 143–
  72
administrative response to,
  untoward, 158, 163–4
Aesculapius, 21, 42, 54, 68, 105
affective neutrality, 34–5
alcohol abuse, 62, 64
Allende, S., 66
almoners, 105
alternative medicine, 42, 63, 64, 72
Amendment Act (1886), 105
American Medical Association,
  200; *see also* United States
anasthaesia, 106, 108
anatomy, 91; cadavers for, 86–7;
  teaching of, 34
Anatomy Act (1832), 34, 86–7
Annual Register (1832), 145
anti/a-septic techniques, 105
Apollo, 42, 192
apothecaries, 20, 94–7, 120, 142,
  183; disappearing role of, 100;
  105; as distinct from doctors,
  109, 141, 206
Apothecaries, Society of, 95–6,
  101, 104

Apothecaries Act (1815), 101, 107,
  129, 139, 206
Apothecaries Company, 97
appeal, right of, 139
Apple, D., 31
Arabia, 88
Aristotle, 47, 48, 195
Arnold, T., 121
Arnott, Dr, 146
art, medicine as, 41, 48, 130, 166,
  172, 192
Arte de Medici, 91
asceticism 43; *see also* Pythagorean
Atiyah, P., 98–9, 143
authority, 152, 153; collective, 186;
  of doctors, 69, 106, 117, 168,
  178; -based medicine, 171
autonomy, professional, 156

Bacon, F., 81
Baker, J., 98–9
barber-surgeons, 94–5
Barber Surgeons Act (1540), 205
Barbers Company, 207
Barbers Hall, 96
bargain theory, 3, 10, 115, 134–6
Barlow, N., 85
Beauchamp, T.L., 169
Beccaria, C., 186
behaviour, compulsive, 62; as
  determinant for health, 57
Bentham, J., 87, 145–6, 186

Berlant, J.L., 112–13, 116–17, 132–3

Berlinguer, G., 62

Bernard, C., 37, 85

Best, C.J., 94–5

Bevan, A., 18, 66

Bioethics Library, 24

biological laws, 189

biomedical ethics (bioethics), 22

biomedicine, xv, 6, 21–2, 34, 162; nature of, 24, 65, 66; regulation of, 6, 67, 149

biotechnology, 22, 32, 35, 172, 180

Birkinshaw, P., 158

Black Report, 32, 40

Bloor, G.W., 59–60

Board of Guardians, 105, 107

Boards of Health, 3, 145

Bobbitt, P., 161

'bodyline', 122, 185

Booth, W., 86

Borough Engineers, 146

Boyle, R., 186

British Medical Journal, 103, 129

British Medical Association, 3, 154, 156; aims of, 109; campaigns of, 104; influence of, 104–5, 129, 135, 157

Brown, L.J., 139

bureaucracy, 3, 4, 29, 110; changes in, 15, 79, 145; organisation of medicine, 9, 77, 178, 179; regulation, 137, 147–53; state health, 144–5, 155

Burt, R.A., on doctor–patient relationship, 73, 173–9; Rule of Opposites, 68–9, 165, 181

Cabanis, 147

Cain, M., 62

Calabresi., G., 161

cancer, 'recovery' from, 21

Cancer Act (1939), 64

Canguilhem, G., 49, 169

cannabis, 67

capitalism, 126

care, *see* health care; primary; secondary; tertiary

Cartwright, F.F., 19, 92, 145

Cassirer, E., 50

Castiglione, B., 117–20, 182

catastrophe, 164

Cave Committee, 106

cell-theory, 85

Cellini, B., 21

Central Board of Health, 145

Chadwick, E., 104, 143, 145–6

Charing Cross Hospital, 102

charity, definition of, 98

Chaucer, G., 209

chemotherapy, 32, 84, 105

Childress, J.F., 65, 169

China, 66

choice, 12, 161, 190–1; individual, 68–9, 176, 178, 188

cholera, 145–6; Regulations/ Prevention Act, 145

chronic illness, 32–3

church, 17, 89, 186; authority of, 38, 84–5, 90; Catholic, 186; control of medicine, 92; mediaeval, 124; as rival to medicine, 20

Churchill, W., 16

Cicero, 90

Civil War, 182

Clark, Sir G., 95, 96, 104, 144

class, social, 66, 161–2

classical (Hippocratic) medicine, 2, 8, 35–61 *passim*, 93, 172; asceticism, 3, 98, 112; current expressions of, xv, 11, 117; disease as natural, 19–20; distinct from economics, 141, 147; in hospitals, 106; in practice, 168–9, 184–5; and professional confidence, 103; and religion, 171; and science, 82, 88–9; *see also* gentleman

clinic, 6, 22, 32–5, 66; development of, 86, 105; Foucault on, 22, 33–5, 45, 147, 180; and role of doctor, 58, 78; and morality, 34; mysticism of, 45, 54

clinical, decisions; 46, 50; encounter, 6; experience, 34; freedom, 155, 167; interaction, 8–9, 22, 47, 56; judgement, 49; procedures, 59; relationship, 47

clinician, 58; *see also* clinic

Code of Ethics, *see* ethics

Coke, E., 81

Coleman, D.C., 118, 120

Coleridge, S.T., 85

Colet, J., 90, 93

collectivism, 30, 48, 127, 180, 190, 191

Colleges, see Royal College

'comfort', 47, 71–3

committees of medical profession, 139

commonalities of individuals, 189

community, doctors' relationship to, 180

Community Health Councils, 157, 164

Company of Physicians and Act (1523), 92, 205

compensation, medical injury, 162, 163, 165

competence, doctors' technical, 30, 110

Comte, A., 82

concern, public, 187

confidentiality, 12–13, 42, 43, 192

consensus between patient and doctor, 12

consent, 29, 30, 168–73, 214; informed consent theory, 35, 62, 69, 176, 177, 180, 184–5; lack of, in treatment, 49; mutual, in healing, 48; rights of, 12

consultants, 105, 183, 184

consumerism, 2, 67, 69, 184; in demand for health care, 73–4, 80; growth of, 10, 132

contract, breach of, 168; freedom of, 143; social, 182

control, of body by individual, 177; bureaucratic, 155; social mechanisms, 158; *see also* sanctions

Corvisant, J.-N., 34

Council on Professions Supplementary to Medicine, 155

Counterblast to Tobacco, 64

court cases, *see* law, litigation

courtiers, 117–18

crash helmet campaign, 104

cricket, 120–3, 185

cultural differences, 31, 72

cure, 11, 35, 47, 50, 72, 135; artificially induced, 20–1; concept of, 20–1, 40, 109; definition of, 18–19; as focus of medicine, 39, 58, 112, 135; natural, 2

custom, 161; of profession, 167

Dahrendorf, R., 191

Dalton, J., 84

damages, payment of, 163, 165

Daremberg, C.V., 88

Darwin, C., xiv, 36, 85–6

Darwin, E., 85

Davis, K.C., 162

death, 18–19, 28, 68, 194; revival from, 20–1; *see also* mortality

Della Casa, 118, 208

democratic theory, 35

Denning, Lord, 140

Department of Health, 157, 163

Descartes, R., 32, 35, 40, 48, 81, 86

deviance, 28; from standards, 123

Dewey, J., xiv

diagnosis, 12, 29, 49

dignity, human, 188

Dioscorides, 88, 89, 91

disciplinary committees/cases, 130, 138–9

disease/illness, 18, 39, 55, 56, 86, 135; aspects of, 25, 48–9, 51, 106; cultural view of, 197; divine cause of, 89, 143; economic cost

disease/illness *cont'd*
of, 146; as focus of medicine,
28–9, 32–5, 39, 47–9, 58–9; as
independent entity, 39–40;
morality of, 32; natural basis of,
20, 85; perception of, 72, 184; as
preventable, 143–4, 146;
requiring state action, 143;
science in, 30; as social
dysfunction, 48; stress of, 178;
supernatural causes of, 41, 89, *see
also* public health
Dispensaries, 183
disputes, 158, 160–1, 172, 178, 179
District Health Authority, 155
doctor, *see* administration;
practice; professionalism; Royal
College; theories
doctor–patient relationship, 9, 12,
22, 48–9, 135, 168–72, 183; and
clinic, 45; and consent, 28–31,
62, 173, 176, 180; and
consumerism, 67; disappointment in, 73; doctor's role in,
153; history of, 109, 215;
inequality in, 161; interdependence in, 177; law and, 178–9;
moral agencies, 182; reciprocity,
58, 154–5; *see also* patients
Donaldson, M.R., 171
Donne, J., 190
Donzelot, J., 98
doubt, 187
drugs, 104, 109; abuse, 62, 64, 65,
therapy, 23, 61, 201
duality of mind and body, 2, 32,
35, 48
Dubos, R., 61
Durkheim, E., xi, 10, 137; on
individual consciousness, 90; on
groups, 95, 123–4, 125–32, 134
duty, of doctors, 2, 11; social, 16

economic liberalism, growth of, 98,
143, 147
economic response to untoward,

loss adjustment, 158, 160–1;
class control, 158, 161–3
economics, xiv, 4, 35, 70–1, 182,
184; and consumerism, 71, 75,
132; medicine distinguished from,
147; and professionalism, 111,
127, 141; and theories of
untoward, 10, 161
Edinburgh Medical School, 111
Elias, N., 57, 118
elite, doctors as, 11, 14, 90, 102,
132
empiricism, 41, 82
*Encyclopaedia of Health Services
and Medical Law*, 4, 138, 157,
167, 168, 170
Enlightenment, 16, 36, 82, 99, 181,
185–7, 198
epidemic disease, 143, 145
epilepsy, 20
Erasmus, D., 60, 89, 90, 93, 118
ethics, 22, 40, 126–7, 130, 198;
codes of, 52, 131, 132, 172; codes
as sanctions, 125, 166, 169;
definitions of, 7, 169;
enforcement of, 105, 110; as
values, 50–1, 110; *see also* morals
etiquette, 7, 167; *see also* courtier;
gentleman
Etzioni, A., 152, 153, 155, 156
Europe, 64, 96, 147, 169; culture
of, 17, 18; in history, 88, 111,
185–6; quarantine, 144
evolution, theory of, 85–6
exotic disease, 143
expectations, of patients, 72; of
society, 51, 66, 91, 93–4, 167
exploitation, 94, 188

faith, power of, 21, 30
Faraday, M., 83
fault, investigation of, 164
financial reward, *see* income
Finucane, R.C., 20, 21, 117
Florence, 91, 93
Forbes, R.A., 100

Foucault, J.B.L., 84
Foucault, M., xiii, 5, 46, 80, 127, 187; on clinic, 22, 33–5, 45, 147, 180; on health, 63; on role of doctors, 33–5, 100; on organisation of medicine, 103, 111
France, 96, 111, 144, 147, 185–6
Frank, J. 23
Frankfurt, H.G., 75
Franklin, B., 83
freedom, 4, 27, 65, 191; clinical, 167
Freidson, E., 2, 116, 123, 142, 182, 188; on autonomy, 125, 156; on organisations, 136; on professions, 14, 18, 71, 90, 110 113–15
Freud, S., 65

Galen, 86, 88, 89, 91, 93, 102
Galileo, 83
Galvani, L., 83
General Board of Health, 146
General Medical Council, 104, 105, 130, 135, 139, 140, 156, 157, 183
general practitioners, 2, 33, 183; changes in, 156; faith in, 21; history, 102, 105; rewards of, 133, 154; status of, 123
genetics, 22, 32
gentleman, ideal/typical, 44–5, 79, 142, 183; attributes of, 117–23; concept of, 132, 182; definition of, 101, 111, 116–23; development of, 90–1; ideology of, 77, 131; morality, 140, 168; recognition in law, 3, 168; status of, 103
Germany, 111
Giesen, I.D., 25, 169
Gilbert, 83
Germain, St, 81
Godel, K., 24
government, *see* state
Grace, W.G., 77, 121, 122–3
Graves, H., 121

Greece, Ancient, 88, 124
Gregory, J., 44
Grocers Company, 94, 95
group practice, 156
groups, 123, 127, 128–9, 130–1, 181, 182; and autonomy, 159; cohesion, 3
guilds, 3, 123, 147, 149, 180; autonomy of, 124–5; early medical, 4, 94–5; as Hippocratic, 43; mediaeval, 210; as organised morality, 132; power of, 95, 172; as social group, 9, 130–1, 134–5, 159
gunpowder, 91
Guy's Hospital, 97, 204

Harvey, W., 83
Hawthorn, G., 17, 86, 123, 126, 185–6
hazard notices, 163
HC81/5, 157
healing, relationship of, 48, 50
health, 6, 28, 56, 59, 60; aetiology of, 18–19; authorities, 154, 157; care, 9, 32, 66; care services, 23, 130, 132, 150, 155; determinants of, 66; improvement of, 72; influence of physician on, 58; interpretation of, 9, 20, 51, 65–6, 135; language of, 67–8; mechanistic model, 32, 40; *see also* National Health Service
Health Advisory Service, 157, 164
Health Service, 148; Act (1977), 149
Health Service Commissioners, 157, 164, 171
Health Service Complaints Act (1985), 164
Health Service Tribunal, 157
health-based theories, 2, 56–79
Henry VIII, 92, 144
hierarchy, professional, 153
Hill, M.J., 152

Hincks et al, ex parte, 148
Hippocrates, 1, 33, 86, 91, 136,
    142; code of ethics, 52; on
    health, 72; legacy of, 41, 88, 89;
    links with Pythagorus, 117
Hippocratic medicine *see* classical;
    oath, 42–3, 44, 107–8, 192;
    recognition of surgery, 90;
    gentleman/physician, *see*
    gentleman
Hirsch, F., 75
Hirschman, A.O., 127, 181, 185;
    on collective action, 76; on
    consumption, 70–1, 73–5; on
    pleasure and comfort, 47, 71, 73,
    77–81; on public–private cycle,
    67, 69, 122, 187; on *vita
    contemplativa*, 117
historico-anthropological response
    to untoward, 158–60
history of medicine, 19, 81–108,
    118
Hobhouse, L.T., ix
Hoby, Sir T., 118
holism, 181
Holmes, G., 111
Horace, 190
Horobin, G., 117, 185
Horobin, M.J., 59–60
hospitals, foundation of, 97–8;
    medical schools, 105, 120;
    nationalization of, 154;
    specialized, 102; teaching, 33,
    106, 107, 129, 156; voluntary, 4,
    102, 105, 107, 183
House of Lords, 153
Hughes, E.C., 1, 129, 142
Hughes, T., 121
Hume, D., 37, 82, 187
Huxley, T.H., 37, 86
Hyde, A., 8
Hygeia, 42, 192

iatocracy, 6, 104, 108, 123, 207
ideal/typical gentleman, *see*
    gentleman

idealism of medical profession,
    116–17
Illich, I., 61, 62, 64
illness, *see* disease
immunisation programmes, 56
income of doctors, 76, 102, 130,
    211; conflict with gentleman
    ideal, 103, 131–2; and
    professionalism, 116–7, 141; and
    status, 132
Independent Broadcasting
    Authority, 64
individuals, commonalities of, 189;
    and relation to others, 185, 190;
    see also self/selves
individualism, 187; as destructive
    of self, 27, 188; growth of, 38,
    99, 186; in United States, 5, 17
industrial growth, 98, 143
Industrial Revolution, 102, 109,
    120; changes in society, 15, 16;
    and institutions, 97, 111;
    technologies of, 20, 83
influence, as authority, 152; of
    doctors, 168
information to patients, 170–1
informed consent theory, *see*
    consent
injury, industrial, 146; 'medical',
    160, 162, 163, 165
inquiries, 163–5, 171
Institute of Advertising, 64
institutions, 4, 5, 136, 188, 191

James I, King, 64
James, C.L.R., 121, 122, 185
Johnson, T.J., 62
Justinian, Roman law of, 124

Kant, I., 36, 55, 6°, 123, 169
Kay, Dr, 146
Kelvin, W.T., 84
Kennedy, I., 166–7; on doctors'
    authority, 61, 131, 171–2; on
    patients' decision-making, 62,
    64; Reith Lectures, 80

Kennedy Institute, 24
Khayyam, Omar, 81
Kings College Hospital, 102

Ladd, J., 117
Lancet, 103, 108
Larson, M.S., 116
Lavoisier, A.L., 84, 99
law, xiii, 4, 7; criminal, 139, 157
law/legislation and medicine, 64,
    105, 145, 154, 166–7; anatomy,
    34, 86–7; apothecaries, 101, 107,
    129, 139, 206; and ethics, 130;
    health service, 149, 164;
    litigation, 4, 80, 138–9, 148–9,
    159, 165–8; mysticism of
    medicine challenged, 55;
    physicians, 92, 205; public
    health, 3, 57, 146, 147; regulation
    in, 36, 136, 140, 147–53;
    theories, 23–5, 152; and
    untoward, 156–7, 159–60, 162–
    5; *see also* Medical Acts;
    National Health; Poor Laws
leadership, 152
Leake, C.D., 7
Leeson v. *General Medical Council*
    (1887), 139
legislation, *see* law
'legitimate domination', 150
legitimation, concept of, 8
Leibnitz, G.W., 99
leprosy, 56, 144
Leyden, 111
liability, 11; criminal/civil, 157,
    165; medical, 4, 11, 167–8
liberty, 68, 190–1; individual, 5
licensing, 113
lifestyles, natural, 185
Linacre, T., 93
Lister, J., 106
litigation, *see* law
Lloyd, G.E.R., 142
Lloyd-George, D., 66
local authorities, powers of, 146
Local Government Board, 144, 147

Locke, J., 17, 186
London, 93, 94, 95, 105, 133, 144
London Hospital, 97
London University, 102
Luther, M., 90

Machiavelli, N., 78, 118, 188
madhouses, 144
magic, 30
Malinowski, B., 30
malpractice, 180, 181; development
    of, 148, 168; Hippocrates on, 1;
    scientific medicine and, 171;
    untoward as, 80, 160, 165; *see*
    also misconduct
Mandle, W.F., 122
Mandrou, R., 16
'manners', 90, 209
Margolis, H., 75–6
Marx, K., xiv, 124
materialism, 84
May, W.F., 133
McDermott, W., 58
Mackenzie, C., 57
McKeown, T., 160; on doctors'
    role, 58, 154; on definition of
    health, 9, 56; on determinants for
    health, 56–7, 64, 66; on medical
    developments, 61, 62
mechanistic view of body, 32, 35,
    40, 86, 201
Medical Acts, 130, 134, 139–40;
    (1511–12), 92; (1542–3), 95;
    (1858), 3, 104–5, 129, 135, 139,
    141, 183; Amendment Act
    (1886), 105
Medical Officers of Health, 146
medical records, 12
medicine, *see* administration;
    practice; professionalism; Royal
    College; theories
Mendel, G., 14
merits, 162
Merrison Report, 134–5
Metropolitan Poor Law Act (1867),
    108; *see also* Poor Law

Michaelangelo, 91
Middlesex Hospital, 97
midwifery, 105
Milgram, S., 174
Mill, J.S., 4–5, 68, 169–70, 176
Ministry of Health, 144
misconduct, 140, 157, 159; *see also*
   malpractice
mobility, upward, 142
Mommsen, W.J., 150
monastic medicine, 88
monopolization, 112
Montesquieu, C.L., 16
moral(s), 7, 126, 185; agencies, 2,
   31, 52, 53, 59, 60, 161, 182, 186;
   choices, 46; and clinic, 34; codes,
   79, 125; medical, 50, 92, 130;
   obligations, 47; power, 127;
   professional, 22, 123, 129, 134,
   140, 167; satisfaction, 165; as
   social concept, 187; *see also*
   ethics
More, Sir T., 90, 93
mortality, infant, 146; trends of,
   56–7; *see also* death
mysticism, 108; challenged by law,
   55; classical theory and, 11, 36;
   in current practice, 21, 54, 80,
   87; degrading patients, 61; from
   Oath, 43, 44–5; rejected, 67, 72–
   3, 86, 91

National Assistance Act (1948), 154
National Health Act (1946), 129,
   153
National Health Service, 9, 130,
   137, 148, 153–6, 183, 213
National Health Service Act (1977),
   164
National Vaccine Establishment,
   144
natural seen as good, 185
negligence, *see* malpractice
neoterici, 91
neutrality, of doctors, 35; of
   science, 38

Newman, J.H., x
Newton, I., 14, 83, 99
Nicot, J., 63
non-intervention, 43
norms, described, 6–7; *see also*
   ethics; law; morality; state
Nuisances, Inspectors of, 146
number of doctors, increase in, 91,
   102, 110, 129–30, 194
nutrition, 66, 72

Oakeshott, M., 182
obligations, of doctors, 167; moral,
   47
Olson, M., 76
opiates, 109
Origin of Species, 85
Ouida, 79

pagan, oath as, 42
Pagel, W., 91
Panacea, 42, 192
pandemic disease, 143
Paracelsus, 91
paraprofessions, 110
Parker, Lord C.J., 140
Parsons, T., 46, 161, 169; on
   affective neutrality, 34–5,
   concept of medicine, 8, 47; on
   disease, 48; model of medical
   practice, 28–32, 45, 53, 58–9, 63,
   154; on professionalism, 132–3
participatory medicine, 2, 8, 35–6,
   39, 45–55
Pasteur, L., 85–6, 106
paternalism, 5, 79, 184, 188, 200
patients, 11, 39–40, 69, 192; co-
   operation of, 41, 170; degraded,
   61, 79, 170, 172; duties of, 2;
   help sought by, 70, 116–7, 154,
   176, 196; helplessness of, 178;
   information to, 170–1, 172, 181;
   moral agency of, 2, 31, 52, 53,
   59, 60; rights, 167; role of, 78,
   180; self-determination, 2, 5, 62,
   63, 69, 73, 80, 168–73, 176, 177,
   178, 181; self-image of, 48, 177,

178; situation liability, 168; view of illness, 169, 197; will of, 33: *see also* consent; doctor–patient relationship
Pearson Commission, 163, 164
Pellegrino, E., 40, 59, 126, 167; on disease and therapy, 48–9; on ethics, 50–3, 131; on health, 9; on clinical interaction, 8, 180; participatory theory, 55; on patients, 43, 52, 53; on philosophy, 46–7
Penty, A.J., 124
Percival, T., 100–1, 110, 131
Permanent Standing Advisory Committee, 130
Pharmaceutical Society, 97
pharmacy, control over, 104
philosophy, of medicine, 46–7
physicians and surgeons, distinction between, 94–5, 109: *see also* Royal College
placebos, 68, 177
plague, 21, 56, 133, 144
Plato, 48, 195
'pleasure', 47, 71–4, 77
Pliny, 88
Plumb, J.H., 111
pluralism, of individuals, 123, 132; of morals, 125, 132
politics of occupations, 1
poor, treatment of, 96–7
Poor Laws, 147, 154; Amendment Act (1834), 106–7, 108; Commissioners, 144, 146; institutions, 86, 107, 108; Unions, 107
Popper, K.R., 14, 36, 128
positivism, 38, 81–7
Posner, R., 160
power, 152, 176; institutionalised, 153; of medical profession, 87, 143, 145, 154, 155, 168; of state, 174
Presthus, R.V., 152
prestige, *see* status

preventative medicine, 72
pride, professional, in U.S., 113
Priestley, J., 84, 99, 186
primary care, 33, 133, 155, 213; choice in, 154; doctors' role in, 62; and pleasure, 47, 72; and scientism, 184; and self, 49
private, action, 69, 78–81; licensing, 113
privilege, professional, 100, 134–5; abuse of, 30
Privy Council, 110, 144, 145
professional/professionalism, 3, 18, 51–2, 61–2, 109–42; autonomy, 114, 115; definition of, 42, 62, 116; economic model of, 110–13; functionalist model of, 115–16; loss of, 155; morality, 22, 123, 129, 134, 140, 167; privilege, 115, 134–6; standards, 65, 136, 140, 167, 168; values of, 185;
prognosis, 49
Protestant(ism), 90, 91, 124, 186; Revolution (1688), 182
Provincial Medical & Surgical Association, 103–4, 109, 129
psychological response to, untoward, 158, 164–5
psychology, 29
public, action, 69, 78–81; licensing, 113
public health, 42, 58, 144–5, 184; institutions, 143–7; legislation, 3, 5, 7, 146, 147
Public Health Acts (1848, 1872 & 1875), 3, 146, 147
Pythagorus/Pythagorean, 42, 43–4; asceticism, 30, 55, 89, 91, 98; gentleman, *see* gentleman

quacks, 20, 142
'Quack's Charter', 95
quarantine, 144

Raleigh, W., 64
Ramsey, P., 169

rationalism, 182, 183, 184, 185
recovery, 29; from death/cancer, 20–1
Regional Health Authorities, 155, 156
Regional Hospital Boards, 156
register of practitioners, 138
regulations, external, 54, 136–43; internal, 137; in law, 36, 140, 147–53
Reith Lectures, 80
relativity, theory of, 5, 193
religion, 37, 89–90, 171; *see also* church
Renaissance, 83, 88, 92–4, 97, 109; changes, 2, 15, 186–7; empiricism, 91; ideas of, 79, 124; individualism in, 99, 181; and manners, 117–8, 209; view of disease, 20
reputation of doctors, 1; of medicine, 36, 92, 100
resources, allocation of, 12, 148, 160–1
Restoration, 182
'revival' from dead, 20
rewards, 116–7, 133, 134, 154, 166
rights, patients', 167
risk, 165
ritual, 28, 128, 152
Roberts, S., 158–9
role of doctors, ix, 40, 57, 153, 178
Romantics, 77, 82, 83
Rome, Ancient, 88, 91, 124; modern, 96
Rousseau, J.-J., 21, 74, 124, 125
Royal College of Nursing v. *DHSS*, 153, 155
Royal College of Physicians, 99–101, 104, 134, 157, 207; and apothecaries, 95–6, 101; criticisms of, 110; as élite, 93; Fellows of, 102, 141; history of, 92–4, 183; influence of, 3, 108, 143, 144–5
Royal College of Surgeons, 87,

157; history of, 95, 102–3, 104, 120, 134, 207
Royal Society, 37
Rueschemeyer, D., 115, 116
Rule of Opposites, 68
Russell, B., 5, 37–8, 40, 44, 191
Russia, 66
Ruthschuh, K.E., 48

St Bartholomew's Hospital, 97
St George's Hospital, 97
St Thomas' Hospital, 97, 204
Saint-Simon, C.H., 82
Salerno School, 88
sanctions, 125, 152, 158, 160; external, 3, 6–7, 40, 54, 180; of group, 3, 135; moral, 128; of state, 10; *see also* law
Sanitary Report (1842), 146
sanitation, 146
Santarcangeli, P., 177
Sartre, J.-P., 78
Scarman, Lord, 171
Schlegel, F., 177
Schools Health Service, 104
science/technology, 30, 168; decisions based on, 54, 105; imperative, 81–7, 150; innovations, 28, 63, 74, 106, 129, 186–7, 201; professionalization, 110; publications, 99; training, 30; *see also* scientific medicine
scientific medicine, theory of, 8, 22, 35–41, 47, 59, 68; history of, 81–7, 102, 111, 181; limitations of, 171; and patients' role, 78, 169, 178
scientism, 77, 111, 133; history of, 85, 90; influence on medicine, 86, 91, 141, 184, 197
Scitovsky, T., 71
Scrutton, L.J., 141
secondary care, 25, 47, 49, 63, 154, 213
secrecy, collective, 99
self/selves, 17, 48, 67, 173–80, 181;

autonomous, 173; awareness, 3; concept in law, 190; self–other distinction, 175
self-determination, *see* patients
self-help, 42, 63, 64
self-image of doctors, 178
self-medication, 63–4
Seneca, 48
Service Committees, 157
sexual mores, 43, 192
Shaw, G.B., 79
Shelley, P.B., 82, 189
Sherwood-Taylor, F., 36, 37
Simmel, G., 71, 188
Simon, Sir J., 146
situation liability, 167, 168, 168–72
Slater v. *Baker*, 170
smallpox, 144, 146
Smith, A., 74, 104, 124
smoking/tobacco, addiction to, 62, 75; as cause of disease, 91, 104, 201; criminalized, 67; production of, 144; virtues of, 57, 63–4, 201
socialism, egalitarian, 183, 184
Société Royale de Medicine, 103, 127
social/society, change, 16; cohesion, 182; environment, 10, 11, 16, 66; organization, xiii, 2, 29, 160, 182, 186; problems, 6; and provision for the untoward, 156–7; order, 158
socialized medicine, 153; *see also* National Health
Southwood-Smith, T., 87, 146
specialization, 130, 188
Spencer, H., 85, 86
sport, 77, 118, 120–2, 195
standards, *see* ethics; professionalism
Stanway, A., 64
state, 3, 104, 110; authority of, 7, 10, 149; bureaucracy, 144–5; duty of, 108; action on illness, 143; intervention of, 134–5, 143, 148–9; policy, 6; power of, 105,

134–5, 174; sanctions of, 10, 158; *see also* public health
stateless society, 158
status/prestige, 102–3, 109, 152, 184; effect on patient, 169; increase in, 107–8, 120, 123; and professionalism, 111, 115
Stein, P., 158
surgeons, *see* physicians; Royal College
Sweden, medical injury in, 160
Sydenham, 33
Szasz, T., 60–1, 64–5

Tawney, R.H., 190, 206
team health care, 55, 77–8, 79
technology, *see* science
Tennyson, A., Lord, 170
tertiary care, 33, 47, 49
theories of medicine, 46–87; health-based, 2, 56–79; *see also* classical; participatory; scientific
therapy, 29, 49, 72
Thomasma, D., 40, 59, 126, 167; on disease and therapy, 48–9; on ethics, 50–3, 131; on health, 9; on clinical interaction, 8, 180; on patients, 43, 52, 53; on philosophy, 46–7
Thompson, V.A., 151, 152
tobacco, *see* smoking
Toryism, 182–3, 184
trade, profession's withdrawal from, 110–11, 142
transplant therapy, 23, 32
tribunals, 158, 202
trust, 116–7, 154, 188

United Company of Barber Surgeons, 95
United States, 111, 153, 161, 194, 204; culture of, 4, 18; ethics in, 100–1; Freidson on, 2; individualism in, 5, 17, 204; institutions in, 17; litigation in, 80; practice in, 133, 136; private

United States *cont'd*
  licensing in, 113; self-
  determination in, 64, 69, 177;
  status in, 132; utilitarianism in,
  169
universities, 147, 156; medical
  study at, 88–9, 92, 102, 111
University College Hospital, 102
unprofessional behaviour, *see*
  misconduct; malpractice
untoward, 4, 10, 156–68;
  mechanisms for response, 158–
  65; rectification of, 162;
  litigation for, 80, 165;
utilitarianism, 10, 82, 196

vaccination, 108, 144, 146
values, *see* ethics
Venereal Diseases Act (1917), 64
Venice, 144
Vesalius, A., 91
Vico, G.B., x
Villerme, 146

Virchow, R., 85–6
vocation, medicine as, 166
Volta, A., 83
Voltaire, F., 81

wages, *see* income
Wakley, T., 103, 121
Webb, B, and S., 86
Webb School of Anatomy, 87, 204
Weber, M., xiv, 78, 158; on
  bureaucracy, 150–1; 153; on
  capitalism, 126, 165; on law, ix;
  on mysticism, 44
Westminster Hospital, 97
Whiggery, 182–3, 184, 186
William of Canterbury, 20
Wisden's Cricketers Almanac, 122
workhouses, *see* Poor Law
World Health Organisation, 6, 56

yellow fever, 144–5

Zola, I.K., 31, 66, 72